The Politics of Health Care Reform

Lessons from the Past,
Prospects for the Future

**Edited by James A. Morone and
Gary S. Belkin**

Duke University Press
Durham and London 1994

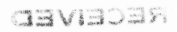
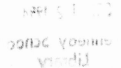

AVP 8002 - 9/1

© 1994 Duke University Press
All rights reserved
Printed in the United States of America
on acid-free paper ∞
Most of these articles were published in volume 18, numbers 2
and 3 of the *Journal of Health Politics, Policy and Law*. The essay
by Colleen Grogan, "Who Gets What? Levels of Care in Canada,
Britain, Germany, and the United States," appeared in volume 17,
number 2, and that by Robert G. Evans, "Canada: The Real
Issues," in number 4 of the same volume.
Library of Congress Cataloging-in-Publication Data
The Politics of health care reform: lessons from the past, prospects
for the future / edited by James A. Morone and Gary S. Belkin.
p. cm.
Articles originally published in the Journal of health politics,
policy and law.
Includes bibliographical references and index.
ISBN 0-8223-1461-4 : $49.95. — ISBN 0-8223-1489-4 (pbk.) :
$19.95
1. Health care reform—United States. 2. Medical policy—
Political aspects—United States. I. Morone, James A., 1951–.
II. Belkin, Gary S.
RA395.A3P635 1994
362.1'0973—dc20 94-10005

Contents

Introduction

James A. Morone

National health insurance has been rising onto and falling off the American political agenda for eighty years. Theodore Roosevelt and the Bull Moose Progressive Party touted a plan in 1912. The reform gathered momentum for almost a decade, then vanished from the political scene. The New Dealers revived the idea while they were drafting the Social Security Act. However, health reform provoked such ferocious opposition that Franklin Roosevelt scrapped even the ritual call for additional study. The debate warmed again when Harry Truman made national health insurance the major domestic issue of his 1948 presidential campaign, roasting the do-nothing 80th Congress for resistance. Despite Truman's unexpected victory, the 81st Congress was no more receptive than the 80th had been. Through the 1950s, liberals whittled down the scope of Truman's reform in order to get it through Congress. A fragment finally passed as Medicare in 1965. National health insurance for everyone else seemed tantalizingly near during the Nixon administration, disappeared from sight in the Reagan years, and, *mutatis mutandi*, is now cheered on many sides as the policy of the 1990s.

The elusive reform has evolved through the decades. What Theodore Roosevelt envisioned was a hardy stock of Anglo-Saxons: national health care would help deliver white America from "race suicide." Later, Progressives pursued their standard blend of efficiency and equity. Harry Truman's rhetoric unabashedly embraced the latter, promising to raze "financial barriers to care." Today the idea that was once condemned as too costly is acclaimed as an internationally proven form of cost control. Here is a reform that has been designed for, among others, the white race, the poor, and the corporate benefits manager. While there are vivid continuities running through the long debate, the American national health insurance saga is not about the fits and starts of a single project. Rather, this is a political story that constantly rewrites itself, one that reflects the institutions, aspirations, and social troubles of each generation.

This rich historical legacy offers us far more than a series of morality tales about successes to emulate and failures to heed. Each reform campaign—whether it wins new policies or not—creates new political conditions; each effort shapes the next generation of proposals and their fate. Even defeated reforms shake up government agencies, revise conventional wisdom, renegotiate political rules, and reorganize the constellation of interest groups primed for the next debate. The commonsensical view is that politics shape policies. The reverse is just as important and less often observed: new policies create entirely new politics.[1]

Consider, for example, how Medicare altered American politics. Medicare helped forge a powerful gray lobby—it was the legislation that made the interest group more than the other way around. The program (with its promises of cash) offered federal health officials a controversial lever for desegregating hospitals. Medicare turned health policy from insuring care to controlling costs; Americans discovered a cost crisis as soon as they started using taxes to fund medical care (a textbook case of problem redefinition in public policy). Medicare produced the Health Care Finance Administration in 1977, reconstructing the federal health bureaucracy and broadly extending its powers. And it sponsored a revolution in the ways we pay doctors and hospitals, introducing reimbursement methodologies such as diagnosis-related groups and relative value scales. These, in turn, helped change the way American health providers do business. Each time national health insurance cycled back into public view—in the mid 1970s, in the early 1990s—it would be fought out in a political setting profoundly influenced by developments in Medicare.

At the other end of the policy spectrum, defeated proposals also shape future politics. For example, when the medical profession and its allies defeated national health insurance, they set in motion an ironic dynamic. Widespread insurance coverage without controls produced inflation; health care costs grew, relative to the economy, in all but three of the past forty years. In other nations, national health programs offer public officials mechanisms with which to cope with inflationary pressures. Without that framework, the American public and private sectors have scrambled

---

1. This is a point developed by Theda Skocpol. See, for instance, *Protecting Soldiers and Mothers* (Cambridge, MA: Harvard University Press, 1992, 57–60).

to respond with a ragged inventory of makeshift programs: they scrutinize (and second-guess) medical decisions, erect new organizations designed to "manage" health providers, fund elaborate research studies designed to identify ineffective procedures, and bury medicine in mountains of paperwork. These efforts add up to a significant—and by international standards, a singular—intrusion into the autonomy of the medical profession. When previous generations defeated government control, they created conditions that led directly to the intrusive policies that the present generation of physicians so bitterly resents.

And the upshot of the new American regime? Not cost control but great gaps in insurance coverage as competing payers discovered the path to success in an unregulated market: insure healthy people, avoid sick ones. The combination of soaring costs and shrinking coverage is what has restored national health insurance, yet again, to the political agenda.

Paradoxically, we face a health reform contest that is both entirely new and long familiar. On the one hand, a swiftly changing medical sector along with the ramifications of past policy choices constantly remake our health politics. We confront new dilemmas, new institutions, new interests, and, as always, new possibilities.

At the same time nothing seems to change. Eight decades of debate are marked by the same ideals, the same tactics, the same rhetoric. For example, as Theda Skocpol shows in her essay, confident reformers again and again propose their neo-Progressive rationalizing schemes. Each time they are ambushed by potent symbols that whip up antigovernment sentiment: the Kaiser, communism, socialism, and those hardy perennial specters, rising taxes and rampant bureaucracy. The following pages offer a long roll-call of recurring themes and legacies—right down to the political results which, as David Rothman argues here, bear a striking resemblance to one another: our reforms solve middle-class problems and strand the poor.

The essays that follow are not the normal stuff of policy studies. Students of health affairs normally parse the latest reform proposals, offer experimental ways to pay doctors, measure the consequences of patient cost sharing—all usually bracketed by public opinion polls and the latest eye popper on the percentage of gross domestic product devoted to health care. To be sure, these matters are all raised in these pages, some repeatedly. But, ultimately, these essays pursue two very different sorts of inquiry.

First, they are all, fundamentally, about politics. This volume is designed to chart the evolution of our health politics infrastructure. Here are the ideas, institutions, and interests that will shape health policy in the 1990s. Some essays place health reform in the context of potent and enduring themes: class, race, political symbolism, American attitudes toward the state, American constructions of social welfare. Others ponder the present state of the policy machinery: Congress, the health bureaucracy, the federal courts, business, state governments.

Second, and more important, we use the politics of health care as a window onto the nature of American politics itself. We comb decades of health policy for evidence about America—its politics, institutions, and culture. We want to ask not just why national health insurance fails but what that failure tells us about the middle class. Not just whether the time is now ripe for reform, but what fatal flaw in the American progressive vision has spoiled the "ripe" moments for eighty years. We explore the insurance industry to discover what is distinctive about American ways of constructing communities and sharing risk. We study public opinion polls, not to measure the latest shift in the political breeze but to explore underlying American attitudes toward government action.

Ultimately, the broad political dynamics illuminate the narrow policy nuances. Our premise is that understanding the enduring dimensions of American institutions and culture will offer a new and more satisfying frame for the details of health care policy. While each essay reflects on reform prospects under the Clinton administration, all aim to engage issues that stretch beyond any one political moment or any single policy proposal.

We begin with the great analytic fault lines of American politics. David Rothman reflects on a century of health care reform and traces an intricate interplay between the middle class, the medical profession, and the underprivileged. Past social politics, he suggests, offer a gloomy prospect for winning equity: the poor have repeatedly been excluded from mainstream health programs and reform coalitions. Deborah Stone roots our insurance dilemmas in the logic of the insurance industry. Ultimately, she argues, the logic of the market and the logic of social community are contending for the "soul" of American health insurance. Theda Skocpol turns to the symbolic politics which have tripped up generations of reformers with their rationalizing policy blueprints and tin political ears. Finally, David McBride reminds us that by every health measure, the African American community is suffering, yet reform debates have moved directly away from the issue. Affirmative action is hotly debated in venues ranging from education to the workplace. In contrast, race-specific policies have vanished from health policy—to the detriment of African Americans' health and wellbeing.

Part 2 turns to the political machinery itself. The current generation of social scientists puts less emphasis on the bald calculation of interest group preferences, still popular among health analysts. Rather, we pay more analytic attention to the organization, biases, and interests of government institutions themselves. Mark Peterson charts structural changes in the interplay between mobilized interests and Congress. Peterson shows how we have moved a long way from the classic iron triangles (that mainstay of introductory political science courses which finds power in the intersection of interest groups, solicitous congressmen, and pliant bureaucrats). My own essay explores the accretion of power in the American health bureaucracy, both public and private. Ultimately, political power over medicine is shifting from the medical professionals to administrators— with deleterious consequences for public accountability. Rand Rosenblatt turns to the evolution of our judicial politics. He suggests that the Rehnquist court has been moving to reverse the patterns that long enabled egalitarian reform: active courts prodding administrative officials to implement statutory promises (in the face of budgetary and political pressures). The emerging pattern, argues Rosenblatt, raises a new and daunting barrier to meaningful reform.

Part 3 addresses the perpetual reform alternative—business. The New Deal embedded the American social welfare regime within the corporate establishment; health inflation (along with other forces such as American deindustrialization) puts enormous pressure on that arrangement. For two decades, observers have suggested that business self-interest will be the key to health care reform. Lawrence Brown suggests that the dogged hope of corporate action flows from a mix of ideology, mythology, and wishful thinking—this giant's slumber rests on a deeply conservative worldview that makes progressive action unlikely. Cathie Jo Martin offers a somewhat more optimistic assessment of corporate will. Business can have a systematic political impact in—but only in—quasi-corporatist partnership with governments. Nancy Jecker challenges the underlying premise. Linking benefits to employment is, she argues, ethically problematic. Joan Ruttenberg seconds Jecker's view; David Rochefort counters with reflections on political feasibility.

Part 4 moves to the force that is most often invoked and least often analyzed, the people. The articles included here use polling data to explore the political dynamics of American public opinion itself. Lawrence Jacobs shows precisely how and why public opinion affects policy results.

In the process, he challenges political scientists who have let a focus on the mobilization of interest groups and the preferences of state actors eclipse the importance of what the public thinks. Schlesinger and Lee turn to that longstanding chestnut: Americans oppose government action. They suggest that health care is different. Over time, Americans show a marked willingness to accept intervention in the health care realm.

Part 5 turns to one of the oldest questions in American politics: the balance between federal and state politics. The classic reform perspective throughout the great national health insurance debate has looked skeptically at state action. Too many health matters are beyond the reach of the states; the states do not have the administrative capacity to sustain effective reform. The increasingly popular alternative rests on the new sophistication and energy in state capitals. In this view, fifteen dry years in Washington have pushed innovation, experimentation, and talent to the state level. Kenneth Thorpe weighs into this debate with evidence that some of the recent state experiments appear to be successful—some innovative states control costs as well as any of the Canadian provinces. Robert Hackey and Michael Sparer each take a careful look at the actual institutional dynamics. Thorpe reports the cost data; Hackey and Sparer look at the policy-making organizations.

We end with the perpetual contrast to American health policy, the international experience. Foreign systems flourish in American scholarship because they offer a world of evidence about the alternatives that we have forgone for the past eight decades. They "stretch the mind" [2] in a nation that is both unique and unhappy in its health care arrangements. Colleen Grogan contrasts the American impulse to organize reform around minutely specified benefits packages with the very different policy practices in Canada, Germany, and Britain. She shows how in all three of these cases, medical services follow from institutional choices about the structure of the health system rather than rationing decisions about the minimum benefits to be provided. Robert Evans and Theodore Marmor turn to the Canadian health experience and its real lessons for the United States. Finally, William Glaser takes a broad view of the lessons that can be learned from the international experience.

Taken together, these articles suggest how our health policies developed and where they are likely to go. But a final reminder is in order. It is easy to imagine that a reform like national health insurance offers a

2. For a discussion of comparative politics see Theodore Marmor, Amy Bridges, and Wayne Hoffman, "Comparative Politics and Health Policies" in *Comparing Public Policies*, ed. Douglas E. Ashford (Beverly Hills, CA: Sage, 1978).

definitive solution, a final policy destination. In politics, there is no such thing. In a field as complex as health care, all reforms produce winners and losers; the losers mobilize to recoup their losses. Innovations solve some problems and exacerbate others. Each political development leads to a new policy debate. Today, both the political developments and the policy debates are carried forward through the institutions, interests, and ideas described in the pages that follow.

Finally, we received a great deal of help in putting this collection together. The Robert Wood Johnson Foundation made the book possible, with generous support and good advice. Special thanks to Alan Cohen, Beth Stevens, and Robert Hughes of the foundation staff. Steve Cohn, the acting director of Duke University Press, offered wisdom, cautions, resources, and a fair chunk of his time. We are grateful to Maura High for her elegant copyediting. And to Anne Keyl who put the book together with her special brand of long patience and high style. Eileen Evans, Marti Rosenberg, and Sauda Said helped organize us in the early going; Leah Pratt—the world's best editorial assistant—kept everything together after that. Finally, many drafts ago, most of these papers were part of an electrifying conference held in Durham, North Carolina. A great many participants helped the paper-writers in a great many ways. There is not room here to name them, but their comments and energy are reflected throughout the papers that follow. Thanks again to all.

Part 1
The Fault Lines of American Health Politics

A Century of Failure: Class Barriers to Reform

David J. Rothman

Abstract To understand fully the persistent failure of the United States to enact national health insurance requires an appreciation not only of the role of government and the dynamics of politics but of underlying social realities. One consideration, which dates back to the Great Depression, is the absence of the middle class from a coalition in favor of such a policy. This absence reflects both the constricted vision of the middle class and the spirited campaigns of groups like Blue Cross to make certain that middle-class needs were met in order to reduce pressure for government intervention. Another critical social feature is the special entrepreneurial character of the American medical profession. Physicians saw themselves as small businessmen and, as such, shared and promoted a suspicion of governmental intervention. All the while, Americans justified the absence of a national program in terms of the ethos of voluntarism, which had a sufficient base in reality for the posture to be maintained without great embarrassment. In fact, the rhetoric that surrounded the enactment of Medicare reinforced these views, making it appear that, the elderly aside, all was well with the provision of medical services in the country. Even as national health insurance assumes a new prominence on the political agenda, it remains unclear whether these several considerations will allow for the enactment of sweeping changes.

There are some questions that historians return to so often that they become classics in the field, to be explored and reexplored, considered and reconsidered. No inquiry better qualifies for this designation than the question of why the United States has never enacted a national health insurance program. Why, with the exception of South Africa, does it remain the only industrialized country that has not implemented so fundamental a social welfare policy?

The roster of answers that have been provided is impressive in its insights. Some outstanding contributions to our understanding of the issues come from James Morone, Paul Starr, Theodore Marmor, and Theda

Skocpol. Their explanations complement, rather than counter, each other. In like manner, the elements that this essay will explore are intended to supplement, not dislodge, their work. A failure in policy that is so basic is bound to be overdetermined, and therefore, efforts to fathom it will inevitably proceed in a variety of directions.

The Liberal State

Morone's frame for understanding American health policy in general and the failure of national health insurance in particular centers on the definitions of the proper role of the state, the acceptable limits for all governmental actions. His starting point is with the fact that the medical profession successfully "appropriated public authority to take charge of the health care field," taking for itself the task of defining the content, organization, and, perhaps most important, the financing of medical practice (Morone 1990: 253–84). This accomplishment points to more than the power of the American Medical Association's lobbying machine; AMA rhetoric, which has seemed to other observers to be bombastic, comical, or even hysterical, in Morone's terms was effective precisely because it drew on popularly shared assumptions about the proper relationship between governmental authority, professional capacity, and professional autonomy. By the terms of this consensus, the government's duty was to build up professional capacity without infringing on professional autonomy—and as long as the medical profession defined national health insurance as an infringement on its autonomy, such a policy would not be enacted. Government was permitted to build hospitals (witness the implementation of the Hill-Burton Act) and to endow the research establishment (witness the extraordinary growth of the National Institutes of Health), but it was not allowed, at least until very recently, to challenge or subvert professional autonomy.

Paul Starr also focuses on conceptions of state authority to explain health policy. Alert to the markedly different course of national health insurance in European countries, he posits that where a spirit of liberalism and a commitment to the inviolability of private property interests in relation to the state were strongest, movements for social insurance made the least headway. Thus, Bismarck's Germany could accomplish what Theodore Roosevelt's or Franklin Roosevelt's United States could not. Put another way, the fact that socialism never put down strong roots in this country, the absence here of a socialist tradition or threat, obviated the need for more conservative forces to buttress the social order through welfare measures.

Starr is more ready than Morone to credit the raw political power of the AMA, but he also reminds us that the AMA found allies among not only corporations but also labor unions. Union leaders preferred to obtain health care benefits for its members through contract negotiation, not through government largesse—even if that meant, or precisely because that meant, that nonunion members would go without benefits (Starr 1982: part 2).

Paralleling their studies are detailed accounts of the legislative histories of various health insurance proposals, the fate of Progressive, New Deal, and Fair Deal initiatives. The work of Theodore Marmor has clarified the political alliances that came together to enact Medicare and Medicaid (Marmor 1982). So too, the writings of Theda Skocpol place health care legislation more directly in the tradition of American welfare policies (Weir et al. 1988). In all, the existing literature illuminates the effects of both conceptions of governmental authority and the realities of constituent politics to tell us why the United States stands alone in its failure to enact national health insurance.

Co-opting the Middle Class

Despite the sophisticated and perceptive quality of these arguments, still other considerations underlie the failure to enact national health insurance. An analysis of them does not subvert the basic contours of the other interpretations but provides a deeper social context for the story.

The starting point for such an analysis is a frank recognition of the fact that what is under discussion is essentially a moral failure, a demonstration of a level of indifference to the well-being of others that stands as an indictment of the intrinsic character of American society. This observation, however, is not meant to inspire a jeremiad on American imperfections as much as to open an inquiry into the dynamics of the failure—not only how it occurred but how it was rationalized and tolerated. Americans do not think of themselves as callous and cruel, and yet, in their readiness to forgo and withhold this most elemental social service, they have been so. This question arises: How did the middle class, its elected representatives, and its doctors accommodate themselves to such neglect? To be sure, Morone, Starr, and others have made it clear that ideas on the proper scope of government were powerful determinants of behavior, that leaders like FDR made strategic political calculations that traded off health insurance for other programs, and that the AMA smugly equated physician self-interest with national interest. But given the signal importance of health care—and, a minority of commentators aside, the ongoing recognition that it is more than one more commodity to be left to the vagaries of the marketplace—there is a need for an even broader framework for understanding these events. The chess moves of politicians, and even the rules of the game of politics, seem somewhat too removed and abstract. Put most succinctly: How could Americans ignore the health needs of so many fellow countrymen and still live with themselves? How could a society that prides itself on decency tolerate this degree of unfairness?

For answers, it is appropriate to look first to the 1930s. As a result of the Great Depression, American social welfare legislation was transformed, as exemplified by the passage of the Social Security Act. Moreover, by the 1930s, the popular faith in the efficacy of medical interventions was firmly established and the consequences of a denial of medical care, apparent. Already by the 1910s, some would-be reformers defined the goal of health insurance not merely as compensation to the sick for wages lost during illness but as the opportunity to obtain curative medical care. Twenty years later, this credo was accepted by almost all reformers, although the efficacy of medical interventions was, at least by current standards, far from impressive. Also by the 1930s, the hospital, which had earlier been almost indistinguishable from the almshouse, had become a temple of science and its leaders, Men in White, widely celebrated. In keeping with these changes, physician visits and hospital occupancy now correlated directly, not inversely, with income.

Why then was national health insurance omitted from the roster of legislation enacted in the 1930s? If medicine was so valued and government so receptive to novel (at least for Americans) social insurance programs, why was health insurance kept off the roster? Although such considerations as FDR's reluctance to do battle with the AMA or to fragment his southern alliance were important, perhaps even more determinative were the tactics, thoroughly self-conscious, that were helping to remove the middle classes from the coalition of advocates for change. And eliminating the middle classes from the alignment successfully deflated the political pressure for national health insurance.

One of the pivotal groups in designing and implementing this strategy was a newly founded, private health insurance company, Blue Cross. Against the backdrop of the report of the Committee on the Costs of Medical Care, urging greater federal intervention in health care, Blue Cross presented itself as the best alternative to government involvement. Its organizers and supporters, such as Rufus Rorem and Walter Dannreuther, held out the promise that enrolling the middle class in its plan would blunt the thrust for national health insurance. Blue Cross, declared Dannreuther, would "eliminate the demand for compulsory health insurance and stop the reintroduction of vicious sociological bills into the state legislature year after year." Blue Cross advertisements, pamphlets, radio programs, and publications insisted that neither the rich nor the poor confronted difficulties in obtaining medical services, the rich because they could easily afford it, the poor because they had ready access to public hospitals. Only the middle classes faced a problem, and unless their needs were met, they were bound to agitate for a change in governmental policy. ("It is the people in the middle income group who often find it most difficult to secure adequate medical and hospital care," declared Louis Pink, president of New York Blue Cross. "It is sometimes said that the very poor and the rich—if there are any rich left—get the best medical care.")[1] The idea was not to buy the middle classes off by expanding the services of public hospitals and persuading them to take a place on the wards to meet emergency needs. Such a solution, as Blue Cross proponents explained, would not only strain the public hospital system beyond its capacity, but would not work because the middle classes considered the public hospitals to be charity, with all innuendo intended, and they were not about to accept charity. As one Blue Cross official insisted: "The average man, with the average income, has pride. He is not looking for charity; he is not looking for ward care. He wants the best of attention for himself and his family. . . . Yet out of his savings, he is very seldom prepared to meet unexpected sickness or accident expenses." Thus, to use the public hospital was not only to get second-best care but to be stigmatized as dependent, incapable of standing on one's own two feet. Like the dole, the public hospital violated the American way. Were this the only choice, the middle classes would push for, and obtain, national health insurance.

The alternative that embodied the American way was a private subscription plan, which, for as little as three cents a day (the Blue Cross slogan), protected members from the high cost of hospitalization. "The Blue Cross Plans are a distinctly American institution," declared one of its officials, "a unique combination of individual initiative and social responsibility. They perform a public service without public compulsion." Another executive asserted that Blue Cross exemplified "the American spirit of neighborliness and self-help [which] solves the difficult and important problem of personal and national health." All of which led inexorably to the conclusion: "Private enterprise in voluntarily providing hospital care within the reach of everyone is solving the public health problem in the real democratic way. The continued growth of the Blue

1. Statements from Blue Cross representatives are taken from Rothman 1991.

Cross Movement might well be considered the best insurance against the need of governmental provision for such protection" (quoted in Rothman 1991).

Blue Cross was notably successful in enrolling middle-class subscribers, serving, as intended, to reduce or eliminate their concern over the payment of hospital bills. To be sure, it took some time to build up a membership, but by 1939 there were thirty-nine Blue Cross plans in operation with more than 6 million subscribers. Indeed, the plans became even more over time, with some 31 million subscribers by 1949 (Starr 1982: 298, 327).[2] In fact, from its inception the impact of Blue Cross was probably greater than even the membership statistics indicate. Its extraordinarily active advertising campaigns made a compelling case that private, as against public, initiatives were more than sufficient to meet the problem, so that even those who did not immediately enroll may have accepted the viability of this alternative. There was no reason to press for political change when the private sector seemed to have resolved the issue. Thus both in rhetoric and in reality, Blue Cross helped to undercut middle-class interest in and concern for national health insurance. The result, fully intended, was that they did not join or lend strength to a coalition for change. Politics could do business as usual, allowing a variety of other considerations to outweigh support for such an innovation.[3]

In fact, the dynamic set off by Blue Cross in the 1930s gained strength in the post-1945 period, not only from its own growth but from the labor movement. Not just private insurance but union benefits served to cushion the middle classes from the impact of health care costs. Over these years, contract provisions negotiated with business corporations provided unionized workers with health care benefits, reducing their felt need for government programs. With that many more middle-class households effectively covered, it would require empathy, not self-interest, to push for national health insurance, and that empathy, for reasons that we will explore further below, was in short supply. As a result, public responsi-

2. In addition, there were another 28 million people enrolled for health care benefits with commercial insurance companies, so the private system was extensive.

3. It may well be that a felt need for health insurance was an acquired, not innate, characteristic. The first Blue Cross advertisements tried to build up a demand for insurance by emphasizing the unexpected character of illness, the sudden and unanticipated strike of disease. One of its popular advertising images represented Blue Cross as a helmet protecting against the club of the hospital bill that lay hidden, waiting to assail the unaware victim; the accompanying slogan read: "You never know what jolt is around the corner." Blue Cross's strategy was to emphasize the unpredictability of health care needs and that illness could strike anyone at any time, suggests that just when it raised consciousness about the need to carry health insurance, it provided an answer as to how best arrange it.

the poor, not the respectable. Coverage was something to be provided for "them," not what "we" needed or were entitled to as citizens.

How this divide between "we" and "they" shaped welfare policy emerges with particular vividness in the history of the almshouse in the 1930s. When the decade began, the institution was still one of the mainstays of public welfare policy, particularly for the elderly and for those considered the "unworthy poor." Although the post–World War II generation associates the almshouse with Dickensian England, it was of major importance in this country even at the start of the Great Depression. Only in the mid-1930s did the almshouse begin to lose its hold on welfare programs, moved aside by such New Deal relief programs as the Works Project Administration (WPA) and the Social Security Act. In fact, WPA regulations prohibited the expenditure of funds to build or enlarge these institutions; the WPA was ready to build roads but not to build or refurbish almshouses. Why this distinction? Why the abandonment, at long last, of the almshouse? Because for the first time, almshouse relief would have had to include the middle classes. With state and city budgets staggering under the burden of relief and private charities altogether unequal to the task, absent a WPA or Social Security Act, many of the once-unemployed would have had to enter the almshouse. The prospect of having respectable middle-class citizens in such a facility was so disturbing as to transform government relief policy.

Imagine this same dynamic at work in health care. Picture the middle classes having no alternative but to crowd into the public hospital, to receive medical services in the twelve-bed wards. It is by no means fanciful to suggest that had this been the case, a different kind of pressure would have been exerted on the government to enact health insurance coverage. Blue Cross, however, self-consciously and successfully short-circuited the process and thereby allowed the play of politics to go on uninterrupted.

The Physician as Entrepreneur

A second critical element that underlay the American failure to implement national health insurance was the character of its medical profession. The speeches, letters, and writings of American doctors over the period 1920–1950 indicate broad sympathy for the positions of the AMA, perhaps somewhat less dogmatic but fully sharing of the organization's commitment to a fee-for-service system. Although some historians have found significant diversity of medical opinion on national health insurance earlier in the Progressive Era, by the 1920s most physicians were profoundly uncomfortable with proposed government intrusions into health care.

Narrow financial self-interest, the fear of a loss of income through national health insurance, was a force in shaping some doctors' attitudes, but it was far from the only consideration. For one, physicians' earnings were not so large as to turn them necessarily into dogged defenders of the status quo. Physicians' average income, for example, was below that of lawyers and engineers; in 1929, of the 121,000 physicians in private practice, 53 percent had incomes below $4,000, and 80 percent, less than $8,000. To be sure, some 12 percent of physicians had incomes over $11,500, but the profession was far from a lucrative one (President's Research Committee 1933: 1104). In strictly financial terms, it would not have been illogical for doctors generally to have supported national programs, particularly in the 1930s. They might have accepted government intervention with some enthusiasm, on the grounds that it was better to receive some payment from Washington than no payment from a patient. But this was not the position commonly adopted, and to understand why requires an appreciation of the essentially entrepreneurial character of American medicine. In more precise terms, the mind-set of physicians was that of the independent proprietor. They identified themselves as businessmen and, as such, shared an aversion to government interference.

It may be that the very differentiation in income among physicians at once reflected and reinforced a scramble for income that is not commonly associated with the practice of medicine. This was the conclusion that the Lynds reached in their portrait of "Middletown" in the 1920s. "The profession of medicine," they wrote, "swings around the making of money as one of its chief concerns. As a group, Middletown physicians are devoting their energies to building up and maintaining a practice in a highly competitive field. Competition is so keen that even the best doctors in many cases supplement their incomes by putting up their own prescriptions" (Lynd and Lynd [1929] 1956: 443). It was not unusual for physicians to invest in proprietary hospitals or to accept fee-splitting arrangements. Doctors also purchased common stocks and invested in local businesses—albeit not always very cleverly. By the 1920s, doctors had such a reputation for being suckers that advice books on business addressed to them devoted large sections to discussions of "Why Do Doctors Fail to Choose the Right Investments?" The answers were generally variations on the theme of "There is a host of people who have found out that the doctor likes to take a chance. . . . He has worked so hard to accumulate his small savings and the possibility of making prodigious returns are presented to him so plausibly by some glib talker that all too frequently this nest egg is frittered away on some unsavory scheme, for he seldom has the time, inclination and facilities to make the essential investigation" (Thomas 1923: 174–75). In effect, the financial dealings that occupy physicians today are far less novel than critics like Arnold Relman might like to imagine.

To account for physicians' entrepreneurial perspective, it is vital to remember that their social world overlapped with that of the local business elite, particularly in smaller towns. When one upper-class resident of "Regionville" was asked by sociologist Earl Koos to list the five most important people in the town, he responded: "I put Doc X on that list because . . . he is one of the best-educated men in town, and makes good money—drives a good car, belongs to Rotary, and so forth. . . . Of course, some doctors aren't as important as others, here or anywhere else, but unless they're drunks or drug addicts, they're just automatically pretty top rank in town" (Koos 1954: 54).

The pattern of recruitment to the profession also encouraged this orientation. Medical school classes in the 1920s and 1930s were the almost exclusive preserve of white, upper-middle-class males. From birth, it would seem, physicians were comfortable, socially and ideologically, in the clubhouse locker room. The image is properly one of Wednesday afternoon off, doctor chatting with town banker, lawyer, and principal store owner about investment opportunities and politics, with a shared antagonism to what all of them considered the evil of Government Control.

Physicians voiced their opposition to national health insurance not only collectively through the AMA but individually as well, in the process helping to mold public attitudes. As Koos aptly observed, in towns like Regionville, especially before 1950 (before the rise of a more national media and greater opportunities for travel), doctors were opinion leaders: "In the small town, the doctor is most often 'a big frog in a little puddle'; what he thinks and does can assume an importance in the community not paralleled in the life of his urban counterpart" (Koos 1954: 150). In brief, the entrepreneurial style of American physicians helps explain much of their own and some of their neighbors' disinclination to support national health insurance.

The Ethos of Voluntarism

But then how did Americans live with the consequences of their decision? How did they justify to themselves and to others their unwillingness to provide so essential a service as medical care to those unable to afford it? The need for pragmatism in politics (we dare do no other) and definitions of the boundaries of state authority (we should do no other) surely mattered. So, too, in health care as in matters of social welfare more generally, they could always fall back on such truisms as "The poor have only themselves to blame for their poverty—they should have saved for the rainy day." And middle-class Americans could also invoke the safety net of the public hospital, noting that its services were available to all comers, regardless of income.

But there were other justifications as well, particularly the celebration of the ethos of voluntarism, the credo that individual and organizational charity obviated the need for government intervention. Individual physicians and community charities ostensibly provided the needy with requisite medical care. This idea was not fabricated from whole cloth, for Americans, and their doctors, had good reason to believe that their own initiatives were sufficient to meet the problem.

Physicians, for their part, insisted that they turned no one away from their offices because of an inability to pay for services. They used a sliding scale for setting fees, charging the "haves" more and the "have-nots" less, so as to promote the social good. The claim was incessantly repeated and undoubtedly had some validity to it. "It was probably true," reported Koos, "that no physician in Regionville would leave a worthy case untreated." The physician, claimed the New York Medical Society in 1939, "has socialized his own services. Traditionally, he is at the call of the indigent without recompense. . . . For those who are self-supporting, he graduates his fees to meet the ability to pay, and extends time for payment over long periods." As late as 1951, a survey of physicians in Toledo, Ohio, found overwhelming support for a sliding scale of fees and widespread agreement that, to quote one response: "It's fair, the fairest thing we can do. If a man is wealthy, you certainly would charge him more than if he didn't have a dime. It's not uncommon for a doctor to call me and say, 'These people don't have any money,' or can pay only a little, and I say, 'Sure send 'em on in. I'll take care of 'em' " (Schuler et al. 1952: 60, 69, 85). Thus, physicians justified their opposition to national health insurance by citing their own altruism. Their charity rendered government intervention unnecessary.

By the same token, community philanthropy often stepped in where the circumstances went beyond the scope of individual physicians. It was not only a matter of a voluntary society establishing not-for-profit hospitals or organizing outpatient dispensaries. Voluntarism seemed capable of meeting the most exceptional challenge. To choose one of the most noteworthy examples, in the case of polio, private charitable efforts helped to make certain that no child, whatever the family's income, would lack for access to an iron lung or to rehabilitative services. By November 1931, only two years after Philip Drinker perfected the iron lung, there were 150 respirators to be found in hospitals across the country. Foundations, including Milbank and Harkness, underwrote the cost of some of the machines, and their efforts were supplemented by the fund-raising work of local ladies' auxiliaries. As for patient rehabilitation, the National Foundation for Infantile Paralysis, founded in 1938 by FDR and directed by onetime Wall Street attorney Basil O'Connor, supported both research and the delivery of clinical services. Several thousand local chapters and one hundred thousand volunteers made certain that no person with polio was denied medical assistance because of economic hardship. And the foundation defined "hardship" liberally, to cover the case where medical expenditures would force a family to lower its standard of living.

The polio experience was particularly important in confirming a belief in the adequacy of voluntarism. With a world-famous patient, in the person of President Franklin Roosevelt, and an extraordinarily successful foundation, a compelling case could be made for the capacity of voluntary action to meet the most unusual and costly health care needs. Moreover, the lesson was felt particularly strongly by the middle classes, because polio was in many ways their disease, disproportionately striking children raised in hygienic, uncrowded, and (epidemiologically speaking) protected environments. Those from lower-class and urban backgrounds were more likely to be exposed to the virus at a young age and had thereby built up immunities to it. Thus the foundation, like Blue Cross, served the middle classes so well that it insulated them from the predicament of health care costs. No wonder, then, that they, and their political representatives, to the degree that they looked out on the world from their own experience, found little need for government intervention and were able to maintain this position without either embarrassment or guilt.

The Dual Message of Medicare

Surprising as it may seem, the rhetoric that surrounded the enactment of Medicare reinforced many of these constricted views. The most significant government intervention in health care did not, the wishes of many of its proponents notwithstanding, enlarge the vision of the middle classes or make the case for national health insurance. To the contrary. The debate around Medicare in a variety of ways made it seem as though, the elderly aside, all was well with the provision of medical services.

In the extensive hearings and debates that Congress devoted to Medicare between 1963 and 1965, proponents of the bill, undoubtedly for strategic political reasons, repeatedly distinguished Medicare from a national health insurance scheme. So intent were they on securing the passage of this act that they went to great pains to minimize the need for any additional interventions once Medicare was in place. And as they offered these arguments, perhaps unintentionally but nevertheless quite powerfully, they reinforced very traditional perspectives on poverty and welfare and the special character of middle-class needs.

The opening statement given in November 1963 to the House Committee on Ways and Means by then secretary of Health, Education, and Welfare, Anthony Celebrezze, laid out the themes that other advocates consistently followed. His goal was to demonstrate that the elderly presented "a unique problem," and thereby warranted special support. Just when their postretirement incomes were declining, they faced disproportionately higher health care costs: "People over sixty-five," Celebrezze calculated, "use three times as much hospital care, on the average, as people under sixty-five." Moreover, the private health insurance system that worked so well for others did not meet their needs: the premiums were too expensive (one-sixth of their medium income), and the policies often included restrictive clauses (for example, ruling out preexisting conditions). Hence, Celebrezze concluded, "this combination of high health costs, low incomes, and unavailability of group insurance is what clearly distinguishes the situation of the aged as a group from the situation of younger workers as a group" (U.S. Congress 1964: 28).

It was a shrewd argument, but it left open several problems. The first was to justify excluding the young from a federal program. To this end, Celebrezze and the other Medicare proponents frankly and wholeheartedly endorsed the status quo: "The vast majority of young workers can purchase private insurance protection. . . . I think for younger employed people, voluntary private plans can do the job" (U.S. Congress 1964: 36). Those below sixty-five were less likely to require health care interventions, and, should they encounter sudden needs, they could always borrow the sums and pay them back through their future earnings. In effect, the Medicare proponents swept under the table the problems of access to health care for those who were outside the net of employer-provided private insurance.

The second and even tougher issue for the Medicare supporters was to explain why the elderly in need should not be required to rely on the welfare system to meet their health care requirements. After all, as one critic noted, these people had been remiss in not saving for the rainy day, and the government ought not to bail them out. They would not have to forgo health care services. Rather, to the opponents of Medicare, which included to the very end the AMA, the just solution was to aid them through a program like Kerr-Mills. Under its provisions, the needy elderly would demonstrate (to public assistance officials) their lack of resources, take a place on the welfare rolls, and then receive their health care services under a combined federal-state program. The counterargument from the Medicare camp was that to compel the elderly to demonstrate their dependency was too demeaning. "We should take into account the pride and independent spirit of our older people," Celebrezze insisted. "We should do better than say to an aged person that, when he has become poor enough and when he can prove his poverty to the satisfaction of the appropriate public agency, he may be able to get help." But if welfare was so humiliating, why should anyone have to suffer such a process? If welfare demeaned the elderly, why did it not demean the young? To which the tacit answer was that if the young were poor, they had only themselves to blame. Those on welfare, the elderly apart, were so "unworthy" that humiliation was their due, at least until they reached sixty-five (U.S. Congress 1964: 31).

The third and probably most difficult question was whether a federal health insurance program for the elderly ultimately rested, as one opponent put it, on the premise that "the federal government, as a matter of right, owes medical care to elderly people." Again Celebrezze backed off a general principle in order to separate out the case of the elderly. Admittedly, he had opened his testimony with the statement that for the elderly, "the first line of defense is protection furnished as a right." But in response to hostile questions, he retreated, declaring that the federal government did not owe anyone "medical attention as a right." Medicare was to be part of the social security system, which meant that beneficiaries had paid for their benefits. And even if the first recipients would not have done so in strictly actuarial terms, still they had made their contributions "on a total program basis" (U.S. Congress 1964: 158). Although the meaning of that phrase was altogether obscure, the gist of the argument was clear: Medicare would not establish a right to health care. Ostensibly, it was not the opening shot in a larger campaign. In some oblique but still meaningful way, the principle remained that you got what you paid for, more or less.

Clearly, all these maneuvers were part of a strategy to get Medicare enacted, and many proponents insisted after the fact that they had been confident, undoubtedly too confident, that Medicare would be the first step on the road to national health insurance. They were, of course, wrong—for all the reasons we have been exploring, along with one other consideration. These Medicare proponents may have been too successful in marking off the case of the elderly. Having taken the pragmatic route, they reinforced older attitudes, afraid to come out in favor of a right to health care, afraid to break out of the mold of a quid pro quo mentality for benefits, afraid to advocate a program in terms that were more universal than middle-class interests. It was the 1930s almshouse dynamic revisited—because the worthy middle class could not be expected to go on relief to gain medical benefits, the system had to change. True, others would benefit from the program, including non-middle-class elderly. But that seemed almost serendipitous. Medicare was to protect the elderly middle classes from burdensome health care costs, not break new ground more generally by changing demeaning welfare policies or rethinking health care rights or the limits of private insurance for those under sixty-five. Thus, it should be less surprising that for the next several decades, Medicare did not inspire a new venture in government underwriting of health care.

Future Prospects

In light of a tradition of narrow middle-class self-interest, the entrepreneurial quality of American medicine, and the tradition of voluntarism, what are the current prospects for a national health insurance program?

Perhaps the most encouraging point is that each of the elements that have been discussed here are in flux. The middle classes, by all accounts, are feeling the impact of rising health insurance costs and are becoming increasingly vulnerable (through periodic unemployment or narrowing eligibility requirements of insurance companies) to the loss of insurance benefits. The weaknesses of a private system are in this way becoming quite apparent to them. At the same time, there are signs that American medicine is becoming less entrepreneurial, witness the increased numbers of salaried physicians employed by HMOs, corporations, and hospitals. And by now, the limits of voluntarism are glaringly obvious: whether the case is kidney dialysis or the future of the voluntary hospital, it is practically indisputable that the not-for-profit sector is incapable of shouldering the burden of health care.

All this would be grounds for optimism, were it not for one final element: the persistence of a narrowed vision of middle-class politics. With no largesse of spirit, with no sense of mutual responsibility, the middle classes—and their representatives—may advocate only minimal changes designed to provide protection only for them, not those in more desperate straits. In policy terms, it may bring changes that are more exclusive than inclusive, serving the employed as against the unemployed, protecting the benefits of those who have some coverage already as opposed to bringing more people to the benefits table. It may also promote schemes that will serve the lower classes in the most expedient fashion. The Oregon model, through which health insurance expands by restricting the benefits that Medicaid patients can receive, may become the standard response. Our past record suggests all too strongly that politics will find a way to protect those several rungs up the social ladder, while doing as little as possible for those at the bottom. Whether we will break this tradition and finally enact a truly national health insurance program remains an open question.

References

Koos, E. L. 1954. *The Health of Regionville*. New York: Columbia University Press.

Lynd, R., and H. M. Lynd. [1929] 1956. *Middletown*. New York: Harcourt, Brace & World, Harvest Books.

Marmor, T. 1982. *The Politics of Medicare*. New York: Aldine.

Morone, J. 1990. *The Democratic Wish*. New York: Basic.

President's Research Committee. 1933. *Recent Social Trends in the United States*. 2 vols. New York: McGraw Hill.

Rothman, D. J. 1991. The Public Presentation of Blue Cross, 1935–1965. *Journal of Health Politics, Policy and Law* 16: 672–93.

Schuler, E. A., R. J. Mowitz, and A. J. Mayer. 1952. *Medical Public Relations: A Study of the Public Relations Program of the Academy of Medicine of Toledo and Lucas County, Ohio, 1951*, Detroit, MI: Academy of Medicine of Toledo.

Starr, P. 1982. *The Social Transformation of American Medicine*. New York: Basic.

Thomas, V. C. 1923. *The Successful Physician*. Philadelphia: W. B. Saunders.

U.S. Congress. 1964. *Medical Care for the Aged*. Hearings before the Committee on Ways and Means, House of Representatives, 88th Cong., 1st Sess. 1.

Weir, M., A. Orloff, and T. Skocpol. 1988. *The Politics of Social Policy in the United States*. Princeton, NJ: Princeton University Press.

The research for this essay was conducted under a grant from the Twentieth Century Fund.

The Struggle for the Soul of Health Insurance

Deborah A. Stone

Abstract The politics of American health insurance is a struggle over which vision of distributive justice should govern: the solidarity principle or the logic of actuarial fairness. Actuarial fairness is central to American private health insurance. It is both an antiredistributive ideology and a method of organizing mutual aid by fragmenting communities into ever-smaller, more homogeneous groups, leading ultimately to the destruction of mutual aid. This fragmentation is accomplished by fostering in people a sense of their differences and their responsibility for themselves, rather than their commonalities and interdependence. Actuarial fairness developed as a business strategy for gaining market share. Medical underwriting, which is far more extensive than commonly known, is the information technology used for implementing actuarial fairness. Despite significant changes in the political context of health insurance which are leading toward restraints on underwriting, the logic of actuarial fairness is so deeply embedded in the structure of competitive markets in insurance and so deeply consonant with social divisions in American society that eradicating it will take more than any current reform proposals contemplate.

In the late 1980s, the trade associations of the health and life insurance industry sponsored an advertising campaign to persuade the reading public that "paying for someone else's risks" is a bad idea. In one of these ads, a photo of a workman in hard hat and tool belt straddling the girders of a steel tower was captioned: "If you don't take risks, why should you pay for someone else's?" Another ad showed a young man and woman playing basketball one-on-one and asked: "Why should men and women pay different rates for their health and life insurance?" The choral refrain at the bottom of each ad in the series went: "The lower your risk, the lower your premium," and the small print explained the relevant facts. For example:

> Women under 55 normally incur more health care expenses than men of the same age, so they pay more for individual health insurance than men. After age 55, women generally have lower claims costs, so they normally pay less for individual health insurance than men of the same age.
>
> That's why insurers have to group people with similar risks when they calculate premiums. If they didn't, people with low risks would end up subsidizing people with high risks. And that wouldn't be fair.

In late 1991, The Prudential Insurance Company ran a very different sort of ad campaign. In the *New York Times*, *Wall Street Journal*, and many newsweeklies, readers saw a photo of a chest X ray with a large white mass in the lower right quadrant. Though most readers couldn't interpret the X ray, the caption explained its significance: "Because he works for a small company, the prognosis isn't good for his fellow workers either." The small-print text went on to explain how one employee's serious illness might cause a small company to be charged "excessively high premiums" come renewal time and how the company might even be forced to drop its health insurance coverage. The Prudential, readers were assured, didn't consider this situation fair and was backing legislation to "regulate the guidelines and rating practices of insurers." Offering a rather different interpretation of fairness from the one in the trade association series a few years back, The Prudential opined, "After all, a small company shouldn't be forced to drop its health plan because an employee was sick enough to need it." [1]

These advertisements have many layers of meaning. On the surface, the issue is how commercial insurers ought to price their health insurance policies. Just below the surface lurks the struggle over health insurance reform proposals in the states and Congress. But the underlying question is whether medical care will be distributed as a right of citizenship or as a market commodity. If, as "the-lower-your-risk-the-lower-your-premium" series commends, we charge people as closely as possible for the medical care they need and consume, then we are treating medical care like other consumer goods distributed through the market. If, like The Prudential,

1. Each advertisement appeared several times in many places. I give here one citation where each may be found: Worker-in-hard-hat ad, *U.S. News and World Report*, 22 June 1987, p. 15; man-and-woman-playing-basketball ad, *USA Today*, 16 February 1987, p. 2A; Prudential chest X-ray ad, *New York Times*, 1 November 1991, p. A29.

we are unwilling to throw sick people and their fellow employees out of the insurance lifeboat, if we think perhaps the healthy should help pay for the care of others, then medical care becomes more like things we distribute as a right of citizenship, such as education. These advertisements symbolize two very different logics of insurance: the actuarial fairness principle and the solidarity principle.

At a deeper level still, these advertisements offer competing visions of community. They suggest how Americans should think about what ties them together and to whom they have ties. Consider hard hats and other workers in dangerous trades who get injuries and diseases doing constructive work for society: no one else, the ads say, should feel an obligation to pay for their risks. Take women of childbearing age, who are daily exhorted to assure the health of their babies, even those not yet conceived: no one else should finance their extra medical care for that purpose, least of all the men with whom they create the next generation (and recreate on the basketball courts). Alternatively, says the Prudential ad, we should not abandon those who are sick or attached in some way to people who are sick; sick and healthy, we are all one community.

Many things go into the making of community. Communities share a common culture and a way of perpetuating it. They establish processes for governance, conflict resolution, and self-defense. Above all, the people in a community help each other. Mutual aid among a group of people who see themselves as sharing common interests is the essence of community; a willingness to help each other is the glue that holds people together as a society, whether at the level of a simple peasant community (Scott 1976), an urban ghetto (Stack 1974), or a modern welfare state. What distinguishes mutual aid in the modern welfare state from that in peasant societies is largely a matter of scale: the number of people encompassed in the network of mutual aid, the degree of elaboration or rules and procedures for conducting mutual aid, and the number and variety of goods and services that are mutually provided.

All mutual aid systems are based on a shared definition of the legitimate reasons for redistribution—why, in what circumstances, and to whom people should give up something of their own and offer help. This is not to say there is no conflict over redistribution in a community; the boundaries of legitimate redistribution are constantly under challenge and always being redrawn (Stone 1988). But there is also a core of stable expectations about when people can expect help from one another.

While in most societies sickness is widely accepted as a condition that should trigger mutual aid, the American polity has had a weak and wavering commitment to that principle. The politics of health insurance can only be understood as a struggle over the meaning of sickness and whether it should be a condition that automatically generates mutual assistance. However, this is more than a cultural conflict or a fight over meanings. The private insurance industry, the first line of defense in the U.S. system of mutual aid for sickness, is organized around a principle profoundly antithetical to the idea of mutual aid, and indeed, the growth and survival of the industry depends on its ability to finance health care by charging the sick and to convince the public that "each person should pay for his own risk."

The central argument of this essay is this: Actuarial fairness—each person paying for his own risk—is more than an idea about distributive justice. It is a method of organizing mutual aid by fragmenting communities into ever-smaller, more homogeneous groups and a method that leads ultimately to the destruction of mutual aid. This fragmentation must be accomplished by fostering in people a sense of their differences, rather than their commonalities, and their responsibility for themselves only, rather than their interdependence. Moreover, insurance necessarily operates on the logic of actuarial fairness when it, in turn, is organized as a competitive market.

The essay begins by explicating the solidarity principle and the actuarial fairness principle as alternative visions of distributive justice. It then describes how actuarial fairness developed as a business strategy for gaining market share and how medical underwriting, the information technology for implementing actuarial fairness, works in practice. Next it describes significant changes in the political context of health insurance that seem to be leading toward restraints on underwriting—not the least of which is The Prudential Company singing the solidarity tune. I argue, however, that the logic of actuarial fairness is so deeply embedded in the structure of competitive markets in insurance and so deeply consonant with social divisions in American society that eradicating it will take more than any current reform proposals contemplate.

The Solidarity Principle

Both social and commercial health insurance are mechanisms for pooling savings and redistributing funds from healthy premium payers to sick ones. They operate by two fundamentally different logics, however. Social insurance operates by the logic of *solidarity*. Its purpose is to guarantee that certain agreed-upon individual needs will be paid for by a community or group. This is the logic of mutual aid societies and fraternal associations, as well as the logic of government social insurance programs. Having decided in advance that some need is deserving of social aid, a society undertakes to guarantee that the need is met for all its members. In the health area, the argument for financing medical care via social insurance rests on the prior assumption that medical care should be distributed according to medical need or the ability of the individual to benefit from medical care.

If medical care were financed like most market goods, by charging people for exactly the goods and services they consume, the ultimate distribution of medical care would be only partially according to need. Those who are sick and need care would come forward to purchase it, but among the sick, only those who could afford it would actually receive care. In addition, some who are not sick but who have resources might try to purchase care as well. People who could not afford to buy care would not receive any, regardless of their need for it or ability to benefit from it.

Social insurance unties the two essential connections of the market: the linkage between the amount one pays for care and the amount one consumes and the linkage between the amount of care one buys and one's ability to pay. Under a social insurance scheme, individuals are entitled to receive whatever care they need, and the amounts they pay to finance the scheme are totally unrelated to the amount or cost of care they actually use. (If there are coinsurance and deductibles in a social insurance scheme, the amount a person pays is slightly related to the amount one consumes.)

Of course, even social insurance does not guarantee that medical care is distributed exactly according to medical need. Need, after all, is a rather elusive concept, all the more so in the area of medicine.[2] Unlike most consumer goods, the value of medical care depends on its being customized. Whether a person can benefit from a particular medical procedure does not hinge on "tastes and preferences," as classical economic theory would have it, but rather on a correct match between a medical procedure and the person's particular pathology. The degree to which social insurance results in allocation of care according to need is mediated by the professional skill of medical personnel in matching procedures to pathologies. Many other factors influence the distribution of care as well, such as local professional norms about the appropriate use of procedures; the supply of

---

2. For an exceptionally insightful and nuanced dissection of the concept of unnecessary care, see Blustein and Marmor 1992.

medical facilities, personnel, and equipment; and ownership of diagnostic and therapeutic facilities, such as imaging centers and dialysis clinics (Hillman et al. 1990). All of these factors mean that even under a system of pure social insurance, medical care will not be perfectly distributed according to medical need. But the *ideal* of the solidarity principle is that we should strive to distribute medical care according to medical need and to limit the influence of ability to pay, past consumption of medical care, or expected future consumption.

At the same time, the solidarity principle does not require that medical care be distributed equally, in the sense that everyone gets the same amount. Social insurance is not a fixed shares arrangement, where each contributing member gets an equal slice of the pie. When people "pool their risks" as well as their savings in social insurance, they are taking their chances that they may never become sick or need expensive care, and that most of their contributions will go to help the members who do need expensive care. As in any lottery, they pay into the pot, regardless of whether they ultimately get to draw out of it.

In fact, only some members of a risk pool will get sick enough to need care. Since only those who get seriously sick will receive a payout, the others necessarily pay to help them. Thus, redistribution from the healthy to the sick is built into insurance. Payouts are made on the basis of need (or loss incurred), not on the basis of contributions to the scheme. Health policy analysts and corporate benefits managers frequently discover with great alarm that a small portion of insured people accounts for a huge proportion of claims expenditures, as though this skewing means that something is amiss. But subsidy from the vast majority of policyholders to a small minority is precisely what is supposed to happen in insurance. Such skewing is what people agree to when they join a social insurance risk pool. They accept it because they don't know, when they join, whether they will be on the giving end or the receiving end, and they want to protect themselves in case they are part of the unlucky minority. They accept it, too, because they believe that sickness is one of those contingencies when society should rally around the individual.

The Principle of Actuarial Fairness

Commercial insurers, that is, private firms selling insurance as a profit-making venture, operate on a deep contradiction. They provide for pooling of risks and mutual aid among policyholders, much as social insurance does, yet they select their policyholders, group them, and price their policies according to market logic. When they speak of equity or distributive justice, commercial insurers espouse the principle of actuarial fairness. It holds that premium rates should be differentiated so that "each insured [person] will pay in accordance with the quality of his risk" (Bailey et al. 1976: 782, citing Mowbray et al. 1969). By quality of risk, insurers mean the likelihood a person will incur whatever loss he or she is insured against. In life insurance, they are principally interested in factors that might affect life expectancy, while in health insurance, they are interested in factors that affect or predict a person's use of medical care. These include one's occupation, hobbies (since some are very dangerous), family medical history, personal medical history, and any medical information that is prognostic of disease, even if disease hasn't yet occurred.

Insurers assert that actuarial fairness requires them to seek the most complete risk information on applicants. An insurer has the "responsibility to treat all its policyholders fairly by establishing premiums at a level consistent with the risk represented by each individual policyholder" (Clifford and Iuculano 1987: 1806). To accomplish this task, insurers must have the "right . . . to create classifications to recognize the many differences which exist among individuals" (Clifford and Iuculano 1987: 1808). People who have diseases or serious risks to their health are in a sense getting a more valuable insurance policy than those with lesser risks, so they ought to pay more for the extra value. Or, to see the matter another way, if insurers did not identify people with higher risks, separate them from the general pool of policyholders, and charge them more, insurers would be causing a "forced subsidy from the healthy to the less healthy" (Clifford and Iuculano 1987: 1811). "An applicant presenting a low risk of loss to the insurer should not be required to subsidize another applicant who presents a higher degree of risk" (Hoffman and Kincaid 1986–87: 717).

Here is the crux of the conflict: the very redistribution from the healthy to the sick that is the essential purpose of health insurance under the solidarity principle is anathema to commercial insurers. Tellingly, insurers virtually never use the word *subsidy* without a pejorative modifier such as *coerced*, *forced*, or *unfair*. Although all insurance entails a subsidy from the lucky to the unlucky (whether for car accidents, diseases, or fires), commercial insurers eschew subsidy from one "class" of policyholders to another. (*Class*, in insurance jargon, means risk class, or a group of people with similar probabilities of becoming sick or, perhaps more accurately, with similar probabilities of generating costs to a company.) To commercial insurers, subsidy is not what they pursue but the *unwanted result* of their failure or inability to segregate people into homogeneous risk classes.

If the actuarial fairness principle could be perfectly implemented, if we had perfect predictive information and precise rating, each person would pay for her- or himself. This, of course, would be the antithesis of insurance. (In fact, in a world of perfect predictive information, there would be no need and no market demand for insurance, because no one would stand to gain by "beating the odds." Since each insurance policy would be priced according to the medical care actually consumed by each policyholder, people would do better to pay for the care directly and avoid paying for the administrative expenses and profit margins of insurance companies. And since the price of insurance would be the same as the price of needed medical care, those who couldn't afford to pay for their own care couldn't afford to pay for insurance either.) Insurers rarely acknowledge that actuarial fairness undermines the solidarity principle of insurance, but the ultimate conclusion of their logic is clear. In the words of Robert Goldstone, vice president and medical director of Pacific Mutual Life Company:

> In theory, every individual should have a different rate, based on a multivariate analysis of every possible health condition and risk factor that can be evaluated. (Goldstone 1992: 26)

Actuarial Fairness as Business Strategy

For all the talk about fairness and equity, tailoring prices to finely differentiated risks is the keystone of insurers' competitive marketing strategy. They seek to gain a larger share of the market for various types of insurance by offering the lowest prices for coverage. A firm can offer lower prices if it can separate the potentially healthy from the potentially sick and offer insurance only to the healthy. Even defenders of the industry acknowledge that market competition and profit seeking drive the pursuit of actuarial fairness:

> Although to a large extent the effect [of increasingly sophisticated risk classification] has been equitable . . . , it must be acknowledged that a motivation equally strong is competition between and among insurance companies. The competitive aspects have long been and remain now very compelling, with the insurance industry striving . . . to attract what are considered the best and most desirable insureds by classification devices which can lead to price advantages. (Bailey et al. 1976: 790–91)

Underwriting is the process insurers use to find "the best and most desirable insureds." In a sense, the customers of life and health insurance companies are not only customers but raw materials. The more durable (long-lived) and well-made (resistant to disease) the policyholders are, the more money the insurance company makes. Underwriting entails gathering information about applicants to determine their risk status and then selecting the better risks to insure. Medical underwriting was first developed in the life insurance business. For most of the nineteenth century, life insurance was sold only to people who could pass a medical examination.[3] People who already had a personal or family history of disease, or for that matter worked in occupations deemed hazardous or unsavory, were refused insurance and labeled by the companies as "uninsurable risks." In the early twentieth century, several companies saw the potential for marketing higher-priced life insurance to people who did not meet the health standards for ordinary (or "standard") insurance, but who still had a very low risk of early death. This market niche was dubbed "substandard" business.

Many life insurance companies saw the substandard market as a way to gain new business. New companies sometimes saw it as a way to attract brokers (who presumably were having trouble placing their high-risk clients elsewhere), and some non–life companies (for example, those selling property or casualty insurance) saw the substandard market as a "way to get their foot in the door" of life insurance (Will 1974: 39–40). As recently as 1985, a British underwriting text said a life insurance company could expect to increase its business by about 5 percent by "accepting substandard lives on a broad basis" (Brackenridge 1985: 45).

To capture the substandard business, life insurers developed a measurement and classification scheme for calculating premium rates for people who normally would not qualify for life insurance. Known as the numerical rating system, it assigns debits and credits to applicants on the basis of their build (height and weight), health history and predictive diagnostic tests, family health history, occupation, and habits. An applicant is assumed to start at 100 percent of the standard risk and so starts with one hundred points. Each disease or abnormal diagnostic finding (such as high blood pressure) is assigned a number of points to be added to the standard risk. If a person has factors that contribute to longevity and health (such as a safe occupation or a good family history), he may receive some credits which will be subtracted from the total. All the points assigned to an applicant are added (or subtracted if they are credits) to

---

3. Some companies, notably The Prudential and Metropolitan Life, developed what was called "industrial life insurance" for the working class. This insurance was generally available without medical examination or with only a very cursory one, but it was available only for very small amounts.

reach a final numerical rating, which is said to be the person's mortality. For example, an applicant who received twenty-five debits for family history, twenty-five debits for excess drinking, and five credits for being in a safe occupation would get a total score of 145, for a mortality of 145 percent, or an "extra" or "excess" mortality of 45 percent. The actuaries then price a policy for someone deemed to have 45 percent excess mortality. Some diseases are considered so likely to result in early mortality that people with them are deemed uninsurable and refused any offer of a policy.[4]

One consequence of the codification of medical and epidemiological knowledge was that both life and health insurers no longer relied so heavily on staff doctors. Most underwriting decisions are now made by lay personnel, based on information disclosed by the applicant as well as information from applicants' physicians and medical records.[5] The underwriting departments of insurance companies use underwriting guides setting forth a detailed list of diseases and diagnostic tests and explaining how each medical finding is to be treated by that company. Many companies also provide their agents and brokers with a simplified version of this guide, often called a rating manual, and agents usually do a preliminary screening at the time they take an application. They are likely to determine on the spot whether a person or group will be accepted by the company.

The numerical rating system, and the underwriting guides and rating manuals it spawned, have all the trappings of scientific objectivity— medical terminology, elaborate matrices of diseases and point values, and numbers—but they often seem to be based as much on social prejudices and stereotypes as on empirical knowledge. For example, a 1930 pocket manual for agents of the Northwest Union Life Insurance Company (1930) begins a section titled "Uninsurable Risks" with the following statement: "Negroes, Chinese, Japanese, Mexicans and more than one-fourth blood Indians will not be considered" (p. 9). In the same guide, pregnant women are not acceptable until three months after "a normal childbirth," and "a married woman who has not borne at least one normal child is uninsurable until she has been married at least five years" (p. 5). A 1931 underwriting guide for accident and health insurance says that "health insurance should not be encouraged" for menopausal women, because "there are disturbed physical functions of many kinds, nervousness being

4. For descriptions of the numerical rating system, see Rogers and Hunter 1919; Shepherd and Webster 1957; Will 1974; Bailey 1985; and Brackenridge 1985.

5. A detailed description of insurers' sources of information in medical underwriting is in Stone 1992.

particularly common" (Hauschild 1931: 83). The same guide has this (and only this) to say about salpingectomy: "Removal of the tube connecting the ovary to the womb. Consider as due to gonorrhea and underwrite accordingly" (p. 83). The "founding document" of the numerical rating system, published in the *Transactions of the Society of American Actuaries* in 1919, uses the following example to demonstrate the importance of letting personal judgment override the numbers when underwriters use the numerical rating system:

> Take, for example, a *clergyman, an occupation which is conducive to longevity*, whose build is most favorable, whose family is very long lived and whose habits are first class. The summation of all of these favorable factors may very well produce a valuation even lower than so favorable a combination would produce in nature. *Undoubtedly the stock from which such a risk springs has expressed its moral and its physical energy in the occupation and the temperate life of this individual.* On the other hand, the rating for a bartender who is known to use alcohol freely or from time to time to excess is not the algebraic summation of the two factors of Occupation and Habits for the reason that *the high mortality incident to the occupation of bartender is in part due of* [sic] *the fact that substantially all bartenders use alcohol freely.* The valuation of all such cases, especially where factors may be interrelated, must always be tempered by the judgment of the medical expert. (Rogers and Hunter 1919: 71–72; emphasis added)

Occupation was always an important aspect of life and health insurance underwriting (the *New York Times*'s alarmed discovery of the phenomenon notwithstanding) (Freudenheim 1990). As the previous quotation illustrates, a great deal of stereotyping went into occupational ratings. Insurers theoretically group occupations into classes with similar average claims costs, but it is striking how the occupational tables of underwriting manuals parallel social class categories. Here are the six occupational categories used in one typical rating system:

5A Professional men (such as doctors of medicine, attorneys, certified public accountants, top management personnel from business, or professional people performing primarily office duties).

4A Sales managers and management-type salesmen dealing with buyers at the management level. The salesman does not carry demonstration equipment with him and does not travel by private automobile.

3A   Real estate agents and salesmen of items usually demonstrated (such as typewriters, adding machines, or hardware). Contractors in the construction industry who do not do actual manual labor.

2A   Self-employed small businessmen, including filling station operators, electricians, and plumbers. Highly skilled technicians and foremen ordinarily employed year-round.

A   Most skilled workers in trades having a relatively light occupational hazard and requiring dexterity rather than strength or lifting ability.

B   All individuals engaged in hazardous occupations, occupations involved in heavy physical work, and substantially all common, unskilled labor. (Closely paraphrased from Will 1974: 122–23)

Insurers use the term *insurability* as though it were a natural property of individuals, rather than a policy decision of a firm.[6] The classic industry textbook on life insurance lists several "reasons why some persons are not insurable." Each of them is a characteristic of applicants—their imminent death, probable short life span, "poor health of such a nature that a premium cannot be computed because of lack of data relating to the risk involved," or their dishonesty (Huebner 1935: 514–15). Contemporary insurance texts often state a numerical criterion for insurability: people are uninsurable for life insurance if their mortality is five or more times the standard mortality (see, e.g., Brackenridge 1985: 33). Insurability for health insurance has no single numerical cutoff point; instead, as insurance magazines and texts are quick to point out, insurability depends on the likelihood of need for expensive medical care for a person with any disease.

Insurance is a social endeavor, however, and insurability is a collective decision about membership, not a natural trait of individuals. A person is insurable if a group (fraternal organization, mutual benefit society, insurance company, government program) *decides* it will extend mutual aid to him or her. Commercial insurers' treatment of insurability as if it were

6. Compare "Applicants for life insurance fall into one of two broad classes, insurable and uninsurable" (Mehr 1983: 458); "Medical insurability is not, however, a phenomenon suffered exclusively by those at risk of developing AIDS. Individuals suffering from developmental disabilities, physical or mental impairments, or chronic health conditions account for a large number of those who are unable to obtain individually purchased health insurance. Estimates place the number of uninsurables in the country today at one million" (Clifford and Iuculano 1987: 1822, footnote omitted).

an individual characteristic, or even a mathematically determined decision based on individuals' natural traits, masks the way insurers create and control membership organizations through which people will conduct mutual aid. Of course, the mutual aid groups within commercial insurance are anonymous statistical communities of "homogeneous risk classes," rather than real social or political communities with a common culture or decision-making structure. Still, this creation of exclusive subcommunities of mutual aid is the essence of insurance as a commercial enterprise.

Insurance underwriting, far from being a dry statistical exercise, is a political exercise in drawing the boundaries of community membership. That insurers always understood they were creating communities of privilege is very clear. When, in 1865, the Connecticut General Life Insurance Company petitioned for a charter to form the Connecticut Invalid Life Insurance Company to specialize in substandard risks, the petition noted that

> as [the business of life insurance in this state and also the United States] is at present conducted, a large class of community is excluded from its blessing and benefits on account of imperfections of health and constitutional weaknesses. (Buley 1953: 113)

The author of a vanity history of the New York Life Insurance Company, who credits the company with invention of the substandard market, notes: "To most life companies there were only two classes of people in the world: one was entitled to all the privileges and benefits of life insurance; the other was entitled to nothing" (Abbott 1930: 279). The significance of the company's development of the numerical rating system was best summed up, he says, by the company's then president, Darwin Kingsley: "This contribution to Life Insurance has taken an innumerable army of men and women out of the Purgatory of the impaired and put them into the Paradise of the insured" (Abbott 1930: 287).

Today's commercial insurance leaders are perhaps less purple in their prose but no less certain in their minds that membership in private sector insurance schemes is a privilege not all can or should share. In response to public controversy and concern over the implications of new genetic knowledge for access to health and life insurance, Robert Pokorski, a vice president and medical director of Lincoln National Life Insurance Company, directed and coauthored a report for the American Council of Life Insurance (ACLI 1989). The report's authors agree that fairness, sound insurance principles, and the public interest will require life and health insurers to use genetic tests to determine insurability and prices. Discussing the topic of "Public and Private Insurance," Pokorski writes:

> Many people believe they are entitled to both private life and private health insurance. . . . The United States has used private means to fulfill certain general social welfare needs such as payment for health care. But private health insurance has never been a completely adequate or universal method of providing access to the health care system, nor has it been a perfect mechanism for covering all diseases. *The poor, disabled, aged or seriously ill cannot always be covered by private means.* (Pokorski 1989: 10–11; emphasis added)

Actuarial Fairness in Practice: Medical Underwriting in Health Insurance

The numerical rating system originally designed for life insurance became the core of the medical underwriting system in health insurance. Though the core technology was the same, however, the dynamics of health insurance competition were just the opposite of those in life insurance. In life insurance, an aggressive insurer would seek to identify relatively *high-risk* people who were being rejected by other companies and offer them insurance at a slightly higher price. In health insurance, if an insurer were able to identify a relatively healthy group of people, a group whose predicted rates of sickness and medical expense were lower than the standard risks on which premium rates are based, the insurer could profitably offer that group insurance at a lower-than-standard rate. As is now well known, this is the dynamic by which commercial companies plucked customers from Blue Cross/Blue Shield plans and thus gained a foothold in the health insurance market which they at first eschewed (Starr 1982: 295–310; Fein 1985: 10–32).

We have long understood how commercial insurers were able to use experience rating to segment the market into more homogeneous risk classes and thus gain market share. Experience rating is simply retrospective underwriting; insurers base their projections of future medical care consumption on how much medical care a group actually used in the previous year, instead of on less reliable personal questionnaires and epidemiological data. To summarize the story briefly, between 1934 and 1945, thirty-five states passed enabling legislation creating Blue Cross plans as hospital service corporations, granting them status as charitable organizations and exempting them from state insurance laws, reserve requirements, and premium taxes. The main justification for this special treatment was their promise to provide health insurance for all people without regard to ability to pay. The Blue Cross plans (and later the Blue Shield plans covering physicians' services) used community rating. They charged the same premiums to all employee groups in a geographic area or industry, thus pooling the risks of illness broadly in a region.

When commercial insurers entered the market, they used experience rating. This pricing was the key to their strategy for gaining market share. By charging different premiums according to a group's actual use of medical services, insurance companies could offer lower rates to occupations, industries, or firms with healthier-than-average employees. Another variation on this strategy is euphemistically called "durational" rating. An insurer offers a small, healthy group or firm a low premium rate for the first year to lure it from another plan; then, as members of the group get sick and incur medical bills, the insurer raises the rates rapidly. Corporate benefits managers and small business owners would naturally choose to buy insurance from companies that offered them cheaper rates, so they would withdraw from the large Blue Cross/Blue Shield (BCBS) community pool, leaving a slightly less healthy group of people (on average) in the pool. BCBS then had to raise its prices to its remaining members. Eventually, most BCBS plans also gave up community rating.

What is less well understood is how commercial health insurers used *prospective* medical underwriting to attract "desirable risks" and screen out undesirable ones and what the impact of these practices is on access to health insurance and medical care. Insurers generally use the term *medical underwriting* to mean examination of *individuals* (or their records) to determine insurability and price a policy, and they consistently maintain that in this sense there is very little medical underwriting. Since most commercial health insurance is sold to large employee groups, and since (they claim) insurers do not screen individuals in large employee groups, very few people are affected by medical underwriting or put at risk of losing access to health insurance on account of their medical histories and prognoses. Thus, a joint report on genetic testing by the American Council of Life Insurance and the Health Insurance Association of America (ACLI-HIAA 1991: 5) asserts:

> Most health insurance is not individually underwritten and so genetic testing would have no effect on the vast majority of health insurance consumers. About 85–90 percent of health insurance is currently purchased through group plans which accept all full-time employees and dependents without evidence of insurability.

This industry assessment of the impact of underwriting is both widely accepted[7] and highly misleading. First, 19 percent of workers who have employer-based coverage work for firms of fewer than ten employees, where individual underwriting virtually always obtains. Another 17 percent work for firms with between ten and twenty-five employees, where individual underwriting is extremely common.[8]

The industry assessment of the extent of medical underwriting is misleading, secondly, because there is a significant amount of individual medical underwriting even in fairly large employee groups. A 1987 survey of health insurer underwriting practices by the Office of Technology Assessment (OTA) (U.S. Congress 1988) found a substantial degree of individual underwriting in groups. Only 44 percent of commercial insurers said they never request a physician statement for some members of large group plans, and only 70 percent said they never use a physical exam for large group plans (i.e., nearly one-third sometimes require physical exams for members of large group plans) (p. 72, Table 2-12). One-third of Blue Cross/Blue Shield plans said they sometimes request an attending physician statement on selected members of large group plans (p. 75). Only 13 percent of commercial insurers said they never use attending physician statements in small group plans (p. 72, Table 2-12). Fully 58 percent of commercial companies and 7 percent of Blue Cross/ Blue Shield plans said they were "using or moving towards" screening individuals for high-risk AIDS status in large employee groups (pp. 80–85).[9]

7. See Clifford and Iuculano 1987: 1809: "In contrast to underwriting for individual insurance, insurers underwriting group life and health insurance consider only the relevant characteristics of the *group*, not of the individuals who comprise the group. . . . Although no screening takes place in most group situations, there are at least three exceptions: (1) small groups; (2) late entrants to a group plan; and (3) large amounts of life insurance that are used to supplement basic coverage." See also footnote 9 below.

8. Figures are from the 1987 National Medical Expenditure Survey, cited in HIAA 1991: 7, Fig. 1. It is striking that the HIAA continues to say that no more than 15 percent of workers are subject to underwriting, when the organization obviously ▪ knows otherwise.

9. Despite the OTA's findings about the prevalence of individual underwriting in group insurance, the Executive Summary of its report repeats the industry's public relations estimate:

Group applicants for health insurance, who comprise 85 to 90 percent of all persons with health insurance and who obtain their health insurance predominantly through the workplace, seldom if ever, are subjected to individual determinations of their health status. (p. 3)

The general discussion prior to the survey results gives the same impression, suggesting that only very small groups of up to fifteen employees are individually underwritten (p. 44). The discrepancy between the OTA staff's own findings and its summary of its whole investigation in the report suggests the extraordinary power of the industry to influence the perceptions of even a scientific staff agency of Congress. Representatives of the commercial life and health insurers, Blue Cross/Blue Shield, and HMOs were members of the advisory panel for the OTA's study and helped design the survey.

A survey of insurers by the Colorado Division of Insurance found an even greater degree of individual medical underwriting in large group policies than the Office of Technology Assessment, in part because the Colorado survey specifically asked insurers about the group size at which they start to underwrite (Yondorff 1990).[10] According to this survey, 11 percent of all commercial accident and health insurers and nonprofits require individual medical underwriting for *all groups*, regardless of size; 18 percent underwrite groups of up to ninety-nine people; 25 percent underwrite groups of up to seventy-four people; 33 percent underwrite groups of up to forty-nine people; and 40 percent underwrite groups of up to twenty-four people (p. 15, Table 8).

A third reason the industry estimate of the prevalence of underwriting is too low is that it ignores a major device for acquiring medical information about employees in large groups *without* obtaining it directly from the employees. Even when employee groups are large enough to escape traditional individual medical underwriting, insurers often require the employer to submit medical information about individual employees and their dependents. This information is gathered through medical questions on the master application for a group, questions called "risk-finder questions" or "gatekeeping questions" in the industry. Typically, one question asks whether, to the best of the employer's knowledge, any employee or dependent had claims over a certain amount (say $2,500 or $7,500) during the previous year or two years. The master application also includes questions about medical problems among employees and their dependents, such as:

Has any employee or dependent had heart disease, cancer, kidney disorder, stroke, or other serious disease?

To the best of your knowledge, during the last 24 months, has any of the employees or dependents to be covered received treatment for cancer,

10. Although this survey covers only insurers operating in the Colorado health insurance market, it is still the best and most important survey on underwriting practices. It asked questions very precisely to elicit clear answers. For example, it asked "What is the smallest group you will cover on a group underwriting basis without individual medical underwriting?" The Office of Technology Assessment survey, by contrast, asked respondents to distinguish their answers to all questions for "individuals" and "individually underwritten groups—i.e., those groups which are too small to qualify for experience rating and whose members must be individually underwritten" (U.S. Congress 1988: Appendix D, p. 184). Thus, the OTA survey was incapable of determining insurer policies about individual underwriting and group size. The Colorado survey also asked many questions about quasi-individual underwriting via "risk fact-finder questions," an important phenomenon discussed below in the essay. Although this was a survey limited to one state, the respondents accounted for 68 percent of the total state insurance market, including nineteen of the top twenty insurers in the state and many large insurers who operate in multiple states.

kidney ailments, diabetes, heart, immune system disorder, psychological, alcohol, or drug disorders?

Are there any employees or dependents with medical conditions that may require hospitalization or surgery within the next 6 months?

Has any of the covered employees/dependents been hospitalized within the last 12 months?

When the answer to any question is yes, the employer is sometimes required to provide the names of employees or dependents and more medical information about them.[11]

Since these group applications request medical information about individual employees and dependents, even though employees do not fill out medical questionnaires, this is really *quasi-individual medical underwriting*, and it is very prevalent. The Colorado survey found that 59 percent of insurers require a risk-finder questionnaire for groups of up to forty-nine people. Nearly half of all insurers (48 percent) require the questionnaire for groups of up to ninety-nine people, and over one-third (36 percent) require it for groups of up to 199 people. Nearly one-third (32 percent) require a risk-finder questionnaire on all groups, regardless of size (Yondorff 1990: 45, Table 15).

In addition to traditional medical underwriting, there is a vast amount of what insurers informally call "underwriting at claims time," after an insurance policy is already in force. When an insured person or the medical provider submits a claim for payment, the insurer must make a decision whether to pay the claim. At this point, individual medical information enters again. The key vehicle here is the *preexisting condition clause*. Preexisting condition clauses exclude payment for any condition the applicant had prior to the insurance contract.[12] They differ from exclusion waivers in two important ways. First, to write an exclusion waiver into a policy, insurers must detect some problem, from either the applicant's medical

11. I am interviewing insurance agents and brokers as part of a larger project. Information about the content and handling of gatekeeper questions comes from these interviews and from health insurance application forms.

12. These clauses vary in three dimensions: (1) the period of time before the policy takes effect, during which a condition must have appeared or been treated to be considered preexisting; (2) the period of time a person must be "treatment free" after the effective date of the policy before the condition is eligible for coverage in the new policy; and (3) the period of time a person must be covered under the policy before the preexisting condition can be covered, regardless of whether the person has received treatment. This is the waiting period. Typically, for each of these three dimensions, the time period can range from three months to two years, depending on the insurer and the policy.

records or the application, *in advance of issuing the policy*. The policy then specifically names the condition (or body part or system) as excluded. With the preexisting condition clause, insurers do not need any information about the applicant. The clause is like a wild card. It allows the insurer to refuse payment (tantamount to not insuring) for any condition the person had prior to the policy issue date, even when no information about the condition turned up in the medical underwriting process.

Preexisting conditions are generally defined in insurance policies as conditions which "manifested themselves," "existed," or "were treated" before the effective date of the policy. These words leave some leeway for interpretation, especially the "existed" criterion. Insurers have insisted on their right to refuse payment even for treatment of conditions which had not been diagnosed prior to the claim and of which the applicant had no knowledge. Courts have often upheld insurers on this point.[13]

Because of the wild-card property of the preexisting condition clause, it is much more potent than the exclusion waiver and can be applied to many more people. Thus, the second key feature of the clause is that, unlike the exclusion waiver, it can be, and is, widely applied to group policies. According to one survey of two thousand employers, 64 percent of firms with fewer than five hundred employees and 45 percent of firms with more than ten thousand employees used these clauses in their policies (Colton 1991, citing a survey by Foster Higgins). Preexisting condition clauses have the same effect as exclusion waivers—denying coverage for precisely those illnesses people have—without insurers having to do any underwriting at all.

Though we still do not know exactly how many people are affected by medical underwriting, the number must be vastly greater than either the insurance industry or the Office of Technology Assessment report suggests. Consider that about *44 percent* of the work force are self-employed or employed in firms of under one hundred employees.[14] Of workers who *have* employer-based health insurance, 36 percent work in firms of twenty-five or fewer employees, and 60 percent work in firms of one

13. Dear v. Blue Cross of Louisiana, 511 So. 2d. 73 (La. App. 1987) (insurer entitled to deny payment for a condition that predated the effective date of the policy, even though there had been no diagnosis or treatment but only symptoms); Hanum v. General Life and Accident Ins. Co., 745 W.W. 2d 500 (Tex. App. 1988) (insurer may deny payment under preexisting condition clause for a condition which, though not diagnosed prior to the policy, manifested itself in symptoms from which one learned in medicine could diagnose such a sickness or illness). See also Goldstein 1988.

14. Citizens Fund 1991: 22, Table 4 (calculated from Current Population Survey, March 1990; figures are for 1989).

hundred or fewer employees, where, incidentally, self-insurance is not prevalent.[15] From what we know about medical underwriting in groups, the number of people subject to medical underwriting is almost certainly much larger than the 10 to 15 percent of people with commercial health insurance claimed by the insurance industry. A more accurate guess, taking into account all forms of individual medical underwriting, including risk-finder questions and preexisting condition clauses, and taking into account family members' dependence on the insurability of breadwinners, might be that at least half of those with commercial insurance are subject to some form of underwriting.

What happens to people who are subject to medical underwriting? When an individual or group is found to have high risks for disease and so not qualify as a standard risk, insurers might do several things. In the individual market, insurers can reject the applicant altogether as uninsurable; accept the applicant but charge a higher premium ("substandard rates"); accept the applicant but exclude coverage for a disease or organ or body system (called an "exclusion waiver"); or apply *both* an exclusion waiver and substandard rates. In the group market, the options are similar but include treating some members of the employee group differently from others. Thus, an insurer can reject a whole group; accept most of the group but exclude individuals who are deemed high-risk; charge a higher rate for the whole group or, alternatively, increase the rates only for the high-risk individuals in the group; limit the conditions or amounts covered either for the whole group or for certain members of the group; or *both* limit coverage and charge higher rates. (In some states, insurers are required to accept or reject an entire group, and it is in these states that they are likely to reject a group with a few sick or high-risk members, because they cannot control the membership of their insured pool.) All of these responses, of course, directly undermine the purpose of health insurance from the point of view of the solidarity principle or the distribution of medical care according to need; they ensure that the costs of care must be borne by those who need it, and they grant access to medical care (via insurance coverage) to the healthiest people instead of to the sickest. Exclusion waivers, moreover, are a major contributor to underinsurance, since they deny coverage for precisely those medical conditions a person has and is likely to need treatment for.

It is very difficult to know what insurers actually do when faced with high-risk applicants. Since underwriting itself is a chief component of

15. HIAA 1991: 7; citing figures from the 1987 National Medical Expenditures Survey.

firms' competitive strategy, insurers are not eager to disclose their practices. An even more important obstacle may be that most insurers do not keep statistics on their underwriting decisions. In the Colorado survey, only 19 percent of respondents said they keep statistics on the number of groups that apply each year and are declined (Yondorff 1990: 20, Table 13).

We can get some indication of the impact of medical underwriting on access to health insurance by looking at the Office of Technology Assessment figures for the individual insurance market in 1987–88, where everyone agrees that individual medical underwriting is universal. The OTA survey found that within the commercial individual insurance market, around 8 percent of applicants are rejected outright for medical reasons. Commercial insurers apply exclusion waivers to another 13 percent, charge higher premiums to 5 percent, and use both exclusion waivers and higher premiums for 2 percent (U.S. Congress 1988: 62). Taking these groups together, fully 28 percent of applicants do not meet the medical criteria to qualify as standard risks. Assuming that people who apply for commercial individual health policies are representative of the population (and they are probably not), we might extrapolate that 23 percent of people would be deemed uninsurable or subject to exclusion waivers if they had to submit to medical underwriting. (Here I have excluded the 5 percent who would have access to insurance if they could afford the higher rates; 23 percent represents the number who would be completely uninsured or underinsured if they had to undergo medical underwriting.) In fact, people who apply for commercial individual health insurance policies are probably wealthier and more educated than average and therefore probably also healthier (if basic epidemiology is right), making the 23 percent estimate *low*.

The Colorado survey asked insurers what actions they took and which action they take most frequently in the group market. Over half the insurers (54 percent) mentioned rejection of the group as the action most frequently taken when underwriting turns up adverse results. Fifteen percent said their most frequent action was to accept the group but exclude the high-risk individuals. Another 15 percent said their most frequent action was to limit coverage of high-risk individuals in the group (Yondorff 1990: 16). Needless to say, each of these actions causes some people to be uninsured or underinsured.

Another way to estimate the impact of medical underwriting on access to health insurance is to determine what portion of the citizenry would be ineligible for standard-risk insurance if they were subject to individual underwriting. The Citizens Fund of Washington, D.C., used the underwriting manual of a large insurance company to identify medical conditions that would lead to denials, substandard rating, or waivers and then estimated the prevalence of those conditions in the general population from epidemiological surveys. Using this method, the study found that 81 million people under age sixty-five would not qualify for standard insurance if they had to submit to medical underwriting (Citizens Fund 1991: 8). This amounts to about 33 percent of the population, quite a bit higher than the estimate yielded by extrapolating from the OTA survey for the individual insurance market. The Citizens Fund estimate also corresponds rather nicely with a *New York Times* survey on "job lock," in which 30 percent of respondents said they or someone in their family had stayed in a job they wanted to leave mainly because they feared losing health insurance (Eckholm 1991).

Where Does It All Lead?

The logic and methods of actuarial fairness mean denying insurance to those who most need medical care. The principle actually distributes medical care in *inverse* relation to need, and to the large extent that commercial insurers operate on this principle, the American reliance on the private sector as its main provider of health insurance establishes a system that is perfectly and perversely designed to keep sick people away from doctors. Many insurance regulators accept this view of insurance as well. A state insurance commissioner defended commercial insurers' use of HIV tests in medical underwriting by saying:

> We encourage insurers to test where appropriate because *we don't want insurance companies to issue policies to people who are sick, likely to be sick, or likely to die*.[16]

The commercial industry needs advertisements like "the-lower-your-risk-the-lower-your-premium" series because it is not easy to persuade the public or its elected officials that the task of health insurers and their regulators is to keep sick people away from medical care. These ads were designed to persuade people that actuarial fairness, not solidarity or subsidy, is what insurance is all about. They are another element in the

16. Statement made at a meeting (17 February 1987) of the Advisory Panel to the Office of Technology Assessment for its study, *Medical Testing and Health Insurance* (U.S. Congress 1988). I was a member of this panel.

campaign, so elegantly described by David Rothman in this volume, to persuade the middle classes to distinguish themselves from the poor, sick, and unfortunate and to feel morally comfortable about refusing to help others.

Nevertheless, despite the heavy public relations conducted by life and health insurers in the 1980s, the political context of commercial insurance has changed, perhaps unalterably. First, we are in a period of extremely heightened concern about health insurance. As every newspaper reader knows, health insurance was the issue that catapulted Harris Wofford to victory in the 1992 Pennsylvania Democratic primary for the U.S. Senate, after which, health insurance reform became a prominent issue in the 1992 presidential race, and a major plank in President Clinton's agenda.

Second, the AIDS epidemic and the development of blood tests for HIV antibodies pushed insurance underwriting practices into the public spotlight. Insurers defeated bills or regulations in four states and the District of Columbia that would have prohibited the use of HIV tests to screen applicants for life and health insurance,[17] but not without the cost of enormous publicity about and research into medical underwriting more generally. The gay community, through its well-organized support groups and legal rights organizations, was instrumental in investigating and challenging medical underwriting. The Office of Technology Assessment report cited earlier was the direct result of congressional fears that commercial insurers would use medical underwriting to avoid paying for care of people with AIDS, leaving these costs entirely to the public sector.

Third, in the late 1980s and early 1990s, when the battle over insurers' use of HIV tests seemed to have been lost, researchers in the congressionally funded Human Genome Project identified a spate of disease-causing genes—for Huntington's disease, some forms of muscular dystrophy, and cystic fibrosis, among many others—and seemed to be on the verge of finding many more, such as a genetic marker for familial breast cancer. Publicity about these discoveries generated enormous popular media speculation about the impact of gene identification on access to health insurance and jobs.

Finally, the presidential election, the HIV epidemic, and the Human Genome Project all happened after a significant political reconceptualization of disability had occurred in the United States. In political and policy arenas, if not the medical community, disability had come to be understood as a problem of discrimination as much as, or even more

17. In California, the prohibition on HIV tests in health insurance underwriting still stands.

than, a medical problem. People with disabilities and their advocates were already well organized in that set of groups and ideas that constitute the disability rights movement, and civil rights legislation protecting people with disabilities was well established at the federal level (in Section 503 of the Vocational Rehabilitation Act of 1973) and the state level (in a variety of Fair Housing and Employment acts, as well as a few specific state statutes protecting people with particular disabilities from insurance discrimination). In this political context, the identification of new diseases and disease-causing genetic defects creates new categories of people who consider themselves deserving of protection under handicap discrimination principles, and the use of any diagnostic tests or genetic information by insurers will inevitably be interpreted through the lens of civil rights. The disability rights community lobbied hard for protection against medical underwriting in the 1991 Americans with Disabilities Act and probably failed (see Rothstein 1992), but the crystallization of the issue around a major new piece of federal legislation only put the spotlight on underwriting once again.

Insurers have faced numerous challenges to their underwriting practices, and the industry has proven extremely resistant and resilient in the past. As early as the 1880s, several states tried to prohibit life insurance companies from charging higher rates to blacks than whites (James 1947: 338–39). In the late 1960s and 1970s, the property insurance field was plagued by the issue of "redlining," wherein racial composition of a neighborhood was an explicit factor in determining the availability of mortgages and property insurance. Also in the 1970s, the use of gender as a factor in pricing life and disability insurance, as well as automobile insurance, was highly contested. Disease-based interest groups (notably for those with Tay-Sachs disease and sickle-cell anemia and DES mothers and daughters) challenged the use of "their disease" as an underwriting criterion in life and health insurance and succeeded in winning protections in several states. In the late 1980s, the dominant underwriting issue was life and health insurers' use of sexual orientation (as a proxy for AIDS risk) and then HIV tests. For the most part, insurers were able to defeat restrictions on their underwriting criteria, either by defeating bills and regulations outright or by inserting narrowing language to permit the use of criteria that are "actuarially sound."

There are reasons to think, however, that the current challenge to medical underwriting is far more serious and pervasive than any earlier challenges. For the first time, the entire system of medical underwriting and the principle of actuarial fairness is being called into question. Several states have begun to prohibit some forms of medical underwriting and push insurers back to community rating. Virtually every proposal for national health reform includes some kind of ban on medical underwriting, whether a prohibition of preexisting condition clauses or a requirement for "guaranteed issue" health insurance. (Guaranteed issue does not mean what it sounds like—guaranteed access to health insurance. Far more modest, it requires that *if* an insurer accepts a small group, it must insure all employees and may not exclude one or a few for medical reasons.) Even President Bush's reform plan of 1992 [18] would have included guaranteed issue and prohibited denial of health insurance for reasons of health, though the plan would have allowed insurers to base their rates on individual health status. The Health Insurance Association of America, too, abandoned some of its attachment to the actuarial fairness principle, and began calling for guaranteed issue and less medical underwriting in the small business market (HIAA 1991).

The election of Bill Clinton shifted the political center of gravity in health insurance reform to the federal level, another major political change. In the past, health insurance (like all insurance) has been mostly a matter of state jurisdiction, and major insurers were able to use this fragmentation to their advantage. Challenges to underwriting practices would necessarily arise in state legislatures or sometimes in insurance departments, which could be picked off one by one. Detail teams from the Health Insurance Association of America and the American Council of Life Insurance could overwhelm local legislators with their technical expertise, and insurance PAC money could buy state votes. Moreover, when regulation of underwriting practices is a state matter, insurers have the potent weapon of the exit threat. (When the District of Columbia tried to stop insurers from using HIV tests, the large companies simply said they would stop writing business in the district. Congress caved shortly thereafter.) Now that underwriting is up for discussion in Congress, the White House, and the Department of Health and Human Services, insurers have a more formidable opponent.

The political actors and alliances participating in the insurance issue have also changed dramatically. Up until recently, commercial insurers were a potent and usually united force, whenever there were public policy challenges to their underwriting practices in the form of proposed regulatory or statutory constraints. The commercial industry is no longer the

18. The President's Comprehensive Health Reform Program, 6 February 1992, Washington, D.C.

political behemoth it once was (Carlson 1992; Garland 1992; Kirk 1992; Kosterlitz 1991, 1992a, 1992b). Several of the largest commercial insurers—CIGNA, Aetna, and Metropolitan Life—have withdrawn from the Health Insurance Association of America, taking millions of dollars in dues and fees with them. They are positioning themselves to be players in any nationally mandated health insurance scheme. Small firms and large brokerage firms oppose many of the small-group market reforms advocated by the larger firms. Insurers are regrouping into new coalitions with other health care interest groups and small businesses. Many firms have ceased writing health insurance, so that there are fewer firms in any coalition to stop health insurance reform. The commercial industry finds itself in competition with some of its old allies—the large corporations who used to be major customers but who now self-insure and, incidentally, are not subject to the state insurance regulation that governs the commercial sector. Indeed, many in the commercial industry promote regulation of the self-insured sector by rewriting some of the ERISA exemptions, a position which creates a deep split between commercial insurers and other big business.

By now, most of the large insurers, as well as the Health Insurance Association of America and other industry trade groups, have acknowledged that underwriting and "cream skimming" are problems to be addressed. The Prudential Company's X-ray advertisement testifies to this rush to the side of the angels. With the fragmentation of the health insurance industry, hastened by the withdrawal of most large employers from commercial markets as they self-insured, and with the simultaneous rise of the health insurance issue to the presidential agenda, imposing public policy goals on private insurers is no longer politically unthinkable. But is it doable? Can a state—or even federal—ban on preexisting clauses or on denials for medical reasons really change the way health insurance operates? Can a few regulations change the balance of human raw materials—middle-class and poor, healthy and not-so-healthy, young and old—between the private sector and the public fisc?

Big change will not come easily. Piecemeal restrictions on underwriting that ban the use of specific medical tests or diseases (such as HIV tests or genetic tests) are clearly not going to be very effective. Though insurers might not be able to ask directly about specific tests or diseases, their network of information sources on any individual is so extensive that they are likely to acquire the information by other means (Stone 1992). They are also likely to resort to cruder, more exclusive proxy measures when they are legally forbidden from using information they believe they need.

(When California banned the use of HIV antibody tests in health and life insurance underwriting in 1985, insurers tested applicants with the T-cell test instead [Battista 1989: 26]; many continued using sexual orientation as a proxy measure for AIDS risk and using occupation, zip code, and beneficiary designations as proxies for sexual orientation.)

Medical underwriting and the belief in the principle of actuarial fairness are so deeply embedded in the structure of business and the mentality of insurance employees that they will be hard to eradicate. Public policy has, for over a century, both permitted and exhorted insurers to compete in the market, on the theory that competition would breed innovation, efficiency, and ultimately public welfare. Insurers quickly discovered that, in health insurance, the most effective competitive strategy was risk segregation and selection. To restrain this kind of behavior while the rest of the competitive economic environment does not change is a tall order. Billions of dollars, millions of jobs, and innumerable organizations depend on the underwriting function. Some examples: The National Association of the Self-Employed, with 165,000 members, probably wouldn't exist but for the fact that it offers health insurance to members. The Council of Smaller Enterprises in Cleveland, a leading opponent of small-group market and national reforms, brokers health insurance coverage for about 8,500 small businesses (Carlson 1992). For small insurance agencies, a substantial part of their business is simply *re-placing* small businesses with new insurers, and these companies would not be looking to move were it not for the competitive underwriting that gives them an incentive to shop.

Even if there were a comprehensive statutory ban on medical underwriting in health insurance, the infrastructure of medical underwriting will remain in place because it will continue to be used for life insurance. Insurers will still have medical underwriting departments and the concomitant capacity to gather medical data. Likewise, the Medical Information Bureau, the industry's central data bank for medical information on insurance applicants and policyholders, will continue to operate for and be financed by life insurers (see Stone 1992).

What risk classification and segregation insurers cannot accomplish through direct medical underwriting they can often accomplish through targeted marketing and through pricing. In 1900, Frederick Hoffman, then chief statistician of The Prudential Company, wrote that many states had passed laws "compelling Industrial [life insurance] companies to accept Negro risks at the same rates as those charged the white population. "Fortunately," he observed, "the companies cannot be compelled to solicit this class of risks, and very little business of this class is now written by Industrial companies, practically none by the Prudential" (p. 153). It is no accident that HMOs and other managed care plans feature their maternity and fitness club benefits when they market their plans to large employee groups: they are appealing to the young and the health-conscious. Through targeting of their sales efforts and tailoring of their benefit packages, insurers can accomplish a great deal of sifting.

Without requiring any medical information or performing any medical underwriting, insurers could offer low-priced policies excluding coverage for various serious diseases, or even excluding only expensive tests and treatments for certain diseases. In the competitive market, customers would shop around for the best deals to suit their budgets and their risk preferences. Those who know (or think) they have a low risk for particular diseases would buy just the policies tailored to their own risk profiles. Through self-selection and pursuit of the almighty bargain, individuals would sort themselves into homogeneous risk classes, albeit perhaps not as refined as the classes achieved through underwriting. The market could accomplish for insurers what government forbids them to do for themselves. Indeed, a great deal of exactly this kind of sorting is already happening within large groups, as insurers and self-insured employers offer employees "freedom of choice" among plans ranging from low-cost, no-frills plans to richer, more comprehensive benefit packages (Kramon 1992).

If risk classification is central to the economic organization of commercial insurance, it is perhaps even more central to the social and political organization of American life. The underwriting criteria that insurers have found so necessary to preserve the fiscal soundness and actuarial fairness of their business dovetail precisely with those identities that have formed our major social cleavages: race, ethnicity, class, and more recently sexual orientation and disability. Underwriting makes and perpetuates a series of internal social divisions, so that, in a far broader sense than insurers usually mean, "likes share their risks with likes." Just as social insurance is a mechanism for implementing mutual aid and a means of defining a diverse and integrated community, the principle of actuarial fairness in all its institutional forms is a marvellously invisible way of creating and perpetuating a segregated society. It explains misfortune as the result of unalterable natural characteristics of individuals, for which the only possible solution is a division of society into the Purgatory of the unfortunate and the Paradise of the blessed.

References

Abbott, L. F. 1930. *The Story of NYLIC: A History of the Origin and Development of the New York Life Insurance Company from 1845 to 1929.* New York: New York Life Insurance Company.

ACLI (American Council of Life Insurance). 1989. *The Potential Role of Genetic Testing in Risk Classification.* Report of the Genetic Testing Committee to the Medical Section of the American Council of Life Insurance, Hilton Head, SC, 10 June.

ACLI-HIAA (American Council of Life Insurance and Health Insurance Association of America). 1991. *Report of the ACLI-HIAA Task Force on Genetic Testing, 1991.* Washington, DC: ACLI-HIAA.

Bailey, H. T., T. M. Hutchinson, and G. R. Narber. 1976. The Regulatory Challenge to Life Insurance Classification. *Drake Law Review* 25:779–827.

Bailey, R. 1985. *Underwriting in Life and Health Insurance Companies.* Atlanta: Life Management Institute of the Life Office Management Association.

Battista, M. 1989. Genetic Data: Impact on Underwriting. In *The Potential Role of Genetic Testing in Risk Classification.* Washington, DC: American Council of Life Insurance.

Blustein, J., and T. R. Marmor. 1992. Cutting Waste by Making Rules: Promises, Pitfalls, and Realistic Prospects. *University of Pennsylvania Law Review* 140:1543–72.

Brackenridge, R. D. C. 1985. *Medical Selection of Life Risks: A Comprehensive Guide to Life Expectancy for Underwriters and Clinicians.* 2d ed. New York: Nature Press.

Buley, R. C. 1953. *The American Life Convention, 1906–1952: A Study in the History of Life Insurance.* New York: Appleton-Century-Crofts.

Carlson, E. 1992. Small Insurers Seek to Block Plan to Widen Coverage. *Wall Street Journal,* 8 April, p. B2.

Citizens Fund. 1991. *Health Insurance at Risk: The Seven Warning Signs.* Washington, DC: Citizens Fund.

Clifford, K., and R. Iuculano. 1987. AIDS and Insurance: The Rationale for AIDS-related Testing. *Harvard Law Review* 100:1806–24.

Colton, P. 1991. Pre-existing Conditions "Hold Americans Hostage" to Employers and Insurers. *Journal of the American Medical Association* 265:2451–53.

Eckholm, E. 1991. Health Benefits Found to Deter Job Switching. *New York Times,* 26 September, p. A1.

Fein, R. 1985. *Medical Costs, Medical Choices.* Cambridge, MA: Harvard University Press.

Freudenheim, M. 1990. Health Insurers, to Reduce Losses, Blacklist Dozens of Occupations. *New York Times,* 5 February, p. A1.

Garland, S. 1992. Health Care Reform: It's Insurer vs. Insurer. *Business Week,* 4 May, pp. 62–63.

Goldstein, C. 1988. Preexisting Condition Medical Exclusion. *For the Defense* 30 (June): 2–7.

Goldstone, R. 1992. Substandard, Not Inferior. *Best's Review* 92 (March): 24–28, 90.

Hauschild, E. 1931. *The Accident and Health Underwriter's Guide*. Cincinnati: National Underwriter Company.

HIAA (Health Insurance Association of America). 1991. *Health Care Financing for All Americans: Private Market Reform and Public Responsibility*. Washington, DC: HIAA.

Hillman, B. J., C. A. Joseph, M. R. Mabry, J. H. Sunshine, S. D. Kennedy, and M. Noether. 1990. Frequency and Costs of Diagnostic Imaging in Office Practice—A Comparison of Self-Referring and Radiologist-Referring Physicians. *New England Journal of Medicine* 323:1604–8.

Hoffman, F. L. 1900. *History of The Prudential Insurance Company of America (Industrial Insurance), 1875–1900*. Newark, NJ: Prudential Press.

Hoffman, J. N., and E. Z. Kincaid. 1986–87. AIDS: The Challenge to Life and Health Insurers' Freedom of Contract. *Drake Law Review* 35:709–71.

Huebner, S. S. 1935. *Life Insurance: A Textbook*. 3d ed. New York: Appleton-Century-Crofts.

James, Marquis. 1947. *The Metropolitan Life: A Study in Business Growth*. New York: Viking.

Kirk, V. 1992. Some Insurers Are Getting Antsy. *National Journal*, 15 February, p. 397.

Kosterlitz, J. 1991. Unrisky Business. *National Journal*, 4 April, pp. 794–97.

———. 1992a. Staking Out Turf. *National Journal*, 15 February, pp. 390–95.

———. 1992b. Insurers Are Gearing Up. *National Journal*, 21 March, pp. 706–7.

Kramon, G. 1992. Medical Insurers Vary Fees to Aid Healthier People. *New York Times*, 24 March, p. A1.

Mehr, R. I. 1983. *Fundamentals of Insurance*. Homewood, IL: Richard D. Irwin.

Mowbray, A., R. Blanchard, and C. Williams. 1969. *Insurance: Its Theory and Practice in the United States*. 6th ed. New York: McGraw-Hill.

Northwest Union Life Insurance Company. 1930. *Premium Rates*. Ottawa, IL: Northwest Union Life Insurance Company.

Pokorski, R. J. 1989. Public Relations and Government Issues. In *The Potential Role of Genetic Testing in Risk Classification*. Washington, DC: American Council of Life Insurance.

Rogers, O. H., and A. Hunter. 1919. The Numerical Method of Determining the Value of Risks for Insurance. *Transactions of the Actuarial Society of America* 20. Reprinted in *Readings in Life Insurance: A Compendium*. New York: Life Office Management Association, 1936.

Rothstein, M. A. 1992. Genetic Discrimination in Employment and the Americans with Disabilities Act. *Houston Law Review* 29:23–84.

Scott, J. C. 1976. *The Moral Economy of the Peasant: Rebellion and Subsistence in Southeast Asia*. New Haven, CT: Yale University Press.

Shepherd, P., and A. C. Webster. 1957. *Selection of Risks*. Chicago: Society of Actuaries.

Stack, C. B. 1974. *All Our Kin*. New York: Harper and Row.

Starr, P. 1982. *The Social Transformation of American Medicine*. New York: Basic.

Stone, D. A. 1988. *The Disabled State*. Philadelphia: Temple University Press.

————. 1992. The Implications of the Human Genome Project for Access to Health Insurance. Working paper, Heller School of Social Welfare, Brandeis University, Waltham, MA.

U.S. Congress, Office of Technology Assessment. 1988. *Medical Testing and Health Insurance*. OTA-H-384. Washington, DC: U.S. Government Printing Office.

Will, C. A. 1974. *Life Company Underwriting*. New York: Life Office Management Association.

Yondorff, B. 1990. *Health Insurance Availability and Affordability in Colorado: A Report on Underwriting and Pricing Practices*. Denver: Colorado Department of Regulatory Agencies, Division of Insurance.

Is the Time Finally Ripe?
Health Insurance Reforms in the 1990s

Theda Skocpol

Abstract Reformers feel certain that the time is now ripe for progressive legislation to ensure universal citizen access to health insurance and to contain rising costs in the health care industry. But history shows us that reformers were equally confident in earlier periods of modern U.S. history, only to find themselves defeated by conservatives willing to deploy ideological, emotionally charged arguments against government-sponsored reforms. Today's advocates of inside-the-beltway bargains for hammering out compromise reforms may be vulnerable to similar conservative counterattacks. Reformers need to engage the U.S. citizenry as a whole in democratic discussion about the ideals of government-sponsored health care reforms. Advocates of single-payer plans can do this more readily than supporters of complex public-private schemes such as play or pay or managed competition, but all those who want inclusive and effective reforms during the 1990s must face the challenge of democratic dialogue.

Right now, in the early 1990s, the time seems ripe for national health care reform. A belief that there are pressing problems about health care access and cost has come together with a sense of *political opportunities* to do something about those problems. This conjuncture of problems and politics is moving the issue of health insurance to the top of the national agenda, and opening a window of opportunity for public policy solutions put forward by experts and policy entrepreneurs who have been lying in wait to change U.S. governmental policies in the health care area. According to political scientist John Kingdon (1984), problems, political opportunities, and proposed solutions must come together before a breakthrough in public policy can occur.

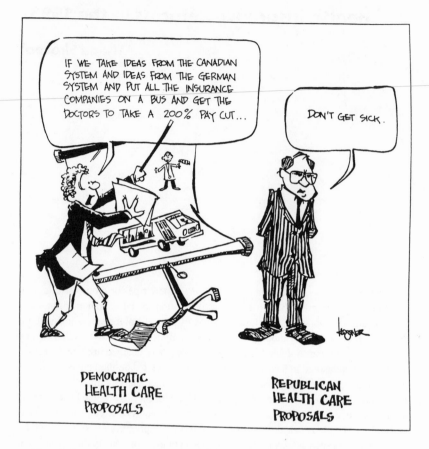

Certainly, we are at a juncture when problems are widely perceived— even by dominant actors in the U.S. health care system and those who, until recently, were quite self-satisfied. Long a strong opponent of reform, the American Medical Association now acknowledges that "our system has its faults," because "over 30 million Americans don't have access to health care" (see AMA 1990; also Todd et al. 1991). Insurance companies are concerned because competition among them is increasingly focused on finding ever-smaller pools of healthier people to insure (Briggs 1992; Jones 1992). Fearing that public resistance to the exclusion of people with preexisting conditions will fuel tough new regulations that further undercut their already tenuous profits, many large insurers are now acknowledging the inevitability of reforms and attempting to influence the terms of new legislation proposed by the Clinton administration. Many employers, too, are willing to join government in a quest for cost containment (Bergthold 1990, 1991; Martin 1993). Large businesses, especially those in unionized industries that already provide employer-sponsored benefits, find their costs rising astronomically and uncontrollably, while small businesses often find it impossible to obtain coverage for their employees at any reasonable cost.

Citizens as well as organized interests are aware of problems. The elderly and poor who are in the public parts of the American health-financing system are experiencing increasing squeezes on their access to care, as efforts at cost containment focus disproportionately on the public parts of the system (Ruggie 1992). The regularly employed middle class, too, is becoming anxious about health insurance (Starr 1991). During the postwar period, from the late 1940s through the early 1970s, stably employed wage and salary earners could feel relatively secure about enjoying generous employer-provided and tax-subsidized health benefits for themselves and their dependents (Stevens 1988). But now, as employers try various expedients to cope with rising health care costs, employees are losing certain health benefits, and dependents are sometimes excluded from coverage. Workers are fearful of losing jobs and coverage altogether, or else are wary of changing jobs and ending up with health coverage that doesn't have as generous terms as before. Unionized workers, moreover, are having to devote much of their organizational energy to defending preexisting health benefits for active and retired workers. Industrial profits and productivity gains often flow into covering rising health care costs, rather than into raises in take-home pay or other benefits.

Even outside of the health policy area, experts are arriving at the realization that reforms in many areas of U.S. economic and public policy may hinge on changes that universalize access and bring rising health care costs under some kind of control. One key to promoting efficiency in the economy may lie in part in finding a way to rationalize the health care system. And certainly some of the most intractable problems in other areas of social policy, such as welfare reform, depend very much on finding a way to allow the working poor to gain access to health coverage (cf. Ellwood 1988: 103–4).

At last it has become politically feasible to do something through government about these problems. Until late 1991, experts and politicians took it for granted that it just was not politically feasible to talk about governmental reforms in health care. Then, suddenly, a new sense of political possibility was kicked off by an entirely unexpected "focusing event" (Kingdon 1984: 99–105) in the fall of 1991. After Republican senator John Heinz was tragically killed in a freak aviation accident, a virtually unknown and seemingly unpromising Democratic party candidate, Harris Wofford, won the ensuing special senatorial election that was held in Pennsylvania. Wofford overcame a forty-point deficit in the polls against well-known Republican Richard Thornburgh, who had recently been attorney general under President George Bush. Airing a television commercial that proclaimed "If every criminal in America has the right to a lawyer, then I think every working person should have the right to see a doctor when they're ill," Wofford's come-from-behind campaign featured calls for "national health insurance." His victory, so unexpected by the Washington and media establishment, signaled that access to affordable health care was an issue on the voting public's mind, an issue on which political capital could be gained by politicians willing to propose governmental solutions (Blumenthal 1991; Russakoff 1991).

Subsequently, Democratic presidential candidate Bill Clinton made calls for health care reform one of the centerpieces of his campaign. Clinton's victory over incumbent George Bush—who had seemed certain of reelection just a year before the November 1992 election—has made it a certainty that major health care reforms will be proposed to Congress during 1993.

Overly pessimistic until recently that health insurance was off the agenda, now many experts—perhaps too many—are blithely optimistic that the 1990s will bring fundamental reforms in health care access and financing. In 1992 I took part in a discussion of health care reform during a session of a conference sponsored by the National Academy of Social Insurance. At one point I suggested that there might be some reforms that were not worth supporting in the short run, that it might possibly be better to hold out for certain more fundamental reforms. Henry Aaron, the legendary health care economist, passed me a note that said: "Don't worry, Theda. No matter what happens now, the issue's going to keep coming up until things are finally addressed in a fundamental way." In a certain sense, of course, Aaron is right (see Aaron 1991 for his rationale). But I wonder if there isn't a certain evolutionary functionalism inherent in this way of thinking. It may fail to take a sufficiently hardheaded look at whether political conditions exist (or could come about) that will ensure changes genuinely for the better. Will the right solutions really come together with felt problems and political possibilities during the 1990s?

At this point, I should say what I mean by changes "for the better." As we all know, in any kind of reforms that occur, the specifics are going to matter a great deal, particular details are going to matter. I don't want to address all that. I simply want to point out that if, in the end, the changes don't move things—promptly and irreversibly—in the direction of genuinely including everyone in health care coverage, both preventive and acute health care coverage, I will not define that change as a change for the better. And if the changes don't lead in the direction of creating a broader regulatory framework for cost sharing and cost containment, that will not be a change for the better. Even incremental reforms will have to be evaluated in terms of whether they change the direction of the dynamics of the health care system. Reforms enacted in 1994 are unlikely to be the last word; there will be further rounds of reform throughout the 1990s. Over several stages of change, we need to ensure full inclusion of all Americans in health insurance. And we need to move firmly away from current patterns of cost shifting that fuel inflation and that formally or de facto exclude many people from adequate care and access to relatively equal care. We must move in the direction of creating some kind of overall control—macro control rather than micro control—on the decisions of medical practitioners and patients about costs and benefits.

It is important to realize that John Kingdon's (1984) model about problems, politics, and solutions applies to "near misses" in the political system as well as to actual or effective changes. In other words, it's a model that explains when possible policy changes come up for debate, not whether anything will actually be enacted. What is more, it is not a model that tells us whether things that are enacted actually solve any problems or just make them worse—perhaps leading to reversals of reforms at a later date.

If we look back historically at earlier attempts at health financing reform in the United States, we will see patterns that should worry us in the present conjuncture. Let us take a small historical detour to see what happened in the past to reformers who were absolutely confident that "the time was ripe" for rational and progressive health care reforms. Then we will return to the present, and I will argue that reformers in the 1990s should pay much more attention than most are doing so far to the requisites of political communication with broad, democratic publics.

Rational Reformers Meet Conservative Ideologues

Repeatedly during the twentieth century, reformers in the United States have been certain that the time had come to enact broad, publicly financed or regulated health insurance. Such confidence bubbled up especially in the late 1910s and at moments during the 1930s and 1940s. But each time, the hopes of advocates of one or another form of public health insurance were dashed on the shoals of the U.S. political system and against the rocks of fervent conservative opposition to this seemingly logical form of public social provision.

From 1916 through 1920, the American Association for Labor Legislation (AALL) campaigned for public "sickness insurance" to cover American workingmen and their dependents (cf. Numbers 1978; Starr 1982: 237–57; Skocpol 1992: chap. 3). Founded in 1906 and devoted to the use of social science research to promote various kinds of "labor legislation" in the United States, the AALL was a small association of reform-minded professionals, mostly university professors, labor statisticians, and social workers. As dozens of U.S. states enacted regulations requiring businesses to provide industrial accident insurance, the experts of the AALL decided that health insurance would be "the next great step" in the march toward comprehensive social insurance. AALL members believed that there would be inevitable progress toward the enactment of public social insurance in all civilized industrializing nations and the United States would have to be part of this worldwide movement. Reformers in the Progressive Era argued that sickness insurance—to be funded jointly by contributions from business, wage earners, and government tax revenues—would help to prevent poverty among wage earners. Health insurance would also promote economic and social "efficiency," because it would encourage employers, employees, and citizens alike to promote healthful conditions at work and in communities.

To the experts of the AALL, the case for the U.S. states to enact health insurance was so obviously rational and the worldwide course of "social progress" so clearly inevitable that they were hardly prepared for the spread of ideologically impassioned opposition to their legislative proposals. Yet there were plenty of potential opponents. Private insurance companies opposed the death benefits that were to be included in health insurance as designed by the AALL. Business associations such as the National Association of Manufacturers looked askance at the new taxes that health insurance would entail. Private physicians and various state and local units of the American Medical Association worried about the imposition of governmental regulation. And certain labor leaders opposed all forms of public social insurance as an intrusion on union autonomy. As the United States entered World War I, ideologues opposed to health insurance highlighted the bogey of German statism, using opposition to "bureaucracy" as an effective rallying cry for the various forces potentially opposed to health insurance. Health insurance was labeled "un-American." What is more, the increasingly hysterical claims of the enemies of health insurance fell upon the ears of middle-class publics that were already skeptical about governmental efficiency and honesty, not to mention wary of new taxes.

The normally cumbersome operations of U.S. governmental institutions—which required reformers to move proposals, state by state, through two legislative houses, past potential vetoes by governors, and around potential constitutional and judicial obstacles—insured that opponents to health insurance would have plenty of time to build coalitions and many institutional points at which to register opposition (Robertson 1989). By 1920, the AALL-sponsored campaigns for health insurance had been deflected altogether in most U.S. states and defeated in pitched battles in California and New York. The progress that had seemed so inevitable a few years earlier was stopped dead in its tracks; and the AALL itself permanently lost momentum after the nationwide defeat of its all-out campaign for health insurance.

During the 1930s and 1940s, efforts to promote public health insurance—now for middle-class as well as working-class Americans—were pursued by various groups of intellectuals and officials located in and around the various administrations of President Franklin Delano Roosevelt and President Harry Truman (cf. Hirshfield 1970; Poen 1979; Starr 1982: 275–89). At first, reform proposals called for federal incentives for optional state-level health insurance, but during and after World War II reformers' hopes shifted toward a comprehensive, national system of health insurance, modeled on contributory old-age insurance. Echoing the faith of the Progressives of the 1910s, many New Dealers were confident that the United States would inevitably "complete" what the Social Security Act of 1935 had begun, building a comprehensive welfare state that would include national employment assurance, unemployment benefits, and health insurance coverage for all Americans. President Roosevelt never gave full backing to health insurance proposals during the 1930s; and they were left out of the legislation for Social Security because of fears that opposition from the American Medical Association might sink the entire bill if health insurance was included. Nevertheless, the hopes of advocates of national health insurance looked as if they might be realized in the 1940s, particularly when Harry Truman featured this reform in his ultimately victorious bid for reelection in 1948.

Once again, reformist hopes were shattered. Throughout the 1930s and 1940s, all proposals for public health insurance were strenuously opposed by the formidable American Medical Association, which from the 1920s had become truly a peak association of private fee-for-service doctors in thousands of local communities and all the states of the United States.

By the 1940s, moreover, private insurance companies had developed an interest in offering health insurance to the middle class. During and right after World War II, major industrial employers were encouraged by wartime controls and provisions of the federal tax code to start offering health insurance as a "fringe benefit" to workers (Stevens 1984, 1988). Thus, not only were industrialists opposed to paying taxes for public health insurance; many of them also became committed to their nascent private systems of health benefits—which had been used as bargaining chips in lieu of higher wages, and which did not seem so costly at that phase of history.

Just as ideological rallying cries against "German statism" brought together potential opponents of workingmen's health insurance during the late 1910s, the various forces ready to weigh in against Truman's plans for national health insurance were brought together in late 1940s by cries of opposition to "communism" and "socialized medicine." The Cold War was emerging, as the United States shifted from its World War II alliance with the beleaguered Russians against the Nazis, toward global superpower rivalry with an imperial Soviet Union. Within the United States, witch-hunts were launched against actually or allegedly pro-Communist public officials and labor union leaders. At this conjuncture, it was simple for opponents of national health insurance to label it "socialist," rapidly shifting public opinion away from public financing of health care costs. Reformers who had thought they were furthering a logical extension of the New Deal and Social Security suddenly found themselves in an ideologically uncomfortable position—appearing to support something un-American, even "subversive." To be sure, the newly powerful CIO unions initially preferred to support Truman's plan for national health insurance. But many CIO leaders were themselves victims of anti-Communist crusades. And strong industrial unions were able, when necessary, to fall back on contract bargaining for employer-provided health insurance coverage. From the 1950s through the 1970s, that is exactly what they did, enabling many unionized workers to enjoy very generous health benefits even in the absence of national health insurance (Stevens 1984).

We see, in short, that both in the 1910s and in the 1930s and 1940s, experts and reformers relied upon rational analyses and arguments about how to solve problems of efficiency or access. Reformers were confident that time was on their side, and that public health insurance (of one sort or another) would "inevitably" be enacted in the United States. But each time, not only were there powerful opponents to reform but debates also quickly took a bitterly ideological turn. This tactic was not expected by the rationally minded experts and led to defeats for proposals that might well have gained broad citizen support, had they been more calmly discussed—or effectively dramatized—in the national political process.

Are Reformers Ready for the Political Debate of the 1990s?

If past battles over health insurance for the United States turned out to be very ideological, leaving the rational reformers mystified and demoralized, it is very possible that this could happen again during the 1990s. Once again, proponents of universal health care coverage may be becoming overly complacent, assuming that rationality and logic will inevitably triumph. Most reformers are placing their faith in technically complicated insider bargaining, overlooking how ideological and politically charged the debates about health care reform are likely once again to become.

From many groups, experts, and politicians, I have gathered statements outlining desirable reforms in U.S. health care access and financing. In the current fashion, I have applied "discursive analysis" to these documents, trying to get a feeling for the audiences that are being addressed. I am interested, in short, in not just what each actor is proposing to do but to whom the actor is talking. More fundamentally, what conceptions of the political process lie behind various proposals? How might changes come about (or be obstructed)? For the most part, I must note, those discussing health care reforms in the early 1990s have remarkably little to say about the civic and governmental processes by which proposals will be adjudicated. One must simply infer who the intended audiences for messages are and how actors think the decision-making process might unfold. What follows are some of my inferences.

Most of today's "rational" reformers in the debates over health care reform are advocates of various schemes that fall under the rubrics of play or pay or managed competition. Supporters of such middle-range, mixed public and private schemes situate themselves in what they feel to be the comfortable center of the spectrum of reform advocates. On the one hand, they want to do much more than merely tinker with the current markets for private insurance; on the other hand, they do not want to go all the way toward universal, government-funded health insurance offering the same basic coverage to all citizens. Middle-range schemes usually aim to build on America's current system of employer-provided health insurance, by requiring and enabling all employers to offer at least basic health insurance to their employees. At the same time, publicly encouraged or subsidized health insurance would be expanded beyond Medicare and Medicaid to include those who are left out of the job-based schemes, as well as those who are dumped from job-based schemes after new regulations on businesses are put into place.

The supporters of middle-range reforms include some very hefty actors in American politics. Along with major unions, a goodly number of major U.S. corporations—such as Xerox, Lockheed, and General Electric— have banded together in the National Leadership Coalition to call for a play-or-pay approach to health care reform (Garland 1991). The Pepper Commission—the U.S. Bipartisan Commission on Comprehensive Health Care, chaired by Senator Jay Rockefeller of West Virginia—called for this approach in its September 1990 report (Pepper Commission 1990; see also Rockefeller 1991; Feder 1992). Building on the Pepper Commission's work, a working group of Democratic party leaders in the Senate— including Senators George Mitchell, Ted Kennedy, Don Riegle, and Jay Rockefeller—then developed a specific legislative proposal incorporating the play-or-pay approach (Peterson 1992). More recently, some politicians and experts have championed "managed competition" approaches that (in some versions) might deemphasize employer-provided health insurance in favor of individual enrollments in plans sponsored by regional health insurance purchasing cooperatives (Starr 1993). During his presidential campaign Bill Clinton at first talked in terms of play-or-pay ideas (Clinton for President Committee 1992); then he switched to speaking, in very general terms, about managed competition (Clinton and Gore 1992). Since Clinton's inauguration, it has become apparent that some sort of mixed public and private scheme will be worked out for the first round of comprehensive health care reform proposed by his administration.

Advocates of either play or pay or managed competition stress the feasibility of a "pragmatic road toward national health insurance" (Pollack and Torda 1991) or a "healthy compromise" (Starr 1993). Perhaps a single-payer, Canadian-style system of universal coverage for all citizens would be ideal, they acknowledge. But doctors, insurance companies, and employers just will not accept this great a change; and American citizens and politicians will not agree to have all health care costs immediately shifted into the system of taxes and governmental expenditures. Proponents of universal health insurance (such as Marmor and Mashaw 1990; Marmor et al. 1990; Kerrey 1991; and Fein 1992) are presented as unrealistic by advocates of the middle-range schemes. Supporters of the universal approach are requested to "back off" from demanding "too much," so that the "realistic" advocates of play or pay or managed competition can at least get half the loaf in the first stage of reform.

Advocates of middle-range reform plans seem to take it for granted that they will be able to get their approaches enacted through congressional brokering, as quiet bargains among major players in the current system—bargains that would not step too much, just a little bit, on established toes. "Political feasibility" in this context thus refers to an interest group arrangement hammered out in Congress, with special attention to the concerns of established economic interest groups. The question remains, though, whether the political premises that lie behind the thinking of advocates of play or pay or managed competition are really true. Let me highlight some of these premises and raise some questions about them.

One premise that lies behind all middle-range schemes for health care reform is that groups such as small businesses, doctors, and private insurers will accept being hurt just a little in order to be brought into a framework of improved access for all citizens. I wonder whether this is realistic. Advocates of managed competition advocate tough caps on costs for health insurance plans. But won't doctors and insurers anticipate such possibilities and maneuver to keep rigorous cost control mechanisms out of any such legislation? Similarly, most supporters of play or pay envisage that once this sort of system is in place, it will probably evolve toward single-payer, publicly funded national health insurance (cf. Pollack and Torda 1991). Faced with paying either private insurance premiums or taxes, businesses will shift more and more of their workers into the public scheme. (The advocates of play or pay apparently do not worry, as I do, that the residual public medical care program may be so underfunded that it will frighten many middle-class people, who will then fight ferociously against being shifted into it.) But if play-or-pay proponents expect their system to propel a gradual transition toward a single-payer public scheme, how can they imagine that the various interest groups they want to bring into the initial bargain won't notice where matters might end up down the road?

Small businesses know very well that, as soon as they're required to pay for health coverage, their costs will escalate, while any initial public subsidies will probably subside or disappear. Even big business is not united in support of reforms (Garland 1991). Insurance companies certainly realize that, over time, public coverage and regulation will squeeze their profits. Doctors certainly realize that calls for cost controls will increasingly lead (especially in a fragmented multiple-payer system) toward ever more microscopic price controls and second-guessing of their day-to-day decisions. In sum, many of the organized interests that advocates of play or pay or managed competition want to propitiate or bring into the initial bargain can surely envisage exactly what sorts of reform provisions might very quickly lead to outcomes they do not want. Since the legislative bargains are going to be very complex, they can fight to prevent such provisions in the initial legislation, or maneuver to evade or reverse them later.

A second premise of middle-range reform approaches is that Congress can hammer out bargains and that legislative gridlock will soon be overcome. This assumption may seem realistic now that we have a Democratic president in place along with a Democratically controlled Congress. Even so, it overlooks pressures that may be brought against congressional representatives by convinced opponents of any fundamental reforms. Proponents of play or pay or managed competition not only need to bargain with advocates of single-payer schemes; they also need to overcome opponents of any tough government-run reforms. And they must face the fact that after initial reforms are enacted in 1994, powerful interests will be lying in wait to eviscerate the implementation of tough cost controls. There will almost certainly have to be subsequent rounds of legislation, some of which might end up taking place in a changed political context, for example, if the Democrats lose in congressional or presidential elections during the rest of the 1990s.

For congressional leaders and other "realists" who are "settling" for middle-range reform plans at this point, the current debate is very much dominated by the fear of repeating what supposedly happened in the early 1970s (see Peterson 1992). Senator Ted Kennedy and some other Democratic congressional leaders believe that they lost the chance in this earlier period to work out a de facto universal access system, because a compromise failed to occur between Democratic party advocates of incremental change and Democratic party advocates of an ideal national health system. In fact, some observers of the health care reform debates of the 1970s (see Starr 1982: 414) argue that *neither* of these Democratic approaches ever had much of a chance of enactment. The later 1970s was a period of perceived budget stringencies and growing public skepticism about the capacities of government to solve social problems. The presidency of Jimmy Carter was, after all, the precursor to Ronald Reagan's victory in 1980.

But even if the problem during the 1970s represented a failure of Democrats to compromise among themselves on less than a purely comprehensive system of health insurance, worrying about repeating that failing now is a little bit like preparing to refight the last war. People are not taking into account that the political context has changed fundamentally from the 1970s to the 1990s. The concern in the 1990s is much more with cost containment and not simply with spreading social access to health care. Single-payer schemes offer a much more credible promise of simplified, uniform, and effective regulation of medical costs than do play-or-pay schemes and many versions of managed competition. Mixed public and private reform plans propose to retain many payers and fragmented, administratively cumbersome methods of cost accounting. Many possibilities for cost shifting may still remain under these plans; and medical cost inflation is virtually certain to continue. What is more, if supporters of middle-range schemes give in to worries about costs right now and decide to "phase in" full coverage for presently excluded groups of Americans over many years, it is possible that continuing cost increases will lead to later reversals of the promise of full access for everyone to health insurance.

During the last two decades, the context for debates over health insurance reforms has changed both ideologically and in terms of partisan balance. In the 1970s, it may very well have been a question of whether Democrats could come up with a compromise in their own ranks. But now a compromise within Democratic ranks is nowhere near enough to ensure enduring and irreversible changes in the way health care is financed in the United States. Back in the 1970s, "conservatives" were mostly moderate, pragmatic Republicans, who could be counted on to be gentlemanly and reasonable about inside-the-beltway bargains over legislation. Now, however, the conservatives who have the edge in the Republican party and beyond are tough street fighters, hostile to brokering in Washington, D.C., and willing to take emotional, ideologically charged debates to the country as a whole.

This brings us to perhaps the most questionable premise tacitly held by advocates of middle-range reforms. These pragmatic practitioners of insider bargaining seem to assume that ideological battles over public opinion will not prove crucial in the coming rounds of the health insurance debate. There has been little attempt by the advocates of play or pay or managed competition to explain their schemes to the broader citizenry. As I mean to indicate jokingly by the cartoon reprinted at the beginning of this article, it is not at all clear that these schemes can be explained very straightforwardly to the American people. Play or pay and managed competition plans are, after all, mind-bogglingly complex, involving adjustments within an already confusing and highly fragmented system of health care financing that involves many, many institutional actors. It is very difficult to come up with simple metaphors that tell the average citizen what the intended changes would do and mean.

Not surprisingly, most of the statements about play or pay or managed competition have so far been directed at business, or the medical profession, or policy experts. Last year, thinking that perhaps the presidential campaign of Bill Clinton might make a stab at a more straightforward message, I asked that campaign to send Clinton's position statements on health care reform. What I received was not reassuring: Clinton's statements as of the spring of 1992 outlined five steps and twelve substeps (Clinton for President Committee 1992). His explanation was very difficult even for someone like me to read through, let alone difficult to incorporate in a speech explaining this approach to the average citizen! Recently, health care reform expert Paul Starr (1993) has written about managed competition as a better middle-range approach than play or pay. Starr writes gracefully, and he presented his views in an article in the *American Prospect* that I am sure was meant to be broadly accessible. But I have read this technically complicated article three times, and I am still not sure exactly what changes managed competition would entail. Nor could I explain them easily to Harvard students, let alone to average citizens.

Speaking to the Citizens of America

Contrary to the assumption that health insurance reform will happen through a series of quiet congressional bargains among established players, the debate is already being taken to the citizens of America. During the final year of his presidency, President Bush started sounding the fundamental conservative themes to shape public opinion and to bring together actors around a defensive position. These themes continue to appear regularly in Republican speeches and in ads run in the media by insurance companies, medical groups, and conservative think tanks.

Advocates of both middle-range reforms and single-payer national health insurance have been accused of "socialism," as conservatives ask why we Americans want to move toward governmental "controls" at a time when the rest of the world is moving away from them. Opponents of strong reforms tell us that any attempt to move in the direction of greater public regulation would simply make bureaucracy worse, stifling innovations in health care that save lives and creating rationing and queues for service. "Governmental coercion" is opposed in conservative rhetoric to such ideals as consumer freedom and technological innovations to save lives (see Gradison 1992). Conservative rhetoric is meant to frighten middle-class Americans—especially those who still enjoy relatively good benefits through private insurance—dissuading them from supporting *any* kind of comprehensive reform. Or if people cannot be dissuaded from accepting initial attempts at comprehensive reform in 1994, such rhetoric is meant to lay the basis for reinterpreting the situation a few years later, when whatever is enacted in 1994 proves not to be successful or socially painless.

In short, during the 1990s, just as in the 1910s and the 1940s, the opponents of any sort of national health insurance have quickly undertaken to create ideological metaphors. They aim to fuel fears of reform among the citizenry and bring together the worries about change of stakeholders in the health economy as it is presently structured. Meanwhile, very little is being done by advocates of fundamental reform to create their own positive ideological metaphors for wide public dissemination.

On the side of those who want reform through an enhanced role for the national or state governments, the problem may be that it would be much easier to explain change in the direction of unified-payer plans of publicly financed health insurance than it is to explain the hoary details of play or pay or managed competition. Both citizens in general and many actors in the present medical care system might find it easier to understand the appeals of an administratively simplified, comprehensive system of health care financing available to every person in America. There may seem to be very little incentive for politicians already in the system—especially representatives in Congress who have to deal constantly with lobbyists for established interests—to declare that they are aiming at such fundamental change as a truly national health insurance system implies. Nevertheless, by not being willing to outline a clear, compelling vision of national health insurance as a desirable end point of reform, the proponents of middle-range reforms in Congress and beyond may actually be undermining their own cause. National health insurance may have to be explained and defended as a desirable goal, before it becomes possible to legitimate lesser reforms that interject greater public control into the health care system. In a climate where conservatives are willing to hammer away against the notion of *any* greater direct governmental involvement in health care, progressive proponents of health care reform may have to face the issue of government's role directly, explaining to the American people why it is not just pragmatic, but actually ideal, to have government increasingly involved in ensuring—and perhaps, in due course, financing—health care for everyone.

Let me close by summarizing some of the straightforward arguments that proponents of single-payer national health insurance can make to the American people about their preferred approach to addressing problems of social access and cost containment.

First and foremost, it is easy to tell people that under national health insurance each individual will have rights as a citizen, rather than through the place he or she happens to be employed. The appeal of equal rights for all citizens can be readily dramatized. Imagine television commercials that feature an unemployed father taking an injured child to the hospital, pulling out the child's "Americare" card, and getting the help that is needed without any complicated forms to fill out.

Proponents of national health insurance can also turn rhetoric about bureaucracy to their advantage, pointing out that the present medical care system has a bewildering variety of rules and paperwork from hundreds of different private insurance companies. The average American citizen knows from experience that the bureaucratic rules and forms are getting more and more complex, as insurance companies increasingly seek to manage and second-guess the care that doctors order. Advocates of play or pay or managed competition cannot easily claim that their approaches would ameliorate this situation; they might well make it worse, especially at first. But supporters of national health insurance can make a credible claim to bureaucratic simplification, arguing that sometimes a greater role for government can actually cut down on rules and regulations. (Parenthetically, doctors might also find this feature of national health insurance quite appealing, for they know that present trends of proliferating insurance regulations are leading to much microregulation of their day-to-day decisions about patient care. Under national health insurance, doctors and hospitals would have to negotiate yearly prices and budgets. But their decisions about individual patients would not be second-guessed by insurance companies.)

Economic efficiency is another goal that could well be furthered by more rather than less comprehensive reform in health insurance. Advertisements and speeches on behalf of single-payer national health insurance could tell Americans how nice it would be to move from job to job without worrying about the loss or diminution of health benefits for themselves or their families. The mobility of the labor force would certainly be enhanced, enabling the United States to compete more effectively in the international marketplace. Many businesses might find it appealing to dump altogether the responsibility of offering expensive health insurance. And single-payer schemes promise to make the capping of health care costs easier, because young and old, the middle-class and the poor, will all be in the same system. Uniform prices can be negotiated and enforced; administrative costs for health insurance will be cut back; and medical care providers will no longer have to deal with uncompensated patients dumped by insurers or other providers.

There are, in short, many advantages to comprehensive rather than incremental governmental reforms of U.S. health care in the 1990s—and these advantages can be easily dramatized to the citizenry as a whole. In my view, today's reform-minded experts need to face the fact that, as in the past, U.S. political battles over health insurance will almost certainly have ideological as well as technical, and emotional as well as rational, dimensions. No matter what happens in the successive elections of the 1990s, it almost certainly will not be possible to rely on purely inside-the-beltway bargains to enact, defend, and build upon truly progressive changes in the American system of access to and financing of health care. Any initial changes will have to be well understood by many Americans, if political support for progress over the 1990s is to be sustained. The access and cost problems of the American health care system will not be solved all at once.

Just as the advocates of Social Security during the New Deal were willing to use compelling metaphors and political rhetoric to explain to the citizenry why it made sense to have new levels of governmental involvement in the provision of old-age security, so will today's advocates of health care reform have to be able to explain their proposals to the American people. Indeed, advocates of health care reforms in the 1990s have more to explain to a skeptical citizenry about why *government* can provide desirable solutions to widely felt problems.

In my opinion, it is easier for supporters of national health insurance to make such a case than it is for advocates of play or pay or managed competition. But whether I am correct about this or not, the challenge of painting a vision of positive changes through government remains for all those who hope that the time finally is ripe to enact full health coverage in the United States. Along with members of Congress who hope to hammer out bargains for reform, health care experts who think about solutions for technical problems need to attend to fundamental processes of political communication. They need to explain to a democratic citizenry where they would like to go and why it is desirable to go there.

If reformers in the 1990s fail to paint an appealing picture of government-sponsored reform, conservatives will—later in the 1990s, if not immediately in 1994—win yet another round in the overly protracted struggle to bring affordable and accessible health care to all Americans.

To avoid the fate of progressive health reformers in the past, today's advocates of universal inclusion and socially managed health costs will have to talk with the people of America. Reformers need to engage in a dialogue with citizens, involving them in a process of reform that is certain to happen, not all at once in a back-room bargain, but over many years of adjustment and learning within a democratic polity.

References

Aaron, Henry J. 1991. Looking Backward: 2001–1991. The History of the Health Care Financing and Reform Act of 1998. *Brookings Review* 9 (3): 40–45.

AMA (American Medical Association). 1990. *Health Access America: The AMA Proposal to Improve Access to Affordable, Quality Health Care*. Chicago, IL: American Medical Association.

Bergthold, Linda. 1990. *Purchasing Power in Health: Business, the State, and Health Care Politics*. New Brunswick, NJ: Rutgers University Press.

———. 1991. The Fat Kid on the Seesaw: American Business and Health Care Cost Containment, 1970–1990. *Annual Review of Public Health* 12:157–75.

Blumenthal, Sidney. 1991. Populism in Tweeds: The Professor and the Middle Class. *New Republic*, 25 November, pp. 10–15.

Briggs, Philip. 1992. A View from the Insurance Industry. In *Social Insurance Issues for the Nineties* (Proceedings of the Third Conference of the National Academy of Social Insurance), ed. Paul N. Van de Water. Dubuque, IA: Kendall/Hunt.

Clinton, Bill, and Al Gore. 1992. *Putting People First: How We Can All Change America*. New York: Times Books, Random House.

Clinton for President Committee. 1992. *Bill Clinton's American Health Care Plan*. Little Rock, AR: Clinton for President Committee.

Ellwood, David T. 1988. *Poor Support: Poverty in the American Family*. New York: Basic.

Feder, Judith. 1992. The Pepper Commission's Proposals. In *Social Insurance Issues for the Nineties* (Proceedings of the Third Conference of the National Academy of Social Insurance), ed. Paul N. Van de Water. Dubuque, IA: Kendall/Hunt.

Fein, Rashi. 1992. Health Care Reform. *Scientific American* 267 (5): 46–53.

Garland, Susan B. 1991. Already, Big Business' Health Plan Isn't Feeling So Hot. *Business Week*, 18 November, p. 48.

Gradison, Bill. 1992. Statement by the Honorable Bill Gradison before the House Ways and Means Committee, 3 March. (Typescript from the representative's office.)

Hirshfield, Daniel S. 1970. *The Lost Reform*. Cambridge, MA: Harvard University Press.

Jones, Stanley B. 1992. What Is the Future of Private Health Insurance? In *Social In-*

surance Issues for the Nineties (Proceedings of the Third Conference of the National Academy of Social Insurance), ed. Paul N. Van de Water. Dubuque, IA: Kendall/ Hunt.

Kerrey, Robert. 1991. Why America Will Adopt Comprehensive Health Care Reform. *American Prospect* 6 (Summer): 81–90.

Kingdon, John W. 1984. *Agendas, Alternatives, and Public Policies.* Boston, MA: Little, Brown.

Marmor, Theodore R., and Jerry L. Mashaw. 1990. Canada's Health Insurance and Ours: The Real Lessons, the Big Choices. *American Prospect* 3 (Fall): 18–29.

Marmor, Theodore R., Jerry L. Mashaw, and Philip L. Harvey. 1990. *America's Misunderstood Welfare State: Persistent Myths, Enduring Realities.* New York: Basic.

Martin, Cathie Jo. 1993. Together Again: Business, Government, and the Quest for Cost Control. *Journal of Health Politics, Policy and Law* 18 (2): 359–93.

Numbers, Ronald L. 1978. *Almost Persuaded: American Physicians and Compulsory Health Insurance, 1912–1920.* Baltimore, MD: Johns Hopkins University Press.

Pepper Commission. 1990. *A Call for Action: Executive Summary.* Washington, DC: U.S. Government Printing Office.

Peterson, Mark A. 1992. Momentum toward Health Care Reform in the U.S. Senate. *Journal of Health Politics, Policy and Law* 17 (3): 553–73.

Poen, Monty M. 1979. *Harry S. Truman versus the Medical Lobby.* Columbia: University of Missouri Press.

Pollack, Ronald, and Phyllis Torda. 1991. The Pragmatic Road toward National Health Insurance. *American Prospect* 6 (Summer): 92–100.

Robertson, David Brian. 1989. The Bias of American Federalism: The Limits of Welfare-State Development in the Progressive Era. *Journal of Policy History* 1 (3): 261–91.

Rockefeller, Jay D., IV. 1991. A Call for Action: The Pepper Commission's Blueprint for Health Care Reform. *Journal of the American Medical Association* 265 (19): 2507–10.

Ruggie, Mary. 1992. The Paradox of Liberal Intervention: Health Policy and the American Welfare State. *American Journal of Sociology* 97 (4): 919–44.

Russakoff, Dale. 1991. How Wofford Rode Health Care to Washington. *Washington Post National Weekly Edition*, 25 November–1 December, pp. 14–15.

Skocpol, Theda. 1992. *Protecting Soldiers and Mothers: The Political Origins of Social Policy in the United States.* Cambridge, MA: Belknap Press, Harvard University Press.

Starr, Paul. 1982. *The Social Transformation of American Medicine.* New York: Basic.

——— . 1991. The Middle Class and National Health Reform. *American Prospect* 6 (Summer): 7–12.

——— . 1993. Healthy Compromise: Universal Coverage and Managed Competition under a Cap. *American Prospect* 12 (Winter): 44–52.

Stevens, Beth. 1984. In the Shadow of the Welfare State: Corporate and Union Development of Employee Benefits. Ph.D. dissertation, Department of Sociology, Harvard University.

————. 1988. Blurring the Boundaries: How the Federal Government Has Influenced Welfare Benefits in the Private Sector. In *The Politics of Social Policy in the United States*, ed. Margaret Weir, Ann Shola Orloff, and Theda Skocpol. Princeton, NJ: Princeton University Press.

Todd, James S., S. V. Seekins, J. A. Krichbaum, and L. K. Harvey. 1991. Health Access America—Strengthening the U.S. Health Care System. *Journal of the American Medical Association* 265 (19): 2503–6.

Black America:
From Community Health Care
to Crisis Medicine

David McBride

Abstract This study traces the major policy shifts in medical care that have affected disadvantaged African-Americans and the response of this community's medical leadership to these changes. Since World War II policy has passed through three major phases. The first—*engagement*—ran from the mid-1960s through the mid-1970s. During this phase a community health policy orientation prevailed as national government targeted resources to health care programs for needy blacks and other poor Americans. From the late 1970s to the mid-1980s the period of *submersion* occurred: black community health professionals and political leaders experienced a new-found inclusion in health policy debate, but, at the same time, broader policy-making circles in government and health care reduced medical resources for the inner-city poor. Finally, in the third phase—*crisis recognition*—a network developed of community health advocates who seek to reorient the health system so that it addresses needs within urban America's "New Ghettos."

Recently a study appeared in the *New England Journal of Medicine*, entitled "Excess Mortality in Harlem" (McCord and Freeman 1990). It showed that, due largely to high levels of homicide, drug- and alcohol-related deaths, and cardiovascular disease, the men of this inner-city community were less likely to reach their sixty-fifth birthday than men in Bangladesh—an impoverished, Third World country. The researchers urge that, given the extraordinarily high death rates of Harlem—and other urban minority communities—the nation treat these neighborhoods with the same consideration given to natural disaster areas (see also Murray 1990).

In this article I take the current crisis in health care as it impacts mi-

nority communities in the context of history and the sociology of knowledge. I ask what national health policy looks like from the vantage point
of a minority population living, for the most part, in the poor, urban sector of American society. One thing is clear: the view has changed, along
with changes in the involvement of black community medical leaders in
national health policies since World War II and with shifts in the health
problems of poverty-ridden black communities. The changes occurred in
three main phases.

The first period—*engagement*—ran from the mid-1960s and carried
over to the Nixon and Ford administrations. During this decade a community health policy orientation prevailed. The federal government trans-
ferred substantial support and resources to advocates for minority health
care who were campaigning to expand health care for the poor and to end
discriminatory medical care and training practices.

The second phase—*submersion*—lasted from the late 1970s to the
mid-1980s, when professionals in black community health care were fan-
ning out into the general health care structure. Ironically, at the same
time, health policies of the Reagan and Bush administrations centered increasingly on reducing overall social spending and medical costs while
expanding the competitive market model and broadening information,
systems management, and medical technologies. Many minority health
professionals and advocates saw—from the inside—health care resources
for the inner-city poor disintegrating. A policy that had once been aggressively pursued was no longer a national political priority, and health
care for underclass and working-poor minorities in urban areas fell into
disorganization.

The third and final phase—*crisis recognition*—spans the late 1980s to
the present. It is characterized by a renewed, though still low-key, focus
on the urban black and Hispanic poor concentrated in the "New Ghetto."
This most recent policy debate on the health crisis of communities like
Harlem is not the result of a major shift in government and large-scale
health care institutions—the sectors that implemented extensive federal
health initiatives for the needy in the 1960s and early 1970s.

Instead, this rediscovery is forged from fragments: from health care
institutions, nonprofit organizations, and communities. It has the form
of an *issue cluster*, a collective message or communication, and is the
by-product of the research and policy recommendations of minority medical activists and small groups of health policy researchers, journalists,
grass-roots community organizers, and independent political voices.

This loose network of health advocates is most vocal about critical care problems associated with social violence, AIDS, teen pregnancy, drug abuse, and homelessness. By the late 1980s, the group managed to gain the attention of both national and black minority media with its "crisis medicine" theme. However, it has not formulated a plan to revamp the intellectual and technological structure of the health care system so that the needs of the New Ghetto can be answered. Nor has it been successful in mobilizing the political support necessary to redirect national health care policy toward this end.

Engagement

1965 marks a turning point in modern American health policy. That year, the Eighty-ninth Congress passed twenty-nine key health laws, which drastically reshaped health care services and the medical work force. Provisions included Medicaid; the Medicare amendments to the Social Security Act; grants for community mental health centers, and community vaccination assistance programs; the "Heart Disease, Cancer, and Stroke" amendments; the Clean Air Act; and vast increases in federal support for the education and development of the health care work force (Forgotson 1967; Neighbors 1987; Brandon 1991).

Behind this federal health legislation package was what Edward Forgotson, a public health physician, described then as the *systems integration method*. Under this paradigm, government directs resources to analyze the social causes of health and environmental problems; then it designs and substantially finances facilities and programs to solve these health problems in their entirety (Forgotson 1967; Wilson 1968). As Forgotson described it in his analysis of the legislation, "The flow paths of planning, organization, money, manpower, equipment, and facilities inputs . . . must be processed and integrated to achieve [for] the American people the most advanced and highest quality of health services" (Forgotson 1967: 935).

These liberal federal health initiatives were largely the product of the antipoverty campaigns of the Kennedy and Johnson administrations and the technical experts nurtured by them, as well as Democratic party congressional elements. The Civil Rights–Health Rights movement that had emerged during the 1960s and early 1970s also had the effect of galvanizing a policy network or "subgovernment" of public agencies and congressional overseers. Wide-scale civil rights and poor people's movements aimed at expanding political participation were being led by such community activists as Martin Luther King and Ralph Abernathy. The liberal health rights advocates, black medical professionals, and social welfare leaders in direct encounter with poverty and health care discrimination joined these political civil rights initiatives. Combined, health and equal rights activists served as the "third leg" alongside Congress and antipoverty agency officials in a three-part "subgovernment"—a quasi-permanent political force that won health care resources for the urban and rural poor (Sardell 1988).

Throughout the mid-1960s and 1970s the long-standing black physicians' organization, the National Medical Association (NMA), was especially active in local and federal political and health-policy-making circles. By this time, the NMA was comprised of both general practice physicians (medical faculty and specialists who traditionally served black communities or black hospitals) and newly trained black physicians educated and employed at predominantly white medical institutions. In its effort to increase general social welfare resources for the nation's black poor, the NMA broadened its financial and political support for national civil rights organizations such as the National Association for the Advancement of Colored People (NAACP), the Congress of Racial Equality (CORE), the Southern Christian Leadership Conference (SCLC), and the Student Nonviolent Coordinating Committee (SNCC), as well as the Congressional Black Caucus (founded in 1970). It also became one of the most vigorous pressure groups on Congress and on the president for civil rights legislation and health reforms like Medicare (Bookert 1977; Keiser 1987).

In addition to its role as a pressure group for liberal governmental health policies, the NMA provided clusters of physicians to serve as medical workers for independent health rights groups, most notably the Medical Committee for Human Rights (MCHR). In the summer of 1964 civil rights organizations in Mississippi, reeling from the murders of James Chaney, Andrew Goodman, and Michael Schwerner, made an urgent appeal for a "medical presence" in their state. Dozens of white and black health professionals based primarily in northern areas responded by organizing the MCHR. Many journeyed south to coordinate health projects with local black medical and community workers. By 1966 the MCHR had branches comprised of physicians, nurses, dentists, psychologists, medical students, and people in other health fields in thirty northern and southern cities (McBride 1991: 154–55).

By the late 1960s, the MCHR had expanded its efforts to raise the public visibility of discrimination in the nation's health system. Its activities grew beyond providing medical and community workers for southern locales into organizing to help expose discrimination in health care throughout the urban North as well. MCHR organizers emphasized that the "insidious and subtle" barriers in health care and politics that existed in northern cities were as much in need of MCHR activism as those in the South. "Of paramount importance to our contribution will be the effectiveness with which we apply medical presence in the Northern ghetto struggle," wrote two major MCHR organizers; "[We] can follow many of the precedents already established in the South" (Bridger and Belsky 1964: 2). Despite losing its national political viability by the early 1970s, the MCHR managed significant initiatives in the North that included establishing child health programs for ghetto neighborhoods, protest marches against discrimination in local hospitals, and support for recruiting black and Hispanic youth into medical work fields (McBride 1991: 154).

Outside of political activism, black and liberal medical leaders were integral to the operation of public hospitals and family practice in the inner city, as well as to the institutionalization of community health centers and the community mental health movement. Utilizing government grants provided through the federal antipoverty health legislation, they resurrected and rebuilt the neighborhood health center model. From 1965 to 1969 the Office of Economic Opportunity (OEO) sponsored 104 comprehensive health services facilities administered by community hospitals, medical schools, health corporations, health departments, and other nonprofit organizations (Sardell 1988; Davis and Millman 1983).

The technical model for community health centers imported by the planners of these centers was that of "community medicine," a new branch of public health and medical administration developed in Third World settings (Sardell 1988: 51–52; Geiger 1984). According to S. L. Kark (1971: 11), an early founder of community medicine and a world authority on it, community medicine is "distinguished from other forms of personal health care in the community in that its interest is centered on the community as a whole and the groups of which communities are composed" (see also Deuschle 1969).

Community medicine, then, like public health, assesses the health of population groups, not of individual patients. But it also provides treatment and allocates resources based on community-level, epidemiological screening. Community medicine programs and facilities are distinct from the neighborhood health centers of early twentieth-century America. Whereas the neighborhood health centers provided only limited service—

exams, immunizations, and hygienic education, for example—the comprehensive community health center includes a variety of ambulatory and multispecialty services (Geiger 1984).

Community medicine principles were widely supported in the 1960s and 1970s by black medical professionals and other activists involved in black community health institutions. They tended to view the health problems of blacks through a "relational paradigm." To these minority health advocates the excessive prevalence of specific diseases in black communities was one dimension in a broad range of erosive, stressful social and economic conditions affecting the inner-city and rural poor (McBride 1991: 85–86).

Moreover, these community health leaders viewed stepped-up primary health care resources for the black poor, together with an end to racially discriminatory policies, as the most important reforms for this medically needy population. Their goal throughout the 1960s and 1970s, in the words of the NMA president, was to "rise above vested interests, and to realize that it is our duty to see that health care is for all" (Bookert 1977: 730). The government's policies of systems integration and comprehensive health care and the black and liberal health sector's relational paradigm linked smoothly in these, the pre-*Bakke* years.

Submersion

In 1976, Atlanta University hosted a national conference, the W. E. B. Du Bois Conference on the health of black Americans. This historically black college had coordinated a pioneering series of conferences from 1897 to 1914 on the social and health problems of post-Reconstruction black Americans. Now, in this period of growing federal conservatism on school desegregation, the dampening of affirmative action programs by the *Bakke* decision, and growing negativism concerning social welfare assistance to the urban (substantially black) poor (Brandon 1991; Wilkinson 1979: 217; Dawson 1980), the university felt compelled to revive those regular gatherings.

One would expect the Atlanta conference organizers to give highest priority to the demise of federal support for school desegregation or to the alleviation of urban poverty. Instead, they held a conference of scholars from public health, the social sciences, and medicine to address "the most serious problem confronting black Americans, the health status of blacks and the lack of adequate health care delivery services" (*Phylon* 1977).

The Atlanta University national health conference of 1976 signaled that those active in black community health care were starting to recognize the early stages of broad psychological alienation and social disorder, spreading throughout lower-income black communities. A most riveting address at the conference was delivered by J. Alfred Cannon, chairman of the psychiatry department at the Charles W. Drew School of Medicine (Los Angeles) (Cannon 1977: 203). "Black America is in deep economic, psychological, social and spiritual distress," Cannon remarked. He described the toll taken on black Americans by the civil rights movement, urban turmoil, and the growing public backlash against the priorities of black urban communities:

> The "highs" of the 1960s, when blacks were at the epicenter of this nation's conscience and led the humanitarian revolution, are over. Blacks who had national and international visibility, relevance and significance are now on the backwaters of progress. Events prior to and following the 1960s have caused severe trauma to the black community, and the depth of the violation is such as to now pose, more seriously than before, the question of the very survival of black America.

Cannon's dire prognosis would seem far-fetched to mainstream health care institutions and policymakers. However, its significance and the importance of several other minority community health issues largely escaped the legislatures, corporations, and large-scale medical associations that were making and institutionalizing health policy in this period.

One such issue was that health care resources for low-income black community residents should go to strengthening community-based health "manpower," as it was then called. To health activists sensitive to black communities, the link between the traditional general practice physician and community hospitals located in black neighborhoods, on the one hand, and black community residents, on the other, was being weakened by new national health policies, just when it needed to be strengthened.

For example, in January of 1977, when Jimmy Carter began his presidency, national health insurance (NHI) appeared to be a possibility again (Coleman 1976). But the NMA cautioned NHI proponents that even if such a policy were implemented, it would not necessarily solve the medical problems of the urban racial minority. During 1977, shortly after Carter's inauguration, Arthur H. Coleman, NMA president, wrote in the association's national journal (Coleman 1977a: 11) that the NMA "would be opposed to a monolithic, government controlled program" sponsored by the new administration, even if it was one based on national health insurance. "We are convinced that any National Health Insurance program which fails to address itself to the socioeconomic aspect of the poor and other minority groups is going to meet with failure for that segment of the population."

More practical to Coleman and the NMA was expanding Medicaid. At the same time Medicaid had somehow to be revised to limit the negative impact that this repayment mechanism might have on traditional doctor-patient relationships in the black community. Finally, some form of government-sponsored catastrophic coverage should be devised. Too many physicians were turning away Medicaid recipients, and those who served them faced an increasing ground swell of dissatisfied "consumers," rather than trusting "patients."

"Practicing medicine in the ghetto can often be a personally rewarding experience for most black physicians," Coleman wrote (1977b: 291). The patients tended to be needy and most appreciative of their physician's care. However, while Medicaid made physician care more affordable for the black community poor, many of these "patients with the purchasing power of the Medicaid card do not remain with 'the old family doctor.' There is a tendency to doctor 'hop,' which lessens the chances of strong physician-patient relationships."

NMA physicians also raised the criticism that too much of Medicaid money went "to administrative and bureaucratic purposes rather than toward services, especially ambulatory services" (Coleman 1977a: 11). Catastrophic insurance was also a paramount need in the black community because the elderly and "the working poor among minorities . . . frequently do not have any or, at most, inadequate insurance coverage" (Coleman 1977a: 11; see also Dillard 1980).[1]

A central feature of national health policy in the 1970s and 1980s was the incorporation of increasingly complex planning techniques and information systems—a "reliance on the technology of planning," in the words of Marmor and Christianson (1982: 209). These technical operations—in offices of health systems agencies (HSAs), for example—were most logical among medical planning experts and academic policy study circles. But they were of little influence in the local world of functionally disconnected health care institutions serving youth, families, and the elderly in impoverished neighborhoods (Marmor and Christianson 1982: 210; McBride 1991: 155–56).

During the 1980s, major health care policymakers were broadening

---

1. A catastrophic health protection measure (the Medicare Extension Act) was proposed by President Reagan and passed by Congress in 1988 but was subsequently repealed.

their dependence on the market model for their policy decisions. Most black medical care advocates criticized this approach from the start. They saw no way for large-scale, market-oriented policy to help eliminate the disparities between white and minority mortality and illness rates.

One analyst of the competitive medical care approach and black community health needs (Winn 1987: 240) pointed out that the existence of "racial barriers to health care is not an issue for advocates of competitive health care." The focus on "market demands means that health care priorities would be responsive to individuals and not blacks as a special group. However, concentrating on individuals ignores the fact that blacks experience shorter life spans, a higher rate of chronic and debilitating illnesses, and lower protection against infectious diseases."

Higher costs for health technology and labor-intensive medical care contributed to the decline of the traditional general practice in the inner city and its social or community role. Consequently, city dwellers became increasingly dependent on public hospitals and community health centers for outpatient and routine medical treatment. At the same time, shifts in demographic and employment patterns, as well as federal-local relations in social welfare programming throughout urban areas, were causing many urban hospitals to close. The remaining public hospitals and health centers lost ground in terms of the quality and quantity of care they were capable of providing (O'Hare 1987; Goff 1980).

Other developments included cuts in medical care for urban neighborhood residents. Federal and employment-based medical benefits were declining, community health centers were underfinanced, and municipalities were decreasing subsidies for free medical services for the poor at city hospitals (Vann 1980; Thompson 1980). For example, in 1982 federal funding for the nation's 872 community health centers was decreased by an average of 30 to 45 percent. This revenue decline resulted in service cutbacks or closings at 239 (28 percent) of the health centers. A study of 5 health centers in Boston attributed a 14 percent reduction in obstetrics visits, a 12 percent drop in pediatric visits, and a significant increase in local infant mortality to the federal aid reductions (Dutton 1987: 48, 49).

Black medical and health policy activists, many holding prominent positions in politics and health agencies, denounced this reduction in health care delivery in inner-city areas. Speaking before the NMA's national conference in 1983, Chicago mayor Harold Washington criticized the federal government for giving financial incentives for the growth of private hospital chains and for-profit medical providers. At the same time, "as health costs run wild, the poor, many of them black, are being shrugged out of private hospitals and being dumped in greater numbers each year on the struggling public hospitals, such as Cook County Hospital here in Chicago" (Washington 1984: 12).

Other city political leaders responding to the decline in hospital services for the poor agitated for more governmental support for transportation of residents living in neighborhoods remote from appropriate medical facilities. These measures included greater government support for emergency city ambulances, incentives to increase voluntary ambulance services in underserved areas, and even repayment for the use of gypsy cabs, frequently the only means for emergency travel in ghetto neighborhoods (Vann 1980).

In addition to retaining and expanding community service, medical care resources, and personnel, the black medical leadership's second primary policy goal for the urban black poor was to promote and develop community health. According to this view, in order for health care resources to reach and benefit needy black community residents, they must be designed and implemented to address both the causes and the effects of past racial exclusion and the growing social and economic isolation experienced by this group. The roots of this isolation were prior patterns of exclusion and mistrust, toughening economic circumstances for the black working poor, and their inability to reverse the federal retreat from subsidizing community-level preventive health care resources.

V. R. Thompson, NMA president for 1980, emphasized that community conditions and ethnic social psychology must be at the center of health planning. He described the priorities of black Americans as being either "micro-community or macro-community in scope." Microcommunity issues affect daily neighborhood life and include street crime, police patrols, garbage collection, transportation services, and physical proximity to community health centers and medical services. Macrocommunity concerns include "broader problems of economic disability, the high rate of unemployment, [the] quality of education and the elementary and secondary school levels, and inequality of access to graduate and professional schools" (Thompson 1980: 833).

In his 1978 study, "Health Policy and the Underserved," S. A. Roman, a Boston public health physician, summarized the roots of social alienation among black community residents. He stressed that the nation's major health policy concerns were increasingly about cost containment and the availability of providers. However, these policy directions ignored the fact that communities can be psychologically distinct—as opposed to distinct on the more narrow grounds of geography and income level—and that they institutionalized racial exclusion.

Underlying this new federal health policy was the false notion of the melting pot. To Roman, this notion that America was essentially prejudice-free obscured the reality that "underserved communities in health care, and in other areas of our society, are those groups lacking in political power" because they constitute racial minorities, women, or the elderly. The social identities of many within these groups clash with the psychological and cultural ideals and norms of mainstream society (Roman 1978: 32).

Roman stressed that the effectiveness of health care plans and institutions was affected by ethnic experiences. The perceptions held by "minority communities about health care providers have implications as to how they utilize health facilities, how they comply with scientific medical recommendations, and how stable a relationship they establish with a given provider of care or institution" (Roman 1978: 33).

A primary cause, Roman continued, for the failure of American health care to achieve equitable distribution and utilization of medical institutions was that the American minority and majority communities had been socialized by having to contend with racial experiences, values, and problems. "We must begin to accept that human beings form attitudes based on early experiences," he emphasized, and "with these attitudes are developed prejudices" (Roman 1978: 33). Unfortunately, he continued, because the new notions of representation were "color-blind" and because consumer networks increasingly dominated large-scale health care policy and governance, health policymakers did not recognize, much less remedy, health disparities tied to broader socioeconomic ethnic inequalities.

Now, in the new age of competitive market-oriented health provision, the size and popularity of health maintenance organizations (HMOs) and preferred provider organizations (PPOs) grew markedly during the 1980s (Starr 1982: 420–49). Black health practitioners and community interest have had a limited role in these new systems (Sampson 1984); early studies had revealed that such competitive provider approaches were ineffective in serving the uninsured, and the community has little influence over the performance of these facilities (Schlesinger 1987: 289).

Crisis Recognition

By the mid-1980s minority health care activists were generally convinced that national reforms to improve financial access to health care—whether they were built on the new medical marketplace model of the unfolding Reagan-Bush administrations or on the recurring NHI ideal—were falling far short of rectifying the health problems of the inner-city black poor. To advocates for the black community, the specific disease problems and access needs of the black poor were intertwined with many general sources of stress in the black community: high unemployment; overburdened community services and public hospitals; drug abuse, fear, and violence in the neighborhood; the overburdening of single mothers; an excess of preventable deaths among black women; and the political self-centeredness of new immigrants and mainstream whites.

In 1984, the NMA published a series of studies on "Health Care Problems in the 1980s from a Black Perspective." Their purpose was to "smoke out" the positions of the presidential candidates and their parties on this issue. Two concerns were raised. One pertained to the crisis in health care delivery: the rising cost of medical care, inadequate distributions of health care facilities, the threat that Medicare was facing bankruptcy, and the overall disorganization of the health care system. The second was about the wide disparity in the health of black and white Americans: black Americans show higher maternal and infant mortality rates, lower life expectancy, and higher death rates linked to cardiovascular disease and cancer. The causes of black America's higher death rates needed to be tackled, they concluded, head on (Sampson 1984; Barber and Sinnette 1984).

The following year the NMA conducted a legislative forum for the House of Representatives Subcommittee on Health and the Environment. The theme of community development was central throughout the testimony of the NMA representatives. While disproportionate instances of cancer among blacks was one of their primary concerns, they stressed the need for a national public school health initiative and an improvement in the quality and quantity of maternal and child medical services.

"If we sincerely believe that children are our greatest national resource for the future," the NMA speakers told the congressional members present, "we must demonstrate our commitment by improving the health of all children and especially children in greatest need. Without special efforts such a phrase will have a hollow ring and future generations will pay the price of our negligence" (Daniel Savage, quoted in U.S. House 1985: 19).

At the same time that this legislative forum was taking place, the *Report of the Secretary's Task Force on Black and Minority Health* was released by then Department of Health and Human Services (DHHS) secretary, Margaret Heckler. The task force was comprised of some of the highest-ranking officials in the nation's federal health agencies (the National Institutes of Health and the Food and Drug Administration, among others). Its report profiled an alarming failure by the health care system to eliminate wide racial differentials in mortality and illness in the nation. It disclosed that blacks were experiencing about 59,000 more preventable deaths per year than white Americans. The six major health problems underlying the much higher mortality rate of blacks were cancer, cardiovascular disease and stroke, substance abuse, diabetes, homicides and accidents, and infant mortality.

Even though the task force delivered shocking data on the lag in minority health, its primary recommendations envisioned no major reorganization of the vast health care resources under DHHS control. It did recommend that DHHS operate outreach campaigns designed to give racial minorities greater access to health information. It also said that DHHS should encourage patient education that would lower the cost of medical care (U.S. DHHS 1985: 9–16). But, as for the area of improving the delivery and financing of health services, the task force stated anticlimactically and vaguely: "The Department should continue to investigate, develop and implement innovative models for delivery and financing of health services, based on current departmental authorizations" (U.S. DHHS 1985: 15).

Critiques by the NMA and the DHHS task force were barely two years old when the AIDS epidemic began to spread rapidly into the black American population. In the DHHS study, infectious disease had not been ranked among the six leading causes of excess minority deaths. But now, as one task force member wrote, while the original six problems had by no means been reduced, "AIDS is a seventh Horseman of the Apocalypse" (Hopkins 1987: 681).

By 1989 the high death rates of blacks tied to preventable diseases (but most especially to AIDS and intravenous drug abuse) resulted in a virtual explosion of criticism from minority health professionals, investigative journalists, and black political and religious activists. Popular magazines, newspapers, academic journals, all flowed with serious and solidly documented indictments of the health system. "The black community is in the midst of a serious survival and health crisis," one magazine journalist wrote (Simon 1989: 48). Community rallies against drug abuse and the AIDS crisis broke out across the nation. In San Francisco, some 1,200 black church and civic leaders held a national grass-roots conference against drug abuse and violence with the theme "The Death of a Race" (*Ebony* 1989, 1990; Gibbs 1988; Dalton 1989).

While the pain and frustration about the excessively high number of deaths in black communities rang loud and clear in the media, a national policy that would address the health, social, and economic conditions behind this calamity was still not formulating in the minds of minority health activists. They seemed stifled by the sheer hugeness and inflexibility of the medical care system. Evidently, neither black community health advocates nor national health care institutions had adjusted to the reality that lower-income black and minority communities have changed radically from the 1960s and 1970s.

Beneath the health epidemics, there has been a steady deterioration of black neighborhood sections throughout large and middle-size cities. The federal and civil rights health and welfare initiatives of the pre-1975 period were geared toward serving the first wave of post–World War II urban ghettos. These were characterized by rapidly expanding black populations in the urban North and West, urban renewal housing projects, high unemployment, and scarce health facilities and physician resources. For example, between 1930 and 1960 New York State's black population more than tripled, from 413,000 to 1,418,000. During this period, the percentage of blacks residing in inner-city sections of urban regions jumped from 30.6 percent to 51.5 percent. The growing black population of New York City and similar cities, such as Chicago, Detroit, and Philadelphia, settled into the low-pay work force and their communities grew impoverished (U.S. Census Bureau 1975: 32). The frustration in urban black communities during the 1960s culminated with a surge of urban riots, documented and brought onto the national agenda by the Kerner Commission (1968).

But in the 1980s and 1990s we witness the rise of the New Ghetto. This is a less politically visible form of ghettoization, characterized sociologically by large neighborhoods with declining populations, high unemployment and homelessness, soaring crime rates, and an overwhelming dependence on emergency-room medical services. Black and Hispanic working-poor districts have been abandoned not only by large-scale private interests but also by long-standing residents unable to cope with the breakdown of neighborhood. The abandonment of single adults, youth, and families in the inner city is directly linked to the decline in these residents' health (R. Wallace 1990; D. Wallace 1990; Birrer et al. 1991).

For example, geographical and sociological health studies of neighborhoods in New York City's South Bronx section reveal that this health district has some of the nation's highest rates of infant mortality, drug and alcohol abuse, and AIDS. These rates vary with this section's level of housing "desertification" and public school transfers. The stressful social circumstances of today's urban poor are manifest inside their households as well as inside individuals and contribute directly to the rapid intensification of HIV infections and AIDS death rates (Birrer et al. 1991; Brown 1990: 54–55).

Finally, intense ghettoization has lowered the already poor health of the children in black and Hispanic inner-city areas. Throughout the 1960s and 1970s, a variety of youth services were operated under Title V of the Social Security Act and OEO. These programs included the neighborhood OEO clinics, Head Start, Medicaid, community health centers, and Title V–funded maternity and child health programs. But as a group of medical researchers at the SUNY Health Sciences Center in Brooklyn has recently stated (Birrer et al. 1991: 339), "The impact of these programs during the late 1970s and 1980s has been significantly reduced because of inflation, restricted eligibility criteria, cutbacks in funding, and an increase in the number of poor immigrant families with children."

These researchers had set up a comprehensive health program at a public elementary school located in Brooklyn, New York. From 1986 to 1989 they conducted health examinations of 1,250 inner-city children (from kindergarten through sixth grade). They discovered that nearly 13 percent of the children had nervous system disease, 9 percent respiratory disease, and 6 percent infectious or parasitic disease. About one-third of all the children needed immediate medical care for these and other conditions (Birrer et al. 1991).

With dedication and expertise, today's minority health policy advocates have unveiled serious health problems unique to large portions of America's racial minority populations, male and female, young and old. They have managed to accomplish this feat during the past decade and a half when federal controllers of national health subsidies and policy regarded facilities such as neighborhood health centers as politically unpopular. Moreover, to these national policymakers, medically needy poor Americans are just a portion of an anonymous mass, a "colorless" marketplace (Brandon 1991: 182).

As this overview of post-1950s health care reform and black America may have suggested, national health programs managed, initially, to direct significant resources to the health problems of minority, low-income communities. But in the last decade and a half, the trend in federal health policy has been to "disidentify" the economically troubled black and Hispanic community, particularly its female sector, and substitute in its place the ideal of the patient-consumer.

This most recent policy direction has come at the same time that health care providers and epidemiologists investigating minority communities are unraveling with increasing technical accuracy severely high levels of preventable ill health and mortality among these populations (Cooper 1991; Kumanyika and Golden 1991; Mays and Jackson 1991). Indeed, since the early 1980s, minority health advocates have produced a "diagnosis" of health care needs in black communities that is as fine-tuned as ever, but follow-up national programming has been woefully muddled. Most recently the Council on Graduate Medical Education (COGME) has issued a report spelling out measures that would greatly improve training and availability of a physician work force that matches more specifically the needs of underserved inner-city communities (COGME 1992). Their implementation would go far in assisting policymakers in the New Ghetto to move beyond crisis medicine.

References

Barber, J. B., and C. H. Sinnette. 1984. Presidential Politics and Minority Health. *Journal of the National Medical Association* 76:969–71.

Birrer, R. B., J. M. Fleisher, L. Cortese, M. Weiner, J. Ferra, F. Richards, and C. M. Plotz. 1991. An Urban Primary School Health Program. *New York State Journal of Medicine* 91:339–41.

Bookert, C. C. 1977. President's Inaugural Address: No Day of Triumph. *Journal of the National Medical Association* 69:729–30.

Brandon, W. P. 1991. Two Kinds of Conservatism in U.S. Health Policy: The Reagan Record. In *Comparative Health Policy and the New Right: From Rhetoric to Reality*, ed. C. Altenstetter. New York: St. Martin's.

Bridger, Wagner H., and Marvin S. Belsky. 1964. MCHR Position Paper: National Committee of Recruitment and Medical Presence. Leonidas H. Berry Papers, Box 5, History of Medicine Division, National Library of Medicine, Washington, DC.

Brown, L. S., Jr. 1990. Black Intravenous Drug Users: Prospects for Intervening in the Transmission of Human Immunodeficiency Virus Infection. In *AIDS and Intravenous Drug Use: Future Directions for Community-based Prevention Research*, NIDA Research Monograph 93, ed. C. G. Leukefeld, R. J. Battjes, and Z. Amsel. Washington, DC: U.S. Government Printing Office.

Cannon, J. A. 1977. Re-Africanization: The Last Alternative for Black America. *Phylon* 37 (June): 203–10.

COGME (Council on Graduate Medical Education). 1992. *Third Report: Improving Access to Health Care through Physician Workforce Reform: Directions for the 21st Century*. Washington, DC: U.S. Department of Health and Human Services, Public Health Service, Health Resources and Services Administration.

Coleman, A. H. 1976. An Era of Accountability. *Journal of the National Medical Association* 68:422–27.

———. 1977a. National Health Insurance and President Carter. *Journal of the National Medical Association* 69:11.

———. 1977b. Medicaid and Malpractice: A Dilemma for the Black Physician. *Journal of the National Medical Association* 69:291.

Cooper, R. S. 1991. Celebrate Diversity—Or Should We? *Ethnicity and Disease* 1:3–7.

Dalton, H. L. 1989. AIDS in Blackface. *Daedalus: Living with AIDS (Part 2)* 118: 205–27.

Davis, K., and M. Millman. 1983. *Health Care for the Urban Poor: Directions for Policy*. Totowa, NJ: Rowman and Allanheld.

Dawson, R. E. 1980. A Meeting with Patricia Robers Harris, Secretary, Department of Health, Education, and Welfare. *Journal of the National Medical Association* 72:431–32.

Deuschle, K. W. 1969. What Is the Role of the Ghetto Hospital in Health Care Delivery? In *Medicine in the Ghetto*, ed. J. C. Norman. New York: Appleton-Century-Crofts.

Dillard, M. C. 1980. Federal Health Policy: New Directions for the 1980s. *Journal of the National Medical Association* 72:1158.

Dutton, D. B. 1987. Social Class, Health, and Illness. In *Applications of Social Science to Clinical Medicine and Health Policy*, ed. L. H. Aiken and D. Mechanic. New Brunswick, NJ: Rutgers University Press.

Ebony. 1989. Ministers Mobilize against "The Death of a Race," August, pp. 160–64.

———. 1990. NMA President Leads National Crusade for Equal Health Care, April, pp. 58, 60.

Forgotson, E. H. 1967. 1965: The Turning Point in Health Law—1966 Reflections. *American Journal of Public Health* 57:934–46.

Geiger, H. J. 1984. The Community Health Center: Health as an Instrument of Social Change. In *Reforming Medicine: Lessons of the Last Quarter Century*, ed. V. W. Sidel and R. Sidel. New York: Pantheon.

Gibbs, J. T., ed. 1988. *Young, Black and Male in America: An Endangered Species*. Dover, MA: Auburn House.

Goff, D. W. 1980. The Plight of the Urban Public Hospital. *Journal of Health Politics, Policy and Law* 4:657–74.

Hopkins, D. R. 1987. AIDS in Minority Populations in the United States. *Public Health Reports* 102:677–81.

Kark, S. L. 1971. *The Practice of Community-oriented Primary Health Care*. New York: Appleton-Century-Crofts.

Keiser, K. R. 1987. Congress and Black Health: Dynamics and Strategies. In *Health Care Issues in Black America: Policies, Problems, and Prospects*, ed. W. Jones, Jr., and M. F. Rice. Westport, CT: Greenwood.

Kerner Commission. 1968. *National Advisory Commission on Civil Disorders Report*. Washington, DC: U.S. Government Printing Office.

Kumanyika, S. K., and P. M. Golden. 1991. Cross-Sectional Differences in Health Status in United States Racial/Ethnic Minority Groups: Potential Influence of Temporal Changes, Disease, and Life-Style Transitions. *Ethnicity and Disease* 1:50–59.

McBride, D. 1991. *From TB to AIDS: Epidemics among Urban Blacks since 1900*. Albany: SUNY Press.

McCord, C., and H. P. Freeman. 1990. Excess Mortality in Harlem. *New England Journal of Medicine* 322:173–77.

Marmor, T. R., and J. B. Christianson. 1982. *Health Care Policy: A Political Economy Approach*. Beverly Hills, CA: Sage.

Mays, V. M., and J. S. Jackson. 1991. AIDS Survey Methodology with Black Americans. *Social Science and Medicine* 33:47–54.

Murray, C. J. 1990. Mortality among Black Men. *New England Journal of Medicine* 322:205–6.

Neighbors, H. W. 1987. Improving the Mental Health of Black Americans: Lessons from the Community Mental Health Movement. *Milbank Quarterly* 65 (Suppl. 2): 348–80.

O'Hare, W. P. 1987. Black Demographic Trends in the 1980s. *Milbank Quarterly* 65 (Supp. 1): 35–55.

Phylon. 1977. Editor's Introduction. Vol. 37 (June), p. iv.

Roman, S. A. 1978. Health Policy and the Underserved. *Journal of the National Medical Association* 70:31–35.

Sampson, C. C. 1984. Health Care Problems in the 1980s from a Black Perspective. *Journal of the National Medical Association* 76:968–71.

Sardell, A. 1988. *The U.S. Experiment in Social Medicine: The Community Health Center Program, 1965–86*. Pittsburgh, PA: University of Pittsburgh Press.

Schlesinger, M. 1987. Paying the Price: Medical Care, Minorities, and the Newly Competitive Health Care System. *Milbank Quarterly* 65 (Suppl. 2): 270–96.

Simon, F. 1989. Countering the Crises. *American Visions* 4 (February): 48, 50.

Starr, P. 1982. *The Social Transformation of American Medicine*. New York: Basic.

Thompson, V. R. 1980. Health Status of Black Citizens. *Journal of the National Medical Association* 72:833–34.

U.S. Census Bureau. 1975. *Historical Statistics of the United States, Colonial Times to 1970, Bicentennial Edition, Part 2*. Washington, DC: U.S. Government Printing Office.

U.S. DHHS (U.S. Department of Health and Human Services). 1985. *Report on the Secretary's Task Force on Black and Minority Health, Vol. I: Executive Summary*. Washington, DC: U.S. Government Printing Office.

U.S. House (U.S. House of Representatives, Committee on Energy and Commerce, Subcommittee on Health and the Environment). 1985. *Health Problems Confronting Blacks and Other Minorities*. Washington, DC: U.S. Government Printing Office.

Vann, A. 1980. Health Care Delivery in America: Major Concerns. *Journal of the National Medical Association* 72:721–22.

Wallace, D. 1990. Roots of Increased Health Care Inequality in New York. *Social Science and Medicine* 31:1219–27.

Wallace, R. 1990. Urban Desertification, Public Health and Public Order: "Planned Shrinkage," Violent Death, Substance Abuse, and AIDS in the Bronx. *Social Science and Medicine* 31:801–13.

Washington, H. 1984. Barriers to Black Physicians and Health Care. *Journal of the National Medical Association* 76:11–12.

Wilkinson, J. H. 1979. *From* Brown *to* Bakke: *The Supreme Court and School Integration*. New York: Oxford University Press.

Wilson, R. N. 1968. *Community Structure and Health Action: A Report on Process Analysis*. Washington, DC: Public Affairs Press.

Winn, M. 1987. Competitive Health Care: Assessing an Alternative Solution for Health Care Problems. In *Health Care Issues in Black America: Policies, Problems, and Prospects*, ed. W. Jones, Jr., and M. F. Rice. Westport, CT: Greenwood.

From Community Health Care to Crisis Medicine: Have We Learned the Right Lessons?

Joan M. Leiman

David McBride's history of health care reform over the past forty years "from the vantage point of a minority population living, for the most part, in the poor, urban sector of American society" (1993: 320) serves as an important reminder that a rising tide does not necessarily lift all ships. The reminder is particularly timely as the Clinton administration prepares its proposals for major reform of the health care system. National health care reform will not reach the inner-city pockets of poverty, where large numbers of black Americans live, unless it takes explicit account of their special circumstances and those of the hospitals and providers that serve them.

McBride rightly charges federal health care policymakers with increasing neglect of the economically vulnerable over the past fifteen years in favor of programs based on the market model of health care and the "ideal patient consumer type." The results have been a failure to deal with the growing incidence of violence and substance abuse in the "new ghettos" and to put in place the public health measures necessary to address the disparities in white and minority mortality and illness rates and, in addition, the withdrawal of resources from the public programs and facilities that comprise the front line of service to the poor and socially troubled.

While McBride points to the lack of support for public hospitals and clinics as one reason for the failure to serve the economically vulnerable, he does not discuss this aspect of the problem in detail, nor does he connect the problem back to Medicare and Medicaid. If we assume, as McBride does, that the "submersion" (1993: 320) of the health care needs of the poor is mainly attributable to the cutbacks of the last fifteen years of federal policy, we risk overlooking an important piece of the explanation for the access and service problems poor black and Hispanic Americans have experienced.

Reliance on a marketplace model of health care did not develop during the last fifteen years. It is deeply rooted in the American political culture. Medicare and Medicaid were built around the principle that the way to assure access to health care is to support individuals, not providers. There is, however, another model that also has deep roots in American political culture, that of local public hospitals and clinics to care for the poor. What happened in New York City following the enactment of Medicare and Medicaid illustrates what can happen when these models are treated as conflicting or competing. It further illustrates the difficulties of relying on a strategy of consumer support to provide the economically vulnerable with needed services.

In 1960 New York operated the largest (but not the only) public health care system in the country, providing care to roughly one-fifth to one-fourth of the city's population and over half of its black and Hispanic population (Klarman 1963). New York City's public system was different in scale but not in kind from other local public services, such as Boston's City Hospital, Chicago's Cook County Hospital, and the Los Angeles County Hospital. Like these others, New York's municipal system existed to provide care to all residents who for reasons of poverty, location, and racial or other forms of discrimination were unable to obtain care from private providers (Duffy 1974). Because they were supported by local tax revenues, public hospitals had more difficulty than private hospitals making the capital investments needed to keep place with rapidly changing medical technology (Klarman 1963). By the time Medicare and Medicaid came along, the New York public hospitals suffered from obsolete facilities, long clinic waiting times, and little or no primary care and were under public attack for making second-class citizens of those New Yorkers dependent on them for their care (Commission on the Delivery of Personal Health Services 1969).

The enactment of Medicare and Medicaid set off a major and bitter debate in New York City over the future of the public hospitals. On one side were ranged private hospitals and "good government" groups who wanted to upgrade the public system by using Medicare and Medicaid to transform them into private hospitals. On the other side were advocates for the poor and supporters of the public hospital who wanted to use the new funds to rebuild the hospitals and establish a network of neighborhood ambulatory centers under public auspices.

The debate ultimately engaged the mayor (John Lindsay) and the governor (Nelson Rockefeller), each of whom established a special commission to deal with the issue. The governor's commission recommended retaining the public system but improving it (New York State 1967). The mayor's commission recommended transferring the hospitals to a new not-for-profit corporation (Commission on the Delivery of Personal Health Services 1969).

By the time these reports were issued, barely two years after Medicare and Medicaid became law, it was apparent that no one could direct or control the flow of the new dollars. Moreover, Medicaid as a welfare program with categorical as well as income eligibility was not providing universal coverage for the poor, not even in New York State, which had one of the most generous programs in the nation. The public hospitals found themselves competing with the private hospitals for Medicare and Medicaid patients and dollars and experiencing an outflow of both patients and dollars (City of New York 1969: 29).

In New York the great debate over the future of the public hospitals was ultimately settled by an uneasy political compromise which moved the hospitals into a publicly controlled public benefit corporation. The idea was to solve the hospitals' deficiencies by freeing the hospitals from the city's overhead controls. Reorganization alone, however, could not compensate for a national health policy that ignored the special role of local public hospitals in providing health care services to economically vulnerable and troubled communities. In 1969 New York State, alarmed by the rapid growth in the cost of Medicaid, cut back its program, returning a portion of the Medicaid population to dependency on public hospitals. With the rapid inflation of health care costs the public hospitals came under increasing financial stress. In 1979 another mayoral commission reported on the financial crisis of the hospitals (City of New York 1979) and today, almost thirty years after Medicare and Medicaid, yet another mayoral commission has found the public hospitals severely overburdened, under serious fiscal pressure, and with long waiting times to see a physician (New York Academy of Medicine 1992).

In the early years of the War on Poverty, McBride points out, federal policy did pay special attention to needs of the economically disadvantaged. There were a plethora of liberal health programs targeted at poor communities, among them, neighborhood health centers, community vaccination assistance, and training for health care professionals. These programs, however, were soon cut back under the pressure caused by the rising costs of Medicare and Medicaid, adding to the pressure on local public hospitals and clinics.

The point here is not to disparage the goal of bringing all Americans into the mainstream medical marketplace or to undervalue the role which Medicare and Medicaid played in enabling millions of Americans, especially black Americans, to gain access to physician and other health care services (Davis et al. 1987). The lesson to be learned, however, from McBride's history and from New York City's experience is that integration of the economically vulnerable into the private marketplace will not easily or automatically occur, even with universal financial coverage. No insurance or managed care program is likely to cover or provide the social and community public health services needed by the economically troubled and vulnerable. In fact, the private medical marketplace may be less willing or able to meet these needs under a national health policy that forces providers to compete for survival by keeping their costs as low as possible. For the foreseeable future, local public services will continue to play a major role in the overall health care system as the safety net and provider of first, and last, resort to the most economically vulnerable and troubled among us. Policy and reform need to recognize, support, and provide for this role and prevent the large needs of the poor from falling financially on the cities and counties, the levels of government least able to bear them.

The Clinton–Rodham Clinton effort gives early signs of recognizing the need to address this concern and respond to it. Reports coming out of Washington suggest that one of the fifteen task teams at the White House is dealing with "health policy initiatives for underserved populations and preventive health," including public hospitals. Let us hope that when David McBride updates health care reform from the special perspective of the inner-city black American, he will be able to label this new phase one of "reengagement" and progress.

References

City of New York. 1969. Executive Budget for 1969–70: Message of the Mayor. Unpublished document. Municipal Reference Library, New York.

———. 1979. A Plan for Improving the Effectiveness of Hospital Services in New York: Report to the Mayor. Unpublished document. Budget Commission Library, New York.

Commission on the Delivery of Personal Health Services. 1969. *Community Health Services for New York City: Report and Staff Studies*. New York: Praeger.

Davis, Karen, Marsha Lille-Blanton, Barbara Lyons, Fitzhugh Mullan, Neil Powe, and Diane Rowland. 1987. Health Care for Black Americans: The Public Sector Role. *Milbank Quarterly* 65 (Suppl. 1): 213–47.

Duffy, John. 1974. *A History of Public Health in New York City, 1866–1966*. New York: Russell Sage Foundation.

Klarman, Herbert E. 1963. *Hospital Care in New York City: The Roles of Voluntary and Municipal Hospitals*. New York: Columbia University Press.

McBride, David. 1993. Black America: From Community Health Care to Crisis Medicine. *Journal of Health Politics, Policy and Law* 18 (2): 319–37.

New York Academy of Medicine. 1992. Report of the Mayoral Commission to Review the Health and Hospitals Corporation. New York: Academy of Medicine.

New York State. 1967. Report of the State Blue Ribbon Panel on Municipal Hospitals of New York City. Albany: New York State Government.

The author wishes to thank Eli Ginzberg and Lawrence Brown, who reviewed an early draft of this piece, for their helpful comments.

Part 2
Political Institutions

Congress in the 1990s:
From Iron Triangles to Policy Networks

Mark A. Peterson

Abstract To assess the prospects of comprehensive health care reform during the Clinton administration, we must examine the changes that have occurred in the political and structural contexts in which reform is debated. The political context includes the status of the health care system itself as well as public attitudes and voting patterns associated with health care reform; it may be friendlier now to reform than it has been in any previous period, but it cannot on its own produce policy change. The structural context, the representational community of organized interests and government institutions, is the means by which politics is either thwarted or translated into action. Changes in these organized interests and in Congress have transformed the health care reform policy community from an "iron triangle" dominated by an antireform alliance of medicine, insurance, and business to a more loosely bound policy network in which a reform coalition may now be able to prevail, especially under the direction of an activist president like Bill Clinton. I consider three hypotheses: The first claims that, despite the apparent structural changes, the core power relationships will remain the same as in the past, and the antireform alliance either will continue to block policy change or will push through a reform program that protects its constituent interests. According to the second, the structural changes produce an atomization of power, making coalition building in support of reform impossible. The third and most plausible hypothesis proposes that the structural changes, in combination with the shift in politics and Clinton's election, have generated new opportunities for fundamental reform.

During one of his frequent trips back to South Dakota, Senator Tom Daschle (D-SD) stopped in at the Good Samaritan Nursing Home, in the quiet community of Canistota, located among cornfields in the southeastern corner of the state. A resident of the home asked, with an air of "outside-the-beltway" innocence, "Tom, why can't we have a health care system like the one they have in Canada?" It is a question that comes up frequently in South Dakota, where proximity to our northern neighbor affords residents more than the usual exposure to news about the Canadian experience. It is natural for people there to wonder why the United States is alone among major industrial nations in having a health care system that neither grants everyone access to care nor keeps health care costs under control. It has become an issue that increasingly occupies the minds of people across the United States.

About nine months after the Canistota visit, on 2 April 1992, Senator Daschle, together with Senators Harris Wofford (D-PA) and Paul Simon (D-IL), introduced the American Health Security Plan (S. 2513), a modified single-payer proposal for the comprehensive reform of the American health care financing system. The moment was laden with symbolism, given Wofford's stunning victory over former U.S. Attorney General Richard Thornburgh the previous November, after a campaign that focused heavily on the need for health care reform cast him as the "poster child" of the reform issue.[1] The American Health Security Plan joined the multitude of proposals and options floating around the nation's capital during the 102d Congress, including but not limited to the single-payer approaches introduced by Senator Bob Kerrey and Representative Marty Russo, the "pay-or-play" employer-based mandated benefits approach promoted by the Senate Democratic leadership, and the voucher and tax credit market-based approach advocated by the Heritage Foundation and then President George Bush (see Blendon et al. 1992).

Major health care reform was strikingly back on the nation's agenda, possible solutions were circulating wildly, and the nation's capital was abuzz with meetings, forums, and press conferences, at which the merits of proposals were earnestly debated. Missing, however, was catalytic leadership from the White House. The election in 1992 of Democratic President Bill Clinton, a proponent of activist government with a campaign commitment to introduce health care reform as one of his first priorities, seems to put a final piece into place. With Clinton in the White House, the momentum toward reform accelerates, even though his adoption of the rhetoric tied to yet another approach—managed competition—complicates the choice about which direction reform might go (see Rosner 1993). But despite all of these activities, the end of divided government, and Clinton's commitment, will the current period of deliberation actually produce reform, unlike all previous periods?

---

1. The "poster child" analogy was coined by a member of Senator Wofford's staff.

The question posed by the nursing home resident implied two others: First, for all the progress that private insurance and public programs have made in expanding the availability of coverage, what explains the absence to date of a universal health care financing system in the United States? Second, is it reasonable to anticipate that we are now at the brink of enacting such a system? Attempting answers to these questions presents the political scientist with an analytical quandary. Explanations of past actions and predictions of future change are predicated on the presence of variance in observable behaviors and outcomes. But comprehensive reform of the system for financing health care in the United States is of interest precisely because it has not happened before (with the partial exception in 1965 of enacting Medicare for the elderly and Medicaid for the poor—see Marmor 1973; Skidmore 1970).

The idea of comprehensive health care reform is not new: it has appeared on the national agenda in one guise or another roughly six times in this century. Between 1912 and 1917, it was tied to the Progressive movement but waned with the advent of World War I and suspicions of "German" ideas like Bismarck's social insurance (Starr 1982: 243–57). Franklin Roosevelt's Committee on Economic Security in 1935 considered it a complement to plans for social security, but his calculation of the political burdens associated with such a national health care program kept the issue on the back burner (Altmeyer 1968; Hirshfield 1970; Witte 1962). During the latter half of the 1940s, President Harry Truman made national health insurance a highlight of his legislative agenda, but established interests were opposed, the public was skeptical, and Congress, especially when in the hands of the Republican party, was anything but receptive (Campion 1984; Poen 1979). Frustrated by these earlier defeats, strategists shifted in the late 1950s and early 1960s to proposing a government insurance program for the elderly as a foundation for a full-scale program for all citizens (Marmor 1973: chap. 1). After Medicare and Medicaid were enacted, however, the follow-through failed to come through. In the 1970s, presidents from Nixon to Carter joined the reform debate with congressional proponents of varying degrees of commitment, from Senator Ted Kennedy to Representative Wilbur Mills, but by the end of the decade no action had been taken, and the idea of major reform disappeared into the social policy black hole of the 1980s defined by the prevailing ideological emphasis on market competition (see Brown 1983; Feder et al. 1981; Starr and Marmor 1984).

Now, in the 1990s, the issue of comprehensive reform is with us again. If all we are interested in is the nature of agenda change, then explaining the political rise and decline of the idea of health care reform is well within our grasp. If, however, we want to answer the tougher question posed by the woman from Canistota and determine why in the past enactment has not followed deliberation and then assess whether the 1990s and Clinton's administration will yield a different outcome, the task is far more vexing. There are three possible approaches. The first is to make a comparative analysis across nations, recognizing that other economically advanced democracies have implemented systematic reforms of their health financing systems, sometimes after political struggles that would sound familiar to U.S. reform advocates (note in particular the Canadian case—see Kudrle and Marmor 1981; Taylor 1987). The comparative approach is valuable, indeed essential, but of necessity it highlights what is exceptional about America, including the unique institutional design of the U.S. government (see Immergut 1990, 1992; Wilsford 1991). We can use comparative analysis to generate convincing explanations for why the outcomes of reform debates in the U.S. have in the past been so different from those of most other societies, but we cannot use it to estimate the evolving probability of enacting reform *given* the generic design of the U.S. government and political system.

The second approach is also comparative. It finds the common ground in the many policy domains that figure in the politics of change in America and draws attention to fundamental reforms that have been both deliberated and executed in this country, such as the creation of the Federal Reserve and the establishment of Social Security. Such comparisons furnish invaluable guidance for explorations of health care politics, but because policy outcomes are influenced by the characteristics of the individual policy domains to which they belong and the substantive issues involved, cross-policy investigations may not furnish much insight into the prospects of health care reform. Few, if any, changes in other policy areas match the scope and significance of a truly comprehensive reform of the now $840 billion health care system (approximately the size of Great Britain's entire economy).

The third approach focuses on the United States and health care policy and emphasizes the attributes of the health policy domain that are both subject to variation and likely to be of consequence to governmental decisions about comprehensive health care reform. The import of these attributes derives from the ways in which they motivate the national policymaking process in the U.S., both individually and in interaction with one another. They provide a framework for assessing the health care debate and the likelihood that President Clinton will prove any more successful as a health care reformer than his predecessors. This is the approach that I adopt in this article.

I review first the politics of health care reform, that is, conditions in the health care system and the role of the public. There is some observable link, however tenuous, between the policy process and conditions confronting society, or more precisely, between policy and the perception that conditions have become problems deserving a collective response. The recognition of conditions as problems depends on how clear they are, how they are interpreted by mediating leaders and institutions, and the breadth and intensity of their impact on the public. But policy proposals and debates about their merits must always refer to objective conditions (see Hall 1986; Heclo 1974; Kingdon 1984).

The public, in expressing its values and opinions, as well as in the actions it takes (or fails to take) as an electorate—determining who has government authority, which partisan coalition is advantaged, whether government is unified or divided—plays a crucial role in framing the constraints on the policy process and the opportunities for substantial policy change. The problems it is responding to may be real or imagined, and political and economic elites may influence its perceptions, but major policy change is unlikely in the face of public opposition or, at least, without its acquiescence. Public sentiment can overpower private interests when its desire for change is unambiguous, when it is clear which policy alternative the public will accept, and when elected officials realize that the issue will affect votes (or when they are voted out of office) (see Bachrach and Baratz 1962; Jacobs 1992; Kingdon 1984, 1989; Marmor 1973; Morone 1990; Page and Shapiro 1992).

After my review of the politics of reform, I turn to institutional structure. I assess changes in the institutional features of the health policy process that potentially turn politics into policy by defining the setting in which ideas are promoted or blocked, options deliberated, first-order decisions made, and cues to other decision makers formulated. My concern is the evolution of the health care reform policy community. It comprises the "representational community" of organized interests and members of the executive and legislative branches of government who turn proposals into policy or orchestrate vetoes of them. As in any policy domain where the public is concerned, the various members of this policy community seek to influence elected officials by stimulating public opinion and action and interpreting the public's positions to their own advantage. They also generate and share information. Of perhaps greater importance, however, is the character of the representational community: it determines which interests project an effective voice and which do not and affects which ideas and perspectives get emphasized in public debate and so gain the most currency among government officials. The way government is organized determines the vitality of the status quo in the face of innovation, shapes the access of private interests to public authority, and establishes the number and availability of "veto points" (see, for example, Gais et al. 1984; Hammond and Miller 1987; Heclo 1978; Katzenstein 1978; March and Olsen 1989; McCool 1990; Immergut 1990; Johnson 1992; Peterson 1990a, 1990b; Skocpol 1992; Walker 1991a; Weir 1992). Previous policy iterations and the outcomes they produce also affect the process. They redistribute the political influence of private interests, reformulate partisan coalitions, transform relationships among institutions, and alter the government's administrative capacity (see Hall 1986; Heclo 1974; Morone 1990; Skocpol 1992; Skowronek 1982; Starr 1982; Weir 1992).

I propose that by the 1990s politics and structure were radically changed. What is especially significant for the prospects of reform—and the success of President Clinton's agenda in particular—is the transformation of the health care reform policy community from an "iron triangle" to a policy "network." The iron triangle was an autonomous policy community, built on close relations between powerful private interests and an oligarchically organized Congress, which organized medicine and its allies could and did thoroughly dominate. The triangle has yielded to a far more diverse and open system, in which a reform coalition has the opportunity to prevail, especially under the direction of an activist president. Serious challenges certainly remain, but never before have the opportunities for reform been as ripe, even during the 1970s, when the hopes of reform advocates last ran high.

Politics

Politics is the process by which a society converts its values into policy. Those values are related to the distribution of resources among society's members. However, since the availability of resources is rarely a static phenomenon, politics is an ever-evolving process of perceptions, decisions, and adjustments: the conditions that underlie a particular policy area are crucial to the process, as are the public's interpretation of those conditions and its response to them.

Objective Conditions

John Kingdon (1984) in his study of the agenda-setting process is careful to note the difference between conditions and problems. Although even large populations may be disadvantaged, their conditions may not be viewed by the public or by policymakers as problems requiring attention (pp. 115–19). Select elites may even possess enough clout to keep specific problems out of the public domain (Bachrach and Baratz 1962). Conditions alone do not an agenda process make. But objective conditions are a necessary precursor to subjective evaluations of them, which in turn must precede the elevation of conditions to the status of problems inviting attention.

There are myriad objective conditions that could be used to characterize the American health care system at any given point in time. With respect to financing medical services, four broad classes of conditions are of particular importance: access to care, the overall cost of delivering health care services, the allocation of financial resources among services and between services and administration, and the administrative burden imposed on providers and patients.[2] Each condition has a status of its own, but they relate to one another in important ways.

Access to Care. Access to care is frequently discussed in the context of the numbers of people without either private insurance coverage or eligibility for government programs like Medicare and Medicaid. Those lacking insurance, however, may actually obtain care, although usually in the most expensive settings (emergency rooms) and once their ailments have been seriously aggravated (see Pepper Commission 1990; Long and Rodgers 1989; Spolar 1991). There is also recent evidence that the uninsured, even when treated, are cared for less effectively and are more likely to die than those with private or public insurance (Hadley et al. 1991).

The access problem is as old as the reform debate itself, but because today the U.S. stands with South Africa as the only industrialized nations not to guarantee access to care, it remains the most embarrassing condition of its health care system. Early in the century, when the cause of

---

2. The quality of care is obviously of central concern, too, and can be affected by the way in which health care services are financed. Because quality of care in the aggregate is not typically cited as a problem with the U.S. health care system and there is not an intrinsic relationship between quality and the financing system (all reform plans seek to address it), I am not including the issue of quality in this discussion of conditions.

compulsory health insurance was championed by the Progressive movement, sickness benefits of any kind covered a mere fraction of the population and only the wealthy could be sure of access to the available healing arts (Starr 1982: 242). The idea of social insurance was relatively new even in Europe. Access, defined as possession of insurance benefits, was not yet a norm, violations of which would constitute a recognized social problem. Even by the end of World War II, only 32 million Americans (less than a quarter of the population) were protected by private insurance (Health Insurance Association of America 1990: 23).

By the 1970s, following the rapid diffusion of employment-based insurance in the postwar period and the introduction of large-scale public programs for the elderly and limited categories of the poor in 1965, the access issue had been fully transformed. The vast majority of people possessed either private or public coverage, and the enrolled population grew as a percentage of the population as a whole, so attention was directed at the shrinking minority who continued to fall outside the access standard, as it was now defined.

In some respects, the access issue is similar in the 1990s. Eighty-five percent of U.S. residents have some kind of insurance protection at any given time, although the percentage of uninsured ranges widely by state, from 8 percent to 26 percent (U.S. General Accounting Office 1991a). Most individuals under sixty-five years old possess private insurance, 70 percent through plans offered by their employers (Congressional Budget Office 1991a: 69). But this progress in enrollment is being reversed. The number and percentage of uninsured individuals under sixty-five (of whom 29 percent are children and 54 percent are full-time employed heads of household or their dependents) have actually increased to the highest levels since 1965 (Foley 1991: 7–8; Pear 1991; Pepper Commission 1990: 22–23). Coverage on paper also no longer necessarily yields coverage in fact.

The reasons for the decline in insurance protection are legion. Responding to everything from the financial pressures of new diseases like AIDS to competitive sales incentives, the private insurance market is unravelling (Stone 1990). Some individuals and families with private insurance are discovering that their insurance benefits are inadequate to protect them against financial ruin in the face of medical catastrophe (Meier 1992). The increasing use of medical underwriting by private insurance companies, excluding those with preexisting medical conditions from coverage, has left myriad individuals without any alternative and has begun to expel the unhealthy from the health insurance market (Kolata 1992). The spread of the HIV virus and the potential for predicting an individual's health through genetic coding will only exacerbate these trends. In addition, employers have been cutting back in their coverage of dependents and, even, of employees and have been supported by the courts in doing so (Freudenheim 1992a). Finally, more physicians are dropping Medicare patients, particularly after the recent implementation of physician payment reform (Freudenheim 1992b).

Cost of the Delivery System. Costs are always a relative matter (and are variously defined; see Marmor et al. 1983). As long as income—personal and national—is on the rise and budgets are flush, a modest escalation in costs can be absorbed without much difficulty or complaint. By the 1970s, however, medical inflation began to hurt both businesses and individuals, with costs rising to almost 10 percent of personal consumption (*Economic Report of the President* 1992: 312; see also Wing 1985–86). The U.S. economy was plagued by the new phenomenon of "stagflation" (high rates of inflation along with slow economic growth and an elevated level of unemployment), expanding federal budget deficits were becoming the norm, and health care costs were outstripping the consumer price index (CPI), often substantially (*Economic Report of the President* 1992: 363; see Marmor et al. 1990: chap. 6).

Despite the considerable attention escalating health care costs received in the 1970s, their impact on policy deliberations was softened by three factors. First, the inflation in the economy and in health costs, in particular, were relatively recent developments. Policymakers could not predict their future course and did not know enough about the full range of mechanisms that could be used to control medical costs. Second, the policies that had been tried, mostly to foster better market incentives—higher cost sharing by patients and expanded availability of managed care, for example—had yet to demonstrate their inadequacy. Third, international comparisons were less illuminating. Throughout most of the 1970s other industrial nations also saw the percentage of their gross domestic product (GDP) committed to health care grow, and while the percentage of GDP spent by the U.S. on health care was consistently higher than that of other countries, the U.S. was not an obvious outlier (the percentage of GDP devoted to health care in the U.S. was less than 10 percent higher than the next highest country, and that difference was arguably the result of more advanced care).

In the 1990s much has changed. Even though the recession of the early 1980s eliminated most of the inflationary pressures in the economy, medical inflation continues to spiral, at 12 percent or more a year, threatening the viability of personal, business, and government budgets (Congressional Budget Office 1991a: 3, 46; Greenhouse 1992; King and Rimkunas 1991: 5; Pear 1993; Rich 1991). The elderly now see a larger percentage of their after-tax income go to health care than before the implementation of Medicare (Rich 1992). Current international comparisons are also far starker. During the 1980s, other industrialized societies implemented far more effective policies and tamed the escalation of their health care costs, leaving the United States the incontrovertible outlier among nations in the world, spending approximately 40 percent more of its GDP on health care than any other nation (Graig 1991: 25–27). The lessons from abroad have also become harder to ignore. By 1971, Canada, in many respects the nation most culturally and demographically similar to the U.S., had consolidated its experiment with a fully implemented single-payer system. During the 1970s, Canada's national insurance program was not yet a useful point of comparison (see Marmor and Mashaw 1990: 19–20; Marmor et al. 1990: chap. 6; Evans 1984). Today, the Canadian health care system (reinforced by the experiences of other nations) offers an example of a financing mechanism that, while ensuring universal access, is far less costly than the U.S. system, and dramatically highlights the excessive administrative costs of the U.S. system (U.S. General Accounting Office 1991b). More than nine out of ten Canadians view their less expensive system as superior to the one in the U.S., even in light of their system's own problems (Blendon et al. 1991). There is no "right" amount of a nation's resources to be devoted to health care delivery, but far more clearly than before, the international arena in the 1990s—where universal access is the norm—reveals the deficiencies of the U.S. health care financing system. The disparities between us and them and the fact that health care is predicted to absorb increasing shares of our national income receive extensive coverage in the mass media.

Allocation of Resources. During times of plenty and when access is unrestricted, it is far less disconcerting if health care resources are misallocated. There are more political dilemmas when costs are growing, budgets fall increasingly into deficit, and a significant portion of the public goes without private or public coverage. In the early 1990s, with costs seemingly out of control and the very integrity of federal and state budgets threatened by massive growth in Medicare and Medicaid expenditures (in 1991, federal expenditures for these programs grew by 13.9 percent and 31.6 percent, respectively—Rovner 1993: 28), two types of misallocation have begun to draw more notice than ever before. First, while all complex health care delivery and financing systems require an expensive administrative apparatus, the General Accounting Office estimates that the United States spends $67 billion more in administrative costs on its current system than it would with a single-payer system; others suggest that the figure may be markedly higher (U.S. General Accounting Office 1991b; Woolhandler and Himmelstein 1991). Second, the development of increasingly expensive high-technology medical procedures raises questions about the allocation of resources among services. So do recent studies revealing that 30 percent of the treatments patients receive may be ineffective or worse and that the use of particular surgical procedures varies widely and does not correlate with actual differences in medical conditions (Callahan 1990; Brook and Vaiana 1989).

Administrative Burden. Under the current system of multiple payers and fee-for-service reimbursements, lacking overall expenditure budgets, all-payer rate regulation, or managed competition, the individual payer has few options in holding down costs. The payer, whether government or a private insurance company, has to conduct case-by-case utilization reviews and deny some reimbursements. Because payers are so numerous and do not adhere to a single standard for claims processing, and because individual treatment episodes are often financed by multiple forms of coverage, the paperwork associated with paying provider bills is often overwhelming. Both aspects of administering the financing of American health care impose tremendous burdens on patients and providers alike, a situation aggravated as escalating costs increase the pressure to scrutinize each medical decision.

Among these deteriorating conditions, cost has become paramount, both for its own sake and because it affects all the others: access, resource allocation, and administrative burden. The increasing cost of health care delivery forces previously covered individuals from the insurance market, dissipates the slack capacity with which misallocation of resources can be tolerated, and leads to a Byzantine and onerous regulatory regime.

Public Values and Attitudes

The American public has historically been suspicious of government involvement in most activities, and that skepticism, encouraged by the American Medical Association and other advocates of private and voluntary approaches, has motivated its attitudes and actions (its voting patterns, for example) with respect to public policy in the health field (see Campion 1984; Morone 1990). In the past, the public has been troubled to see millions of fellow citizens go without proper insurance coverage, and most Americans endorsed the concept of Medicare (see Jacobs 1992: 194), but even in the 1970s that altruistic impulse was not sufficient to overcome serious reservations about the suitability and practicality of significant government action and to send elected officials a clear message that reform would be encouraged.

Twenty additional years of unrelenting growth in the cost of health care have not shaken the public's generic contempt for government (see Fuchs 1991: 14), but it has recast the health care debate, especially among the crucial middle class (Starr 1991; see also Knox 1992a; Matthiessen 1990; Rich 1991). Worries about continued access to care, today or in the near future, and frustration over the mounting administrative hassles generated by the current financing system, have made people rethink private health insurance and the role of government in this domain. Middle-class individuals, protected by employer-provided insurance in the past, now find themselves losing benefits and subject to "job lock," that is, being unable to change jobs, for fear they will lose insurance. As Rashi Fein notes, "People with insurance want change because *they* are hurting" (Fein 1992: 158). Surveys and focus groups conducted by the American Association of Retired Persons (AARP) captured the public's view of insurance companies as the embodiment of "efficient greed," while the government represented "bumbling benevolence"; with one pitted against the other, it preferred bumbling benevolence.[3] As Robert Blendon testified before the Senate Finance Committee in 1991, we have reached a forty-year high in the level of public support for major government involvement in health care financing (see Blendon and Donelan 1991).

What kind of federal action would be appropriate, however, is far from settled in the minds of most U.S. citizens. Although large majorities agree that fundamental change is required, about as many, for example, favor employer-mandates as favor government as a single payer (*Health Cares* 1992: 85). Some surveys do show that an increasing proportion of the public, up to 66 percent in 1990, express a preference for the Canadian

---

3. Based on conversations with AARP lobbyists. See Daniel Yankelovich Group, Inc. 1990. Note, too, that the public misperceives the efficiency of the private market. Administrative overhead for private insurance is far higher than for government programs. Figures reported by the General Accounting Office show that overhead accounts for 12 percent of private insurance costs, but only 3 percent of Medicare's and 1 percent of Canada's provincial programs.

system, even among high-income groups (Blendon et al. 1990: 187; Blendon et al. 1991: 172). Most polls, however, portray a public that is thus far unwilling to commit many additional tax dollars to financing major reform (see Blendon and Donelan 1991). That might be changing. The AARP's most recent studies suggest that in the area of long-term care, when respondents are told the actual trade-offs of different courses of action, people support government involvement and are willing to pay for it, as long as the revenues are earmarked for the program (Daniel Yankelovich Group, Inc. 1990).

These public attitudes toward health care represent significant departures from the 1970s. They found vivid expression in Senator Wofford's 1991 election, where people were "voting their fears" (Fein 1992: 158; see James and Blendon 1991; Petts 1991; Turner 1992) and in the support that Bill Clinton received in 1992 (67 percent versus 19 percent for President Bush) from the significant proportion of voters ranking health care reform as one of the most important problems facing the country (Pertman 1992). For the most influential segment of the voting public, the debate has thus been transformed from one of altruism to the far more powerful motivation of self-interest. The very fact that they have not settled on a preferred solution gives President Clinton and other reform proponents room for maneuver and an opportunity to bring the public to their side.

Structure

Changes in conditions and public attitudes, even if they affect elections, do not have a direct bearing on the course of public policy, especially if the public is not decided on which direction policy should go (see Jacobs 1992). Conditions become perceived as problems, problems attract attention, and popular sentiment motivates adjustments in policy only through mediating institutions, which are, additionally, players in their own right (see March and Olsen 1989). We can demonstrate that health care conditions are conducive to major policy change and that widespread perception of health care problems indicates that the public is ready to engage a serious political discourse on possible solutions, but this is only part of the story. If representational institutions, such as interest groups, reflect primarily the perspectives of those with the most to lose from adjustments in the status quo and if the structure of governmental institutions leaves them dominated by those very interests, no amount of variation in "politics" will result in policy innovation that is more than symbolic, except under extraordinary circumstances (such as a distinct electoral mandate from the public when the government is unified by a strong political party). The second and central part of my story, however, is that as the politics has changed, so has the health policy domain, with respect to both the representation of interests and their access to policymakers. The result is an entirely new type of policy community.

The Health Representational Community

A representational community comprises the organized interests in a particular policy domain. At any given time, one or both of two types of interests may be represented within a policy community: first, the "stakeholders," the interests that benefit by the status quo, or at least are more threatened by revisions in it; second, the "stake-challengers," the interests that want to change the status quo because they either do not benefit from it or are actually harmed by it.

Representational communities vary, both over time and across policy domains, according to the characteristics of these organizational representatives. Stakeholders, for example, may agree on the optimal public policy, creating the conditions for a strong alliance, or they may be divided enough to engender a competitive environment. Stake-challengers may be an effective presence in the representational community, able to compete against the stakeholders' interests, or they may be absent or ineffective.

This simplified view of the variegated world of interests is summarized in Table 1. The different attributes of stakeholders and stake-challengers combine to produce four distinct kinds of representational communities. When stakeholders are allied and stake-challengers are not effectively present, the community is homogeneous and one can label it a *block*. If stake-challengers remain absent but the stakeholders are competitive with one another, the community is made complex, revealing a less uniform and cohesive *amalgam* of interests. On the other hand, effectively organized stake-challengers confronting allied stakeholders creates a polarized community, a *dyad* of opposed coalitions. Finally, where stakeholders are competitive with one another and stake-challengers are vigorous, the community is heterogeneous and loosely structured, creating a *network* whose broad boundaries are defined by the shared attentiveness of participants to the same issues in the policy domain.[4]

---

4. This typology, of course, is a major simplification of reality. For example, current stakeholders might eventually lapse into open conflict, losing all cohesiveness. Further, when stake-

Table 1 Types of Representational Communities

	Stake-Challengers Present	
Characteristics of Stakeholders	No	Yes
Allied	Block	Dyad
	(Homogeneous)	(Polarized)
Competitive	Amalgam	Network
	(Differentiated)	(Heterogeneous)

In most policy domains, representational communities typically begin as blocks, with allied stakeholders unencumbered by stake-challengers. Business interests, for example, organize to secure government protection in certain markets or in response to unwanted government intervention (see Stigler 1971). Membership associations formed early in the development of a policy domain traditionally organize around occupational categories, which may not yet be prone to the kind of specialization that would stimulate meaningful competition over the definition of interests (see McConnell 1966). The interests most readily organized are those for whom the costs (or benefits) they incur from government action are concentrated and thus easily recognized (Wilson 1973: chap. 16). The consequences of government action are often significant enough for an individual stakeholder to attempt political influence on its own, if necessary. The interests of stake-challengers, however, are generally more diffuse and thus less likely to prompt mobilization. An individual stake-challenger cannot justify unitary action, and organized representation is achieved only if barriers to collective action are overcome (Olson 1965; see Walker 1991a: chap. 3).

Early in this century, the health care domain was a block-style representational community. Stakeholders were represented by large peak associations, such as the American Medical Association (formed in 1847) and the American Hospital Association (1898). The numbers of stakeholder organizations began to grow as the medical community grew more specialized (with the foundation of the American College of Surgeons in 1913, the American College of Physicians in 1915, and the American Academy of Family Physicians in 1947); the health insurance industry

---

challengers are effectively present, it makes a difference whether they are competitive with one another and whether a single policy advocacy group emerges with the influence and recognition necessary to lead a cohesive coalition against stakeholders, such as the labor movement can do in European settings.

emerged as a major player; and, after World War II, business became the major purchaser of health insurance. All these stakeholders held very similar views of optimal government policy: Government should protect their interests, including favorable tax policy but not intervene in the delivery and financing of health care (see Starr 1982; for later periods, see Wilsford 1991).

Representational communities, however, are rarely static. Fluctuations in the larger political environment, such as the emergence of patrons of political action supporting underrepresented constituencies, can foster new opportunities for stake-challengers to organize (Walker 1991a: 48–51). By the mid-1970s, business interests were finding themselves increasingly challenged by environmental, consumer, civil rights, and women's groups, creating a redefined polarization in many policy domains (Schlozman and Tierney 1986; Walker 1991a). In the case of health care reform, it was with the battles over Medicare in the 1960s and the return of health care reform to the nation's agenda in the 1970s that the stakeholder alliance began to be confronted by a more forceful and expansive set of stake-challengers. Some organizations had always been advocates of reform (the National Farmers Union, Americans for Democratic Action, and the AFL-CIO, for example), but the 1970s witnessed the development of a broader-based reform coalition. Nevertheless, the close alliance of the stakeholders and the relative weakness and inexperience of the emergent stake-challenger organizations helped to reinforce the political influence of the old powers (see Alford 1975; Wilsford 1991).

The 1990s, Challenges to the Stakeholder Alliance, and the Special Role of Business. The period since the last reform debate has brought new pressures to bear on the alliance of stakeholders (for an analysis of similar patterns at the state level, see Imershein et al. 1992). Changes in health care conditions have compelled all of them to recognize the utility of reform and, in some cases, to lead the call for innovation. Even the American Medical Association now views the status quo as unacceptable and has offered a plan for improving access and holding down costs. In this spirit, in May 1991, it devoted one issue of all of its publications to consideration of reform needs and options.

However, even though the provider community as a whole recognizes the need for reform, it has lost its cohesiveness and its capacity to dominate health care politics and the course of policy change (Morone 1990: chap. 7). The previously stalwart AMA no longer enjoys autonomy in medical decision making or a political monopoly within the community of practitioners (Morone 1990; see also Campion 1984; Brown 1979). The American College of Physicians and the American Academy of Family Physicians, for example, appear prepared to accept more dramatic reform and government promotion of change than the AMA (see Greenberg et al. 1990; Ginsburg and Prout 1990). The American Hospital Association is split by rifts between the nonprofit and for-profit sectors.

On the purchaser side, the constituency of the Health Insurance Association of America (HIAA) pursues increasingly incompatible interests. Reacting to the gathering momentum of reform, the trade association itself announced at the end of 1992 its support for mandated universal health coverage with a standard benefits package and uniform reimbursement rates (Pear 1992c). This plan, however, is unacceptable to many in the HIAA membership, which is sharply divided between the small firms who profit from the current insurance market distortions, on the one hand, and Blue Cross/Blue Shield and other large carriers, who are more accepting of increased market regulation, on the other, as well as among the large companies, according to their level of participation in the managed care business.

Reflecting this factionalization of the old medical/insurance/business alliance, more and more people and groups with stakes in health care policy have in recent years organized and financed their own lobbies in Washington (Pear 1992a). They are expressing divergent messages. The Louis Harris survey (1991: 35) of stakeholders, commissioned by the Metropolitan Life Insurance Company, exposes some of these differences, such as the 67 percent of major insurers who want to maintain an insurance system offering numerous plans and benefit packages, contending with the 55 percent of hospital CEOs who prefer limiting the set of available policies.

Perhaps more important, however, are the gathering tensions between providers and carriers on one side and the business consumers of health insurance coverage on the other. As long as the cost of providing health benefits remained stable and predictable and insurance practices were not exclusionary, many businesses benefited from collective bargaining with labor by offering extensive health care coverage and saw little reason to disrupt the status quo. Government intervention in the financing of health care was anathema. When conditions changed, however, the commercial and political calculations of some employers had to adjust as well (see McLaughlin 1991). Around 1975, in the midst of the last reform debate, businesses providing health care coverage to employees began to witness steep inclines in premium payments (U.S. Congress 1978: 56).

During the 1980s, much of business's invigorated participation in health care politics occurred at the state level, as represented by the explosion in the number of business coalitions in just a few years. A primary objective of these coalitions, often working in collaboration with state government, was to control costs by enhancing market forces in the private sector, such as increased reliance on health maintenance organizations and other managed care schemes. This strategy required challenging the autonomy of physicians and hospitals (Bergthold 1987). So too at the national level. Willis Goldbeck, then executive director of the Washington Business Group on Health, stated that "our biggest job is . . . to *break business away* from the *providers*" (quoted in Bergthold 1987: 11; emphasis in the original).

The original concerns of the 1970s have sprouted into full-scale alarm in the 1990s, as costs have escalated, despite the range of competitive market approaches tried in the 1980s. Representatives of businesses large and small have brought their concerns to one congressional committee and subcommittee after another. Companies providing comprehensive insurance coverage for their employees watch as health care costs consume more than 50 percent of their pretax profits and place them at a competitive disadvantage. Insurance is completely unavailable to many smaller firms because of preexisting condition restrictions or skyrocketing premiums that can increase more than threefold in a three-year period, as one small business owner testified to the Senate Finance Committee on 9 April 1991 (see also Edwards et al. 1992). Most large companies and increasing numbers of smaller businesses are turning to self-insurance in an effort to cut costs and avoid state insurance mandates (Freudenheim 1992a). By 1991, 80 percent of both large and small employers reported their belief that the health care system required more than minor modifications in order to perform effectively; nearly a third of small employers agreed that "we need to completely rebuild it" (Edwards et al. 1992: 169).

None of these trends bodes well for the continuation of a mutually supportive, dominating stakeholder alliance among doctors, hospitals, insurance companies, and businesses in favor of maintaining the status quo (see Ginzberg 1990). Indeed, at the national level businesses are now joining in unusual coalitions: among themselves (e.g., the Alliance of Business for Cost Containment), with unions (e.g., the steelworkers and steel companies task force), and with consumer and other activist groups (e.g., the National Leadership Coalition for Health Care Reform) (Kosterlitz 1991: 66). If business interests were to reach consensus on policy, the impact could be dramatic. As Cathie Jo Martin notes, "When business is unified and clear about its interests, it usually gets what it wants" (Martin 1992: 196; see also Vogel 1989). But the business community is more typically diverse in its outlook and fragmented in organization (Bergthold 1987: 8; Martin 1992: 35). On the issue of health care, it is split along deep internal fault lines. Small businesses, represented by groups like the National Federation of Independent Business, will not accept any form of employer mandates, while the large firms already providing coverage for their employees are more sympathetic; half of them (almost twice the percentage of large firms) could support single-payer national health insurance (Edwards et al. 1992: 169). Whichever direction business ultimately pursues, it will no longer be part of a coherent opposition to change.

The 1990s and the Health Reform Representational Network. At the risk of oversimplifying a complex evolutionary process, one can describe the health care representational community as having traveled through three distinct stages of development. Until the 1940s and probably through the 1950s eras of reform debate, it conformed with the definition of a block community. The 1960s and 1970s saw it become more dyadic, as new stake-challenger groups increasingly polarized health care politics while stakeholders maintained their old alliance. The stresses produced by the 1980s and early 1990s have made the stakeholders more competitive with one another, while time and opportunity have increased the number and resilience of stake-challengers, creating a heterogeneous representational network (see Salisbury 1990).

This pattern of change in the health care representational community is consistent with the findings of Jack Walker's 1985 survey of national voluntary associations concerned about public policy (Walker 1991b). He found that even in 1985 fully 36 percent of national membership organizations in America indicated that they were "very interested" in federal involvement in health and human services; a total of 58 percent were at least "somewhat interested." Given the first- and second-order consequences of redesigning the health care financing system, a considerable percentage of these organizations is likely to have a significant interest in the issue of health care reform itself.[5]

5. Unfortunately, the most detailed question in the survey about health care includes health with other social services. This categorization casts a broad net, and captures a number of groups

Table 2 Changes in the Representational Community of Groups "Very Interested" in Health and Other Human Services (row percentages)

| Year by Which Group Was Founded | N | Sectors Represented | | | | |
		Profit	Mixed Profit/ Nonprofit	Nonprofit	Citizen	Union
1945	130	30%	3%	37%	19%	11%
1970	226	25%	4%	42%	22%	6%
1985	310	23%	6%	38%	28%	5%

Note. Percentages are rounded and may not sum to 100.
Source. Walker 1991b.

The surveys from the Walker study also furnish corroborating evidence about how and why the policy orientation of the organized interests concerned with health policy have changed and diversified over time.[6] One can begin by reviewing the distribution of groups according to the sectors they represent (see Walker 1991a: chaps. 3, 4) and assess differences in that distribution based on the periods during which the organizations were founded. Table 2 presents the percentage of groups within each sector that were founded by 1945 (when Truman was beginning his efforts to launch compulsory social health insurance), by 1970 (right before the last flurry over comprehensive reform was played out), and by 1985 (the year of the survey and the latest responses available before the start of the current reform debate). To the extent that the initial imperatives that prompted a group to organize continue to carry weight within the organization and the extent to which these organizational imperatives differ by era, one can identify meaningful changes in this representational community.

Of the groups formed by 1945, 30 percent represented the profit sector of the economy and included most physicians, for-profit facilities, pharmaceutical and insurance companies, and other non-health-related businesses. Another 37 percent derived from nonprofit enterprises, in-

that are also very interested in education, civil rights, and housing and urban policy, as well as other concerns (Walker 1991a: 72). One wishes the specific issue of health care reform had been addressed.

6. For a rigorous assessment of long-term change in the representational community, of course, one ideally requires comparable data collected from organized interests in the health domain from several points in time, and the inclusion of lobbying entities that do not have enrolled members, such as law firms, corporate public affairs offices, advocacy centers, and think tanks. Such data do not exist.

cluding public hospitals and schools of medicine and public health. Very few organizations represented memberships from both the profit and non-profit sectors. Less than a fifth were citizen groups, associations not organized according to occupational or professional backgrounds but rather around a particular cause. Labor unions, of course, were also present, although they are underrepresented in the data set, due to an especially poor response rate. As one progresses to groups organized by 1970 and then by the mid-1980s, the composition of the representative community shifts. Both profit-making enterprises and labor unions decline in their proportional significance, while the mixed profit-nonprofit organizations double and citizen groups increase by nearly 50 percent as a proportion of national voluntary associations very interested in health and human services. The current array of groups is quite different from what it was in the past. Almost all the unions (93 percent) and over half of the relevant profit sector organizations were founded by 1945 and, by 1970, 80 percent of today's profit and nonprofit sector associations were established. For citizen groups and mixed-sector organizations, on the other hand, four in ten arrived on the scene following 1970, and many of them were not founded until after the last round of reform debate. It is likely that if the survey had been done in 1990 instead of 1985, these trends would be reinforced.

This transformation of the representational community matters, of course, only if there are distinct differences among these various types of groups in how they view federal action in the health domain. As Table 3 shows, the overall set of groups that were active in 1985 shows a majority in favor of "much more" expenditure and provision of services by the federal government in health and human services, compared to the 1985 status quo. Only 40 percent of the groups organized before 1946 held the same position, compared to nearly two-thirds of those established since 1970. Far more important, however, are the shifts within certain sectors of groups and differences among types of groups. Support for the expansion of federal services is substantially higher among nonprofit sector groups founded since 1945 than those established earlier, a pattern repeated for the small number of mixed profit and nonprofit associations. These changes indicate a growing tension in the health domain between nonprofit enterprises, which include some providers, and profit-making providers and other businesses who remain (at least in the mid-1980s) far more antagonistic to government involvement. Here we see how the interest of the stakeholders has diversified—a trend that undoubtedly has

Table 3 Group Support for the Expansion of Federal Expenditures/
Services and Regulation in Health and Other Human Services, by Sector
and Founding Date

Sector Represented	Year by Which Group Was Founded	N	Percentage Favoring "Much More" Federal Expenditure or Service	N	Percentage Favoring "Much More or More" Federal Regulation
All	1945	106	40	100	43
	1970	189	51	171	43
	1985	260	53	229	45
Profit	1945	28	21	30	10
	1970	44	30	44	11
	1985	54	26	56	14
Mixed Profit/	1945	2	0	2	50
Nonprofit	1970	6	33	6	66
	1985	13	54	12	50
Nonprofit	1945	40	38	35	43
	1970	80	59	70	39
	1985	101	59	82	38
Citizen	1945	22	64	19	63
	1970	45	62	37	70
	1985	77	64	64	72

Source. Walker 1991b.

intensified in the 1990s (see also Heinz et al. 1990; Salisbury et al. 1987).

Citizen groups make up another essential element of the transformation of the representational community. No matter when they came into existence, the vast majority of them favor much more federal spending on health and human services and support increases in federal regulation, as measured against the 1985 status quo. They polarize the representational community. Two additional attributes of citizen groups contribute to their importance. First, the groups formed prior to 1946 include various associations promoting disease prevention and cures who traditionally have not been confrontational, unlike the organizations spawned in the 1960s and 1970s. Groups founded since 1970 are about twice as likely as their pre-1945 counterparts to be enmeshed in intense and regular conflict in their policy domain and to view the distinctions between the Democratic and Republican parties as being relevant to their concerns. Second, because of the emergence of supportive patrons of political action and new communications technologies, these later, cause-oriented organizations found it much easier to overcome collective action problems and grew dramatically in number compared to the other types of groups (see Schlozman and Tierney 1986: 74–82; Walker 1991a: 62–64). These new groups not only disagreed with the status quo favored by the stakeholder alliance, they actively challenged it in an effort to effect policy change (Walker 1991a: chap. 6; see Salisbury et al. 1987).

Access to Government Authority

The transformation of the health care representational community from a block to a network is only one half of the structural equation. If access to government officials, especially elected officials like members of Congress, were tightly restricted, then stakeholders could continue to dominate the influence structure, assuming they retained the capacity to cultivate a policy consensus among themselves. At the very least they could defeat challenges to their essential stakes in the status quo. But government itself, and thus the paths of access to U.S. government authority, changed in some ways as markedly as the representational community, albeit somewhat later. The most significant of these changes occurred in Congress, many of them beginning in the 1970s but not taking full root until after the health care reform debate of that decade had waned without bringing about reforms.

The General Transformation of Congress. In many respects, the Congress of the 1960s would have been recognizable to any congressional scholar or participant whose personal perspective dated back as far as World War I. By then, for example, the House had rebelled against the "Reed Rules" and their application by Reed's successor as Speaker, Joseph Cannon, ending the centralizing power of the Speaker of the House (Galloway 1969: 52–56). That paved the way for an institution dominated by baronial committee chairmen, selected on the basis of seniority on the committee (often favoring Southern Democrats from safe districts), who had a firm grasp of independent sources of influence. In the House in particular, the authority structure was as oligarchical as the external representational community was cohesive.

This convergence of the representational and governmental structures —one of consensual and largely unchallenged stakeholders and the other of baronial policymakers on Capitol Hill—allowed the relatively impregnable "iron triangle" policy communities to take over a variety of policy domains (see Gais et al. 1984; McConnell 1966; McCool 1990; for an alternate account, see Johnson 1992). The American Medical Association and its allies, in such a constricted policy community, could maintain control of the policy process and stymie efforts at state intervention, even if a single political party—typically the Democrats—maintained control of both the executive and legislative branches of government (see Immergut 1990).

By the late 1960s, congressional committee chairs had grown increasingly out of step with the other members of the House, whose ranks were significantly transformed, in particular by the elections of 1958 and 1964 (Bolling 1966). Starting in 1971, a series of reforms, manifest mostly in rule changes promoted by the Democratic Caucus, challenged the power and autonomy of the sitting committee chairs (see Ornstein 1975; Smith and Deering 1984). A few chairs were eventually actually deposed, but most of the reforms left chairs in place while dispersing their power to newly invigorated subcommittees. Under the new rules of procedure, implemented between 1971 and 1975, members could chair only one subcommittee, subcommittee chairs were to be elected by the full committee caucus, and every committee had to have standing subcommittees with permanent jurisdictions, their own staffs, and their own budgets. Professional staff resources expanded rapidly throughout Capitol Hill, in new institutional settings like the Congressional Budget Office (CBO) and the Office of Technology Assessment (OTA), on the committees and subcommittees reinforcing their independence, and in the members' personal offices, all of which enhanced the entrepreneurial spirit in Congress (Ornstein et al. 1987: 135–49; Malbin 1980; Price 1971). New "sunshine" provisions also opened previously closed-door meetings. The oligarchy had been changed into a remarkably decentralized institution. Some of the reforms of the 1970s and other procedural changes witnessed in the 1980s reinforced certain aspects of control of the House by party leaders (see Davidson 1992; Sinclair 1983; Smith 1989), but Congress as a whole generally became a more permeable and less manageable institution than ever before.[7]

Since in many policy domains, both representational communities and

7. The reforms of the 1970s had a much greater impact on the House than the Senate, largely because the Senate was already an extensively decentralized, if not atomistic, institution. For a discussion of the Senate in particular, and how it has become a more egalitarian and open institution, see Sinclair 1989.

congressional structure evolved, iron triangles had to give way to looser, less stable, less predictable, and more diverse patterns of interaction and decision, eventually yielding "policy networks" (Heclo [1978] uses the term "issue networks"; Walker [1981] discusses "knowledge communities"; see also McCool 1990 and Salisbury 1990). In this setting, policy deliberation and change occur in the context of fluctuating "advocacy coalitions," to use Sabatier's term—variable factions made up of both government officials and organized interests that may or may not have a partisan basis to them (Sabatier 1988). Significant events, such as major electoral shifts or crises, can alter the size, composition, and distribution of these coalitions (Jenkins-Smith et al. 1991).

Health Care Sites Then and Now. The first-order effects of these structural changes can be seen in the health policy domain by examining the four authorizing committees that have a jurisdictional claim over initiatives to reform the health care financing system: in the House, the Ways and Means Committee and the Energy and Commerce Committee (until recently called Interstate and Foreign Commerce); in the Senate, the Finance Committee and the Labor and Human Resources Committee (previously Labor and Public Welfare). Important contrasts are to be found in Congress before and after the congressional reforms of the seventies and between the Congress of the 1970s and the 1990s.

The committees of 1959, the first year of the Bobbs-Merrill *Congressional Staff Directory*, offer a point of departure. What we see is committee oligarchy. The Ways and Means Committee was chaired by Representative Wilbur Mills of Arkansas, who retained full control over the committee, its legislative jurisdiction, and its staff (see Manley 1970). The committee had no real subcommittees, so all issues had to be deliberated, marked up, and voted upon solely in full committee sessions under Mills's supervision. Because the Democrats on Ways and Means also served as the committee-on-committees for making Democratic committee assignments and because Ways and Means had a tradition of securing closed rules from the Rules Committee, Mills possessed unusual influence within the chamber. Health care reform built on the Social Security program or requiring federal revenues would have to go through the Ways and Means Committee, and Mills was deeply skeptical about such a major government health care financing program.

The situation in the Senate was similar. The Finance Committee, chaired by the archconservative Harry Byrd of Virginia, also had no standing subcommittees. And in both cases, although far more for Finance, the committee members voted more conservatively than their chambers as a whole (Ornstein et al. 1992: 206–11).[8] Both the Interstate and Foreign Commerce Committee in the House and the Labor and Public Welfare Committee in the Senate and their health-related subcommittees were also chaired by Southern Democrats, although the Labor Committee is the only one of the four overall to have an average voting record decidedly less conservative than its parent body and to have a chairman, Lister Hill of Alabama, identifiable as an "economic liberal" (Barone et al. 1977: 10).

Congress in the 1940s and 1950s (especially during periods of Republican control, 1947–48 and 1953–54) was not an institution whose committees took easily to major social programs in health. As powerful "veto points" accessible to the dominant interests of organized medicine and its allies, the committee system afforded the opponents of comprehensive reform a distinct structural advantage.

As the 1970s opened, the committees of Congress would hardly seem any more conducive than before to moving major health care reform legislation. Wilbur Mills remained at the helm of Ways and Means, and wily Russell Long, a Louisiana conservative, rose to chair the Finance Committee, still sans subcommittees. Only the House Interstate and Foreign Commerce Committee and Senate Labor Committee were more inviting. Each now had more liberal chairs (Harley Staggers and Harrison Williams, respectively) and health subcommittee chairs (Paul Rogers, less so, and Ted Kennedy).

Then the institutional reform revolution hit the House of Representatives. By 1975, Al Ullman (D-OR) had replaced Mills as chair of Ways and Means, giving its leadership post a more liberal cast. But other changes occurred as well. The committee was expanded from twenty-five to thirty-seven members, it lost its Democratic committee-on-committees responsibilities, and standing subcommittees with permanent jurisdictions, including health, were imposed upon it (the Senate's Finance Committee also created a Subcommittee on Health in 1973). Renewed debate over major health care reform bills in the 1970s came to a head just as the House committees, in particular, were grappling with the effects of significant institutional dislocations. In the meantime, the representational community was becoming polarized, with nascent stake-challengers confronting the still rather strong alliance among stakeholders in a govern-

8. This assessment of ideology is based on the percentage of times members supported the "conservative coalition" (the voting alignments of a majority of Southern Democrats joining a majority of Republicans against a majority of Northern Democrats) when it was present, with all the attendant problems associated with such measures.

mental setting experiencing considerable flux. Despite the arrival in 1977 of a Democratic president and the continuation of Democratic majorities in Congress, the majority party was divided and unable to bridge the unpredictable institutional fragmentation of Congress in the 1970s. Although committee barons no longer automatically stood in the way of reform, the changes also meant that congressional "whales" no longer existed with whom a president might possibly have negotiated successful coalitions. All the elements of this situation could be exploited by the still relatively united stakeholders against their less numerous and less endowed challengers.

So what is different in the 1990s? Congress remains a highly decentralized institution (Hook 1992). Nevertheless, there have been changes in the last decade and a half. First, committee and subcommittee structures, as well as most power relationships in the legislature, have stabilized. Second, if the 1970s was the decade of subcommittee government, the 1980s brought growth in the leadership's capacity to manage the floor proceedings in the House (Davidson 1988; Smith 1989). Third, the increase in staff has permitted a wider range of members to generate serious proposals for reform. Personal staffs have been responsible for crafting almost every major bill under consideration, even, for the most part, the Senate Democratic leadership plan.[9]

Finally, perhaps most importantly, unlike any time in the past, all of the relevant House and Senate committee and subcommittee chairs, as well as members of the Democratic leadership in each chamber, are committed to some version of comprehensive reform of the U.S. health care financing system, as are a number of their ranking Republican counterparts.[10] They are also individuals with either long or concentrated experience in the health domain: Senate Majority Leader George Mitchell, for example, has chaired the Health Subcommittee on Finance. Daniel Patrick Moynihan, the new chair of Finance, following Lloyd Bentsen's departure, has a long intellectual and practical association with social policy, as well as lengthy service on this committee. Jay Rockefeller, chair of the Finance Subcommittee on Medicare and Long-Term Care, recently led the U.S. Bipartisan Commission on Comprehensive Health Care (the Pepper Com-

9. The leadership initiative was produced by the personal staffs of Senators Mitchell, Riegle, and Rockefeller, working in cooperation with Kennedy's health policy staff from the Labor Committee.

10. The two Democratic leaders who have been the most cautious on the issue of reform are House Speaker Thomas Foley and Lloyd Bentsen, former chairman of the Senate Finance Committee. Foley, however, will go along with President Clinton's program and the appointment of Bentsen as secretary of Treasury removes him as a serious legislative barrier.

mission) and the National Commission on Children. Ted Kennedy now chairs the full Labor Committee and has abolished its health subcommittee (while retaining its staff as the health policy staff on the committee) so as to maximize his influence on health concerns. In the House, Dan Rostenkowski, former chair of the Health Subcommittee of Ways and Means, is now chair of Ways and Means. Pete Stark, current chair of its subcommittee, joined the health fold more recently, but with no lack of energy and immersion; in the summer of 1992, he accepted Majority Leader Dick Gephardt's charge to forge an interim Democratic consensus bill (Rovner 1992). Over on the Energy and Commerce Committee, the chair, John Dingell of Michigan, is both a supporter of national health insurance and a power to be reckoned with. Henry Waxman has chaired the Energy and Commerce's Health and Environment Subcommittee since 1979. All of these committee and party leaders have either authored their own bills for reforming the health care system or have been active participants in collective bill-writing efforts. Although as a party more reactive and less comprehensive in their approach, Republicans in both houses have sought to meet the Democratic challenge (see Peterson 1992b).

It would be difficult to identify any other period when so many members of Congress in pertinent leadership roles were as intimately associated with the health care reform issue, or when so many relatively junior members could be so involved. The structure of the prereform Congress would not have allowed these activities; the 1970s Congress had not stabilized enough to motivate them. At the same time, the huge influx of new members in 1993—110 in the House and 11 in the Senate, the highest turnover since 1948—may enable new coalitional strategies. The impact on the Ways and Means Committee is particularly pronounced, where 39 percent of its members from the 102d Congress—and over half the ranks of the Health Subcommittee—have departed due to retirement, seeking other offices, or defeat (including Marty Russo, the Democrat from Illinois, who was a major advocate of single-payer reform). Unless the infusion of new members sets in motion significant changes in the legislature's organization and procedures, Congress should not revisit the institutional turmoil of the 1970s. It is also possible that, on average, freshmen members of the House and Senate elected in the "anti-gridlock" atmosphere of 1992 may be more supportive than their predecessors were of both comprehensive health care reform and streamlining congressional procedures to facilitate action.

Moreover, neither the leaders nor new members face the same old dominating stakeholder alliance. Today, a broad spectrum of the representational community in the health domain enjoys similar levels of access to Congress, at least with respect to the number and quality of reported contacts. In the 1985 Walker survey (Walker 1991b), 49 percent of the profit sector groups very interested in health and other human services acknowledged communicating with five or more congressional subcommittees in the previous year, but so did 41 percent of both nonprofit sector organizations and citizen groups. A slightly higher percentage of citizen groups than for-profit organizations actually reported frequent contact with these subcommittees, 45 percent to 41 percent. Equal percentages revealed that these communications were "normally cooperative" (70 percent); only the nonprofits were higher, at 77 percent. About seven out of ten of all types of groups said that their interactions with congressional subcommittees were both frequent and normally cooperative. Organizations representing the profit sector differed from the others in only one respect: a mere 8 percent indicated that the switch of the Senate to Republican control after the 1980 election decreased the cooperation they received from Congress, compared to a quarter of the nonprofit sector groups and a third of the citizen associations. After the 1986 election returned Democratic majorities to the Senate (affecting relationships two years following the Walker survey), it is possible that citizen groups would now even show some advantage over the profit sector organizations, at least in the context of these measures.

These data and the changes that they reflect—a representational community of both competitive stakeholders and plentiful stake-challengers, a Congress decentralized and more open—indicate that in the health care realm the policy community has all it needs to be a policy network. There are no strict boundaries or barriers. The scope of the community is defined by a shared interest in the subject, but with divergent views, shared information and expertise, and competing stakes in the outcome of the policy process (for a detailed empirical assessment of the structure of health policy networks in the 1980s, see Laumann and Knoke 1987).

The Impact of Structural Change

We can now turn our attention to what impact these structural changes—which replace the iron triangle with a policy network—may have on the prospects for comprehensive health care reform in the 1990s, given concomitant shifts in politics and President Clinton's election. There are three hypotheses: first, that the transformations of the representational community and Congress are of little consequence; second, that they reduce the likelihood of reform; and third, that they create previously unavailable opportunities for enacting reform.

Hypothesis 1: The Structural Changes Are of Little Consequence. There are strong and weak versions of this hypothesis. Proponents of its strongest formulation would argue that my analysis has left out two of the most important political ingredients. One is campaign financing. Although stake-challengers enjoy some access to government, the stakeholders (by sector and collectively) channel huge sums of money through political action committees (PACs) toward precisely the most central players in Congress. In what might be dubbed the "Common Cause" hypothesis (more precisely, conclusion), major policy change will continue to be stymied by members of Congress who are directly or indirectly bought off by campaign contributions from the insurance industry and the medical community.

A second missing consideration is that the business community, erstwhile ally of organized medicine and the insurance companies, will not change. Employers large and small decry the current financing system and the cost increases it generates and their role in subsidizing care for the uninsured, but as a matter of ideology many will not accept the cost containment provisions most proponents of reform believe are necessary. Senate Democrats, for example, striving during 1992 to craft a consensus reform proposal acceptable to small businesses, grew frustrated by the National Federation of Independent Business and other groups when their representatives insisted on cost controls, but rejected all the mechanisms (enforceable budgets and price regulation) that they themselves agreed stood the best chance of working, because they saw it as government intrusion. In this context, business representatives cannot join in active support of any particular reform initiative and instead may thwart those presented by other participants. So the old politics lives on, only with new clothing.

Is this hypothesis persuasive? The effects of PAC money are certainly to be considered in any evaluation of the policy-making process. But there are counterarguments to be made. First, social science research has uncovered few instances or circumstances in which PAC contributions actually change congressional voting behavior, especially when policy issues are subject to extensive public debate (see, for example, Grenzke 1989; note, however, Hall and Wayman [1990], who argue that "moneyed interests" do influence the levels of legislative involvement by members). Second, contributions have influence mostly because of their capacity to strengthen campaigns for garnering votes. In the end, politicians are more concerned about votes than dollars. If the two are in conflict, the electorate can overcome well-financed "special" interests (but not necessarily—see Hall and Wayman 1990). For better or worse, the repeal of the Medicare Catastrophic Coverage Act in 1990 had more to do with fears of a block of antagonized voters than with campaign financing (Rutledge 1992). How this set of competing forces will break on the issue of comprehensive reform will depend in part on the clarity and robustness of the public's message to members of Congress and the president in the 1992 (and perhaps subsequent) elections.

The impact of business's philosophical intractability is more difficult to assess. If enacting comprehensive reform requires an active alliance of employers with stake-challengers, then the prospects of reform remain dim. But the fact that business interests themselves lack coherence and that the past alliance of business with other stakeholders is strongly challenged means that for the first time groups advocating change—and their collaborators in government—confront a far less influential coalition of opponents. The parameters of the 1990s are nothing like those of the 1940s and 1970s.

The weaker version of the hypothesis that structural change does not matter, articulated mostly "inside the beltway," is that comprehensive health care reform may be enacted, but the traditional patterns of influence will shape the reform policy to comport with the interests of the stakeholders, just as Medicare's Part A, for hospital care, and Part B, covering physician services, were crafted in ways perfectly compatible with the interests of hospitals and doctors, by preserving their traditional payment practices and autonomy. The political analysis offered by Henry Aaron (1991), an Urban Institute team (Holahan et al. 1991), Families USA (Pollock and Torda 1991), and the Senate Democratic leadership pay-or-play initiative all work on this hypothesis.[11] So does the latest strategy of the AFL-CIO and several of its member unions, promoting employer mandates instead of national health insurance as they had in the 1970s and earlier. Some would suggest that Clinton's embrace of managed competition reveals a similar strategy for achieving reform by avoiding direct attacks on the insurance industry and other interests perceived to be too powerful to defeat. In this scenario, reform can be achieved, but only if the interests of stakeholders—especially private insurance and medical

---

11. For a description of the process that led to the Democratic leadership initiative sponsored by Senators Mitchell, Kennedy, Riegle, and Rockefeller, see Peterson 1992b.

providers—are well accommodated in the reform. As one senior senator reportedly stated in private, 80 percent of the public would support a different kind of reform than pay-or-play employer mandates, but the other 20 percent have the political influence. Efforts to promote more extensive government involvement are doomed, it is argued, because of the continuing power of the stakeholders and the relative frailty of and lack of consensus among the stake-challengers.

This version of the hypothesis may be born out by subsequent events, but it, too, must be probed and debated. It ignores a few compelling features of the current reform debate. First, while most people respect their physicians, there is no love lost between the public and their insurance companies. Only 29 percent of the public believes health insurance offers good value for the money. Private insurance companies lead the public's list of suspects responsible for the high cost of medical care (Blendon et al. 1991: 172, 174). The increasingly prevalent insurance practices of experiential rating, medical underwriting, and termination of coverage for individuals once they get sick have raised suspicions further about the efficacy of private health insurance. Insurance interests have the weakest base among the public of all past stakeholders. Second, while a unified insurance industry with powerful friends might have the resources and influence to overwhelm any effects of such popular disdain, it is weakened by being deeply divided internally over acceptable strategies of reform. In addition, the whole alliance among stakeholders shows signs of severe strain, between representatives of the profit and nonprofit sectors and especially between business interests and the combination of insurers and providers. Employment-based plans may be especially vulnerable, particularly if opposed by small businesses, the firms most compromised by the imposition of any mandated health insurance coverage. They are numerous and scattered across every state and located in each House district.

Hypothesis 2: Structural Change Has Reduced the Likelihood of Reform. This hypothesis proposes the same conclusion as the strong variant of the first hypothesis, but for a quite different reason. It recognizes the dramatic shifts that have occurred in the representational community and the rearrangement of power in Congress. Both types of change, however, are viewed as contributing to the fragmentation of power and authority in the United States, making it nearly impossible to forge majorities on any policies of any consequence. To use Anthony King's terms, the American system has been "atomized," and as a result, leaders are reduced to "building coalitions in the sand" (King 1978). Samuel Kernell suggests that we have moved from a system of "institutionalized pluralism" to one of "individualized pluralism," destroying the stable building blocks necessary for coalition formation (Kernell 1986: 10–35). Recent reports about the rapid escalation in the number of lobbyists representing parochial interests in the health policy domain, each committed to protecting its own narrow slice of policy turf, may lend credence to this view (Pear 1992a). No wonder Congress has settled into a policy gridlock, given this fragmentation of authority, stimulating calls for the next generation of institutional reform (Hook 1992). And there is little President Clinton can do about it, according to proponents of this hypothesis, other than watch his initiative succumb to the death of a thousand cuts.

In this context, the decline of organized labor in the U.S. is especially significant (see Goldfield 1987). Labor—with its extensive and active national memberships in associated unions—customarily led the charge for comprehensive health care reform. But, while new potential partners have emerged among stake-challengers and the stakeholder alliance has degenerated, the labor union movement has suffered an organizational crisis. National union membership peaked in the early 1950s at around 25 percent of the entire labor force; today, after a precipitous drop in the 1980s, it is about 16 percent nationally (only 25 percent of manufacturing jobs) and well under half that in the South (Goldfield 1987: 10; U.S. Bureau of the Census 1991: 424–25). The AFL-CIO, viewed now by members of Congress as "just one more PAC," has not been able to claim a single legislative achievement among its priorities in four years (Sammon 1992: 1810).

During the present health care debate, labor's influence has been further eroded by divisions among the AFL-CIO's affiliated unions that prevent labor from extending its full endorsement to any particular reform plan (see Peterson 1992b). Activists in union locals may also have realized that because health care benefits have become so central to collective bargaining and represent such a signal achievement of the labor movement, an entirely publicly funded or even a mandated system of health care financing, whether or not guided by managed competition, might rob the union movement of its raison d'être during this period of evaporating union membership. As yet no other broad-based organization with a coherent reform plan has appeared to fill what was labor's role.

The fragmentation argument is worrisome, but it, too, ignores—or perhaps misinterprets—significant features of American politics. It identifies increasing numbers of actors with increasing numbers of interests and, thus, fragmentation. But there is a political structure lying below the numbers that can be exploited. There are "special" interests, to be sure, but substantial numbers of groups have common or at least over-lapping interests. Ideological and partisan fault lines cleave the interest group system just as they divide the electorate (Peterson 1992a; Walker 1991a: chaps. 2, 8). These divisions are certainly not European in their depth or consistency, but they provide one basis for coalition building that is available to President Clinton (Peterson 1992a). The more obvious the deficiencies in the health care financing system, the more public the debate over policy change; and the greater the media coverage, the more significant these cleavages become and the harder it is for parochial interests to achieve their objectives behind the scenes in what is now a far more open legislative process.

Hypothesis 3: Structural Change Has Introduced Previously Unavailable Opportunities for Reform. The institutional transformation of the representational community and Congress produces a challenge for any reform coalition, but as long as the structure of American politics and government lent enormous advantage to the original and often unified alliance of medicine, insurance, and business, reform was either impossible or almost entirely dictated by the long-established interests. This hypothesis is the optimistic one for reformers, because it suggests that the previous barriers to comprehensive change have been breached. That provides an opportunity, an opening, for reform where perhaps none ever existed before.

The health care reform policy community, now a policy network, is more complex than ever. Perhaps along the lines suggested by hypothesis 2, the reform effort will consequently collapse under its own weight, aided by the weakening of labor's influence and continuing confusion among the public. But in the current system, new ideas and new players have an entrée and, with them, so do previously unseen alignments of advocates for reform. Not only are leaders of the traditional type active in the reform campaign, but so too are far less senior members, like Jim McDermott in the House, and Tom Daschle, Bob Kerrey, Harris Wofford, and James Jeffords in the Senate (see Kerrey 1991; Peterson 1992b).[12] In combination with conditions in the health system that are increasingly difficult to ignore and the public's attraction to at least the notion

12. As the pool of serious participants expands and includes less senior members, there is also greater risk that influential proponents of reform will become the victims of electoral vagaries, such as occurred with the 1992 defeat of Representative Marty Russo, the result of redistricting, in the Illinois primary.

of major reform in the health care area, reform proponents may be able to cultivate enough cohesion in the policy network to obtain a workable majority in Congress. That is where Clinton's election becomes so important. Although even reformist Democrats have substantive disagreements among themselves, all turn to President Clinton to take the lead in mastering a coalition they each can join. They are more willing to compromise with him than with each other.

Entrepreneurs and Leaders

Ironically, the foremost threat to the reform agenda may be the effects of a "perceptual drag" evident in some of the most influential members of the reform coalition, from Senators Mitchell and Kennedy to, possibly, President Clinton (see Peterson 1992c). Just as military officers always find themselves fighting the last war, employing tactics and weapons suited for past campaigns, not the current one, policy leaders tend to fight the battle they just lost, not the one at hand. Originally philosophically linked to single-payer approaches to reform, Senator Kennedy and others, including the major labor unions, have aligned themselves behind the very employment-based schemes they had rejected years before. The reasons are clear and understandable. In the 1970s, national health insurance seemed within reach, but then the opportunity collapsed. Perhaps the advocates pushed too hard, the argument goes, and should have settled on the employment-based plan offered by President Nixon and others in the 1970s. The experiences of that decade, it is thought, proved the folly of bolder reform. President Clinton's submission of a complex employment-based plan, wrapped up in the rhetoric of health alliances and managed competition—all of which is intended to retain the image of a largely private, rather than government-dominated, system—is also consistent with this view. But this line of reasoning assumes that little has changed between the 1970s and 1990s, especially with respect to the coherence and influence of stakeholders, the character of stake-challengers, and the structure of Congress.

The 1990s are, in fact, distinctly different from the 1970s. Following the voluminous scholarship produced by health policy analysts, I have argued that both the health conditions the country faces and the public's attitude about reform have undergone major shifts, all favoring the prospects of reform. Even more importantly, the reform policy community has transformed itself from one of iron triangle entanglements that a unified antireform alliance of medicine, insurance, and business could use to defeat change into a more expansive and open policy network in which reform proponents, especially with presidential leadership, have an unprecedented opportunity to forge a winning coalition. Much of this change has been accomplished since the 1970s. (For assessments of the remaining barriers to reform and their significance, see Brown 1992; Marmor and Boyum 1992.)

Because coalitions and institutions do not act without direction, what actually happens as a result of these changes in politics and structure—whether reform is enacted or we replay once again the scenario of opportunity denied—will largely rest on the presence, skills, and strategies of three types of leaders (Peterson 1992c). First, there are the policy entrepreneurs, the authors and promoters of particular approaches to reform, who help define the issues of the debate. This leadership is well established and, in the process, those in Congress and elsewhere who are not health specialists are being educated about our problems and the possible solutions. Second, there are the *political* entrepreneurs, who help define perceptions of the political landscape. Their major responsibility is to persuade the major players to see clearly the circumstances of the 1990s and realize that they are indeed not a reprise of the 1970s or earlier configurations of politics and structure in the U.S. The newer players, untainted by the tempering experience of the 1970s, may have to be the ones to play this role. However, given the extent to which the single-payer alternative has disappeared from coverage in the media, despite explicit support for it from a third of the Democrats in the House of Representatives, and the Clinton administration's forthright rejection of a publicly financed plan, it appears that politics entrepreneurship continues to be dominated by those most fearful of the past and least imaginative about the possibilities of the present.

Finally, there are the major political leaders, those with the resources and influence to mobilize the broad coalitions necessary to enact legislation in a heterogeneous policy network and the larger legislative process. This role is typically borne by presidents. Truman tried, at least symbolically, in the 1940s. Johnson was there for Medicare in the 1960s. Nixon and Carter joined the effort, albeit reluctantly, in the 1970s. Other than LBJ, none enjoyed the overlapping of politics and structure that would permit or at least facilitate comprehensive reform. Such a favorable alignment of factors finally began to happen, however, during a period in which there was no mobilizing leadership from the president. President Bush tepidly offered his tax- and voucher-based plan to counter the Democrats only when political dynamics rendered his failure to participate untenable (President's Program 1992; *New York Times* 1992; Pear 1992b). After the introduction of his plan, he all but disappeared from the scene (Knox 1992b). With President Clinton ensconced in the White House, for the first time in the long history of comprehensive health care reform debates, major attributes of politics, structure, and leadership appear to have come together simultaneously. Clinton's program would probably be defeated if politics and structure had not changed—particularly if the reform policy community had not evolved—and the prospects of reform would be far more uncertain had Clinton not been elected. It is fair to conclude, therefore, that we are in the midst of the greatest test yet of the proposition that the United States lacks the capacity to secure a major reorientation of its health care financing system.

References

Aaron, Henry J. 1991. *Serious and Unstable Condition: Financing America's Health Care.* Washington, DC: Brookings Institution.

Alford, Robert R. 1975. *Health Care Politics: Ideological and Interest Group Barriers to Reform.* Chicago: University of Chicago Press.

Altmeyer, Arthur J. 1968. *The Formative Years of Social Security.* Madison: University of Wisconsin Press.

Bachrach, Peter, and Morton S. Baratz. 1962. The Two Faces of Power. *American Political Science Review* 56 (4): 947–52.

Barone, Michael, Grant Ujifusa, and Douglas Matthews. 1977. *The Almanac of American Politics, 1978.* New York: Dutton.

Bergthold, Linda A. 1987. Business and the Pushcart Vendors in an Age of Supermarkets. *International Journal of Health Services* 17:7–26.

Blendon, Robert J., and Karen Donelan. 1991. Public Opinion and Efforts to Reform the U.S. Health Care System: Continuing Issues of Cost-Containment and Access to Care. *Stanford Law and Policy Review* 3:146–54.

Blendon, Robert J., Jennifer N. Edwards, and Andrew L. Hyams. 1992. Making the Critical Choices. *Journal of the American Medical Association* 267 (18): 2509–20.

Blendon, Robert J., Jennifer N. Edwards, and Ulrike S. Szalay. 1991. The Health Insurance Industry in the Year 2001: One Scenario. *Health Affairs* 10 (4): 170–77.

Blendon, Robert J., Robert Leitman, Ian Morrison, and Karen Donelan. 1990. Satisfaction with Health Systems in Ten Nations. *Health Affairs* 9 (2): 185–92.

Bolling, Richard. 1966. *House out of Order.* New York: Dutton.

Brook, Robert H., and Mary E. Vaiana. 1989. *Appropriateness of Care: A Chart Book.* Report prepared for George Washington University, National Health Policy Forum. Washington, DC.

Brown, E. Richard. 1979. *Rockefeller Medicine Men: Medicine and Capitalism in America.* Berkeley and Los Angeles: University of California Press.

Brown, Lawrence D. 1983. *Politics and Health Care Organization: HMOs as Federal Policy.* Washington, DC: Brookings Institution.

———. 1992. Getting There: The Political Context for Implementing Health Care

Reform. In *Implementation Issues and National Health Care Reform*, ed. Charles Brecher. Washington, DC: Josiah Macy, Jr., Foundation.

Callahan, Daniel. 1990. *What Kind of Life: The Limits of Medical Progress*. New York: Simon and Schuster.

Campion, Frank D. 1984. *The AMA and U.S. Health Policy since 1940*. Chicago: Chicago Review Press.

Congressional Budget Office. 1991a. *Rising Health Care Costs: Causes, Implications, and Strategies*. Washington, DC: U.S. Government Printing Office.

———. 1991b. Trends in Health Expenditures by Medicare and the Nation. Washington, DC: Congressional Budget Office.

Congressional Quarterly Weekly Report. 1992. Congressional Departures, 1 August, p. 2299.

Congressional Staff Directory. 1959 and later editions. Indianapolis: Bobbs-Merrill.

Daniel Yankelovich Group, Inc. 1990. Long-Term Care in America: Public Attitudes and Possible Solutions. Executive Summary. Prepared for the American Association of Retired Persons, Washington, DC.

Davidson, Roger H., ed. 1988. The New Centralization on Capitol Hill. *Review of Politics* 50 (3): 345–64.

———, ed. 1992. *The Postreform Congress*. New York: St. Martin's.

Economic Report of the President. 1992. Washington, DC: U.S. Government Printing Office.

Edwards, Jennifer N., Robert J. Blendon, Robert Leitman, Ellen Morrison, Ian Morrison, and Humphrey Taylor. 1992. DataWatch: Small Business and the National Health Care Reform Debate. *Health Affairs* 11 (3): 164–73.

Evans, Robert G. 1984. *Strained Mercy: The Economics of Canadian Health Care*. Toronto: Butterworth.

Feder, Judith, Jack Hadley, and John Holahan. 1981. *Insuring the Nation's Health: Market Competition, Catastrophic, and Comprehensive Approaches*. Washington, DC: Urban Institute.

Fein, Rashi. 1992. National Health Insurance: Telling the Good from the Bad. *Dissent* 39 (2): 157–63.

Foley, Jill D. 1991. Uninsured in the United States: The Nonelderly Population without Health Insurance: Analysis of the March 1990 Current Population Survey. Washington, DC: Employee Benefit Research Institute.

Freudenheim, Milt. 1992a. Employers Winning Right to Cut Back Medical Insurance. *New York Times*, 29 March, pp. 1, 26.

———. 1992b. Doctors Dropping Medicare Patients. *New York Times*, 12 April, pp. 1, 26.

Fuchs, Victor R. 1991. National Health Insurance Revisited. *Health Affairs* 10 (4): 7–17.

Gais, Thomas L., Mark A. Peterson, and Jack L. Walker. 1984. Interest Groups, Iron Triangles, and Representative Institutions in American Government. *British Journal of Political Science* 14 (2): 161–85.

Galloway, George B. 1969. *History of the House of Representatives*. New York: Thomas Y. Crowell Company.

Ginsburg, Jack A., and Deborah M. Prout. 1990. Access to Health Care. *Annals of Internal Medicine* 112:641–61.

Ginzberg, Eli. 1990. *The Medical Triangle: Physicians, Politicians, and the Public.* Cambridge, MA: Harvard University Press.

Goldfield, Michael. 1987. *The Decline of Organized Labor in the United States.* Chicago: University of Chicago Press.

Graig, Laurene A. 1991. *Health of Nations: An International Perspective on U.S. Health Care Reform.* Washington, DC: Wyatt Company.

Greenberg, Norton J., Nicholas E. Davies, Edwin P. Maynard, Ralph O. Wallerstein, Eugene A. Hildreth, and Linda Hawes Clever. 1990. Universal Access to Health Care in America: A Moral and Medical Imperative. *Annals of Internal Medicine* 112:637–39.

Greenhouse, Steven. 1992. Wider U.S. Deficits Are Now Forecast for the Mid-1990s. *New York Times*, 23 March, pp. A1, D6.

Grenzke, Jane M. 1989. Shopping in the Congressional Supermarket: The Currency Is Complex. *American Journal of Political Science* 33 (1): 1–24.

Hadley, Jack, Earl P. Steinberg, and Judith Feder. 1991. Comparison of Uninsured and Privately Insured Hospital Patients: Conditions on Admission, Resource Use, and Outcomes. *Journal of the American Medical Association* 265 (3): 374–79.

Hall, Peter. 1986. *Governing the Economy: The Politics of State Intervention in Britain and France.* Oxford: Oxford University Press.

Hall, Richard L., and Frank W. Wayman. 1990. Buying Time: Moneyed Interests and the Mobilization of Bias in Congressional Committees. *American Political Science Review* 84:797–820.

Hammond, Thomas H., and Gary J. Miller. 1987. The Core of the Constitution. *American Political Science Review* 81:1155–1174.

Health Cares. 1992. *Public Opinion and Demographic Report*, March/April, pp. 85–89.

Health Insurance Association of America. 1990. *Source Book of Health Insurance Data.* Washington, DC: Health Insurance Association of America.

Heclo, Hugh. 1974. *Modern Social Politics in Britain and Sweden.* New Haven: Yale University Press.

———. 1978. Issue Networks and the Executive Establishment. In *The New American Political System*, ed. Anthony King. Washington, DC: American Enterprise Institute.

Heinz, John P., Edward O. Laumann, Robert H. Salisbury, and Robert L. Nelson. 1990. Inner Circles or Hollow Cores? Elite Networks in National Policy Systems. *Journal of Politics* 52 (2): 356–90.

Hirshfield, Daniel. 1970. *The Lost Reform.* Cambridge: Harvard University Press.

Holahan, John, Marylin Moon, W. Peter Welch, and Stephen Zucherman. 1991. *Balancing Access, Costs, and Politics: The American Context for Health System Reform.* Washington, DC: Urban Institute.

Hook, Janet. 1992. Extensive Reform Proposals Cook on the Front Burner. *Congressional Quarterly Weekly Report*, 6 June, pp. 1579–85.

Imershein, Allen W., Philip C. Rond III, and Mary P. Mathis. 1992. Restructuring

Patterns of Elite Dominance and the Formation of State Policy in Health Care. *American Journal of Sociology* 97 (4): 970–93.

Immergut, Ellen M. 1990. Institutions, Veto Points, and Policy Results: A Comparative Analysis of Health Care. *Journal of Public Policy* 10 (4): 391–416.

————. 1992. Institutions of the Welfare State and Professional Power: The Case of Health. Paper prepared for presentation at the Eighth International Conference of Europeanists, Chicago, IL, 27–29 March, and at the Center for European Studies, Harvard University, 27 April.

Jacobs, Lawrence R. 1992. Institutions and Culture: Health Policy and Public Opinion in the U.S. and Britain. *World Politics* 44 (2): 179–209.

James, Matt, and Robert J. Blendon. 1991. Poll Shows National Health Insurance as Pivotal Issue in Pennsylvania Race. Press release. Menlo Park, CA: Henry J. Kaiser Family Foundation.

Jenkins-Smith, Hank C., Gilbert K. St. Clair, and Brian Woods. 1991. Explaining Change in Policy Subsystems: Analysis of Coalition Stability and Defection over Time. *American Journal of Political Science* 35 (2): 851–80.

Johnson, Cathy M. 1992. *The Dynamics of Conflict between Bureaucrats and Legislators*. Armonk, NY: Sharpe.

Katzenstein, Peter J. 1978. Introduction: Domestic and International Forces and Strategies of Foreign Economic Policy. In *Between Power and Plenty: Foreign Economic Policies of Advanced Industrial States*, ed. Peter J. Katzenstein. Madison: University of Wisconsin Press.

Kernell, Samuel. 1986. *Going Public: New Strategies of Presidential Leadership*. Washington, DC: Congressional Quarterly Press.

Kerrey, Robert. 1991. Why America Will Adopt Comprehensive Health Care Reform. *American Prospect* 6 (Summer): 81–91.

King, Anthony. 1978. The American Polity in the Late 1970s: Building Coalitions in the Sand. In *The New American Political System*, ed. Anthony King. Washington, DC: American Enterprise Institute.

King, Kathleen M., and Richard V. Rimkunas. 1991. National Health Expenditures: Trends from 1960–1990. Congressional Research Service Report to Congress. 91-588 EPW. Washington, DC: Congressional Research Service.

Kingdon, John W. 1984. *Agendas, Alternatives, and Public Policies*. Boston: Little, Brown.

————. 1989. *Congressmen's Voting Decisions*. 3d ed. Ann Arbor: University of Michigan Press.

Knox, Richard A. 1992a. For Most, Top Fear Is Medical Bills. *Boston Globe*, 8 April, p. 3.

————. 1992b. Bush Stalls on Health Reform. *Boston Globe*, 15 March, pp. 1, 21.

Kolata, Gina. 1992. New Insurance Practice: Dividing Sick from Well. *New York Times*, 4 March, pp. A1, A15.

Kosterlitz, Julie. 1991. Softening Resistance. *National Journal*, 12 January, pp. 64–68.

Kudrle, Robert T., and Theodore R. Marmor. 1981. The Development of Welfare States in North America. In *The Development of Welfare States in Europe and*

America, ed. Peter Flora and Arnold J. Heidenheimer. New Brunswick, NJ: Transaction Books.

Laumann, Edward O., and David Knoke. 1987. *The Organizational State: Social Choice in National Policy Domains*. Madison: University of Wisconsin Press.

Long, S., and J. Rodgers. 1989. The Effects of Being Uninsured on Health Care Service Use: Estimates from the Survey of Income and Program Participation. Paper presented at the annual meeting of the Allied Social Sciences Associations, Atlanta, GA, 28 December.

Louis Harris and Associates. 1991. Trade-offs and Choices: Health Policy Options for the 1990s. New York: Metropolitan Life Insurance Company.

McConnell, Grant. 1966. *Private Power and American Democracy*. New York: Knopf.

McCool, Daniel. 1990. Subgovernments as Determinants of Political Viability. *Political Science Quarterly* 105 (2): 269–93.

McLaughlin, Loretta. 1991. A Tide-Turning on Health Care. *Boston Globe*, 17 November, p. 83.

Malbin, Michael J. 1980. *Unelected Representatives: Congressional Staff and the Future of Representative Government*. New York: Basic.

Manley, John. 1970. *The Politics of Finance*. Boston: Little, Brown.

March, James G., and Johan P. Olsen. 1989. *Rediscovering Institutions: The Organizational Basis of Politics*. New York: Free Press.

Marmor, Theodore R. 1973. *The Politics of Medicare*. Chicago: Aldine.

Marmor, Theodore R., and David Boyum. 1992. American Medical Care Reform: Are We Doomed to Fail? *Daedalus* 121 (4): 175–94.

Marmor, Theodore R., and Jerry L. Mashaw. 1990. Canada's Health Insurance and Ours: The Real Lessons, the Big Choices. *American Prospect* 3 (Fall): 18–29.

Marmor, Theodore R., Jerry L. Mashaw, and Philip L. Harvey. 1990. *America's Misunderstood Welfare State: Persistent Myths, Enduring Realities*. New York: Basic.

Marmor, Theodore R., Donald A. Wittman, and Thomas A. Heagy. 1983. The Politics of Medical Inflation. In *Political Analysis and American Medical Care: Essays*, ed. Theodore R. Marmor. New York: Cambridge University Press.

Martin, Cathie Jo. 1992. *Shifting the Burden: The Struggle over Growth and Corporate Taxation*. Chicago: University of Chicago Press.

Matthiessen, Constance. 1990. Bordering on Collapse. *Modern Maturity* 33 (3): 30–82.

Meier, Barry. 1992. A Growing U.S. Affliction: Worthless Health Policies. *New York Times*, 4 January, pp. 1, 46.

Morone, James A. 1990. *The Democratic Wish: Popular Participation and the Limits of American Government*. New York: Basic.

New York Times 1992. Bush on Health: Smart, Gutless. 7 February, p. A28.

Olson, Mancur. 1965. *The Logic of Collective Action*. Cambridge, MA: Harvard University Press.

Ornstein, Norman J., ed. 1975. *Congress in Change: Evolution and Reform*. New York: Praeger.

Ornstein, Norman J., Thomas E. Mann, and Michael J. Malbini. 1987. *Vital Statistics on Congress, 1987–1988*. Washington, DC: American Enterprise Institute.

———. 1992. *Vital Statistics on Congress, 1991–1992*. Washington, DC: Congressional Quarterly, Inc.

Page, Benjamin, and Robert Shapiro. 1992. *The Rational Public: Fifty Years of Trends in Americans' Policy Preferences*. Chicago: University of Chicago Press.

Pear, Robert. 1991. 3.47 Million Lack Health Insurance, Studies Say; Number Is Highest since '65. *New York Times*, 19 December, p. B17.

———. 1992a. Conflicting Aims in Booming Health Care Lobby Help Stall Congress. *New York Times*, 18 March, p. A17.

———. 1992b. President Leaves Many Areas Gray. *New York Times*, 7 February, p. A15.

———. 1992c. In Shift, Insurers Ask U.S. to Require Coverage for All. *New York Times*, 3 December, pp. A1, A22.

———. 1993. Health-Care Costs Up Sharply Again, Posing New Threat. *New York Times*, 5 January, pp. A1, A10.

Pepper Commission (U.S. Bipartisan Commission on Comprehensive Health Care). 1990. *A Call for Action*. Washington, DC: U.S. Government Printing Office.

Pertman, Adam. 1992. Democrats Scored with Most Groups, Exit Polls Report. *Boston Globe*, 4 November, p. 24.

Peterson, Mark A. 1990a. *Legislating Together: The White House and Capitol Hill from Eisenhower to Reagan*. Cambridge, MA: Harvard University Press.

———. 1990b. Institutions, Networks, and the Development of National Health Care Policy in America. Paper prepared for delivery at the annual meeting of the American Political Science Association, San Francisco, CA, 30 August–2 September.

———. 1992a. The Presidency and Organized Interests: White House Patterns of Interest Group Liaison. *American Political Science Review* 86 (3): 612–25.

———. 1992b. Report from Congress: Momentum toward Health Care Reform in the U.S. Senate. *Journal of Health Politics, Policy and Law* 17 (3): 553–73.

———. 1992c. Leading Our Way to Health: Entrepreneurship and Leadership in the Health Care Reform Debate. Paper prepared for delivery at the annual meeting of the American Political Science Association, Chicago, IL, 3–6 September.

Petts, David. 1991. Wofford and the Middle Class Squeeze. *The Polling Report*, 2 December, pp. 1, 7–8.

Poen, Monte M. 1979. *Harry S. Truman versus the Medical Lobby*. Columbia: University of Missouri Press.

Pollock, Ronald, and Phyllis Torda. 1991. The Pragmatic Road toward National Health Insurance. *American Prospect* 6 (Summer): 92–100.

President's Program (President's Comprehensive Health Reform Program). 1992. Washington, DC: The White House.

Price, David E. 1971. Professionals and 'Entrepreneurs': Staff Orientations and Policy Making on Three Senate Committees. *Journal of Politics* 33 (2): 316–36.

Rich, Spencer. 1991. Health Costs Will Further Crimp Family Income by 2000, Study Predicts. *Washington Post*, 11 December, p. A15.

———. 1992. Despite Medicare, Elderly Health Costs Up, Study Says. *Washington Post*, 26 February, p. A3.

Rosner, Jeremy D. 1993. A Progressive Plan for Affordable, Universal Health Care. In *Mandate for Change*, ed. Will Marshall and Martin Schram. New York: Berkley Books.

Rovner, Julie. 1992. Democrats Agree on Road Map, If Not Direction, for Overhaul. *Congressional Quarterly Weekly Report*, 20 June, p. 1802.

———. 1993. A Job for the Deficit Bomb Squad . . . Defusing Exploding Health-Care Costs. *Congressional Quarterly Weekly Report*, 2 January, pp. 28–29.

Rutledge, Peter B. 1992. Prescription for Repeal? Unpublished senior honors thesis. Harvard University, Department of Government.

Sabatier, Paul A. 1988. An Advocacy Coalition Framework of Policy Change and the Role of Policy-oriented Learning Therein. *Policy Sciences* 21:129–68.

Salisbury, Robert H. 1990. The Paradox of Interest Groups in Washington—More Groups, Less Clout. In *The New American Political System*, 2d version, ed. Anthony King. Washington, DC: American Enterprise Institute.

Salisbury, Robert H., John P. Heinz, Edward O. Laumann, and Robert L. Nelson. 1987. Who Works with Whom? Interest Group Alliances and Opposition. *American Political Science Review* 81 (4): 1217–34.

Sammon, Richard. 1992. Fall of Striker Bill Spotlights Doubts about Labor Lobby. *Congressional Quarterly Weekly Report*, 20 June, p. 1810.

Schlozman, Kay Lehman, and John T. Tierney. 1986. *Organized Interests and American Democracy*. New York: Harper and Row.

Sinclair, Barbara. 1983. *Majority Leadership in the U.S. House*. Baltimore, MD: Johns Hopkins University Press.

———. 1989. *The Transformation of the U.S. Senate*. Baltimore, MD: Johns Hopkins University Press.

Skidmore, Max J. 1970. *Medicare and the American Rhetoric of Reconciliation*. University, AL: University of Alabama Press.

Skocpol, Theda. 1992. *Protecting Soldiers and Mothers: The Political Origins of Social Policy in the United States*. Cambridge, MA: Harvard University Press.

Skowronek, Stephen. 1982. *Building a New American State: The Expansion of National Administrative Capabilities, 1877–1920*. Cambridge: Cambridge University Press.

Smith, Steven S. 1989. *Call to Order: Floor Politics in the House and Senate*. Washington, DC: Brookings Institution.

Smith, Steven S., and Christopher J. Deering. 1984. *Committees in Congress*. Washington, DC: Congressional Quarterly Press.

Spolar, Christine. 1991. For Uninsured, Medical Care a Luxury. *Washington Post*, 27 December, pp. A1, A4.

Starr, Paul. 1982. *The Social Transformation of American Medicine*. New York: Basic.

———. 1991. The Middle Class and National Health Reform. *American Prospect* 6 (Summer): 7–12.

Starr, Paul, and Theodore Marmor. 1984. The United States: A Social Forecast. In *The End of an Illusion: The Future of Health Policy in Western Industrialized Nations*, ed. Jean de Kervasdou'e, John R. Kimberly, and Victor G. Rodwin. Berkeley and Los Angeles, CA: University of California Press.

Stigler, George J. 1971. The Theory of Economic Regulation. *Bell Journal of Economics and Management Science* 2:3–21.

Stone, Deborah A. 1990. AIDS and the Moral Economy of Insurance. *American Prospect* 1 (Spring): 62–73.

Taylor, Malcolm G. 1987. *Health Insurance and Canadian Public Policy: The Seven Decisions That Created the Canadian Health Insurance System and Their Outcomes*. Toronto: McGill-Queen's University Press.

Turner, Robert L. 1992. The Man out Front on Health-Care Reform. *Boston Globe*, 2 February, p. 63.

U.S. Bureau of the Census. 1991. *Statistical Abstract of the United States, 1991*. Washington, DC: U.S. Government Printing Office.

U.S. Congress (Senate Select Committee on Small Business). 1978. *Hearings on the Impact of Inflation on the Economy and Small Business—Health Care*. 95th Cong., 2d sess. Washington, DC: U.S. Government Printing Office.

U.S. General Accounting Office. 1991a. *Health Insurance Coverage: A Profile of the Uninsured in Selected States*. HRD-91-31FS. Washington, DC: U.S. General Accounting Office.

———. 1991b. *Canadian Health Insurance: Lessons for the United States*. HRD 91-90. Washington, DC: U.S. General Accounting Office.

Vogel, David. 1989. *Fluctuating Fortunes*. Berkeley and Los Angeles: University of California Press.

Walker, Jack L., Jr. 1981. The Diffusion of Knowledge, Policy Communities, and Agenda Setting: The Relationship of Knowledge to Power. In *New Strategic Perspectives on Social Policy*, ed. John Tropman, Milan Dluhy, and Roger Lind. New York: Pergamon.

———. 1991a. *Mobilizing Interest Groups in America: Patrons, Professions, and Social Movements*. Ann Arbor: University of Michigan Press.

———. 1991b. *Activities and Maintenance Strategies of Interest Groups in the United States, 1980 and 1985*. Ann Arbor: University of Michigan, Institute of Public Policy Studies, 1985, and Inter-University Consortium for Political and Social Research, 1991.

Weir, Margaret. 1992. *Politics and Jobs: The Boundaries of Employment Policy in the United States*. Princeton, NJ: Princeton University Press.

Wilsford, David. 1991. *Doctors and the State: The Politics of Health Care in France and the United States*. Durham, NC: Duke University Press.

Wilson, James Q. 1973. *Political Organizations*. New York: Basic.

Wing, Kenneth R. 1985–86. American Health Policy in the 1980s. *Case Western Reserve Law Review* 36:608–707.

Witte, Edwin. 1962. *The Development of the Social Security Act*. Madison: University of Wisconsin Press.

Woolhandler, Steffie, and David U. Himmelstein. 1991. The Deteriorating Administrative Efficiency of the U.S. Health Care System. *New England Journal of Medicine* 324:1253–58.

Much of this article is based on research and experiences made possible by my 1990–91 affiliation with the Brookings Institution as a guest scholar in the Governmental Studies Program and by the 1990–91 American Political Science Association Congressional Fellowship that afforded me the opportunity to work as a legislative assistant on health policy in the office of Senator Tom Daschle. Senator Daschle, Rima Cohen, and Peter Rouse have my deepest appreciation for making it such an enriching experience. Special thanks are also owed Robert Blendon, James Brasfield, Morris Fiorina, William Glaser, John Kingdon, Mary Hale, Theodore Marmor, Cathie Martin, James Morone, Theda Skocpol, and Joseph White for their extremely helpful comments on an earlier version of this article.

The Bureaucracy Empowered

James A. Morone

Abstract Administrative changes have been reshaping health policy for the past decade. One consequence is a more constrained medical profession. Another is a more powerful health care bureaucracy. Most industrialized nations have called on democratic principles to balance professional norms; in contrast, Americans are developing a distinctly bureaucratic health care regime. This article suggests why and explores the ramifications for both the politics of health care and the practice of medicine.

The usual American health politics story describes long seasons of stalemate punctuated by sudden moments of reform. Bold innovations are long contested, rarely won. The national health insurance debate, for example, is now in its ninth decade, the health care cost crisis in its third. However, a focus on health care bureaucracy yields a sharply different plot. A decade of quiet, incremental reforms have transformed our administrative politics, reshaping the organization, expectations, and distribution of authority in medical policy.

There are at least three working models of authority in health care politics: professional, democratic, and bureaucratic (with an additional handful of largely theoretical alternatives, most notably the free market). Each locates accountability for health care in different hands.

The traditional view (which proved particularly resilient in the United States) placed authority over health policy squarely in the hands of the medical profession. Physicians, drawing on their expertise, operated as health care trustees. Legislators were solicitous, government bureaucrats deferential, patients obedient, payers passive. The profession defeated the legislation it opposed, won the policies it supported, and guided the administration of existing health programs.

Most nations eventually developed a second model, the social democratic one, in an effort to constrain the power of the medical profession. The principles of democratic representation offered a counterweight to the authority of professional norms and knowledge. The state could set overall economic and social policy, then leave the professionals alone to practice within its frame. Although health care systems vary enormously from nation to nation, two key features characterize the social democratic model: Public officials, acting as monopsonists, bargain with professional groups over the health economy. And the economic bargains they strike (as well as the social rules they promulgate) are explicit, visible, and political.

Like most representative institutions, this model claims legitimacy by offering citizens a public accounting for the choices made in their name. The analytic ideal is a public process in which officials act, explain, and are held to account (Thompson 1988; Pitkin 1967). Though political practice often falls short, this is the underlying basis of legitimacy for health policy across most of the industrialized world (Abel-Smith 1992; Hsiao 1992).

The great exception, of course, is the United States. Here, the profession was too powerful and the state too weak for the creation of a bluntly political countervailing power. Instead, Americans coped by concocting a long string of modest, fragmented, piecemeal programs. Over time, the programmatic pieces have begun to add up. The argument I make in this essay is that Americans are unreflectively developing an entirely new model of health care policy-making—one that places power in bureaucratic hands.

The emerging American health politics increasingly operates with the language, methodology, and mind-set of bureaucratic actors. Even highly politicized judgments are coded in dense, complex, technical constructions—what Daniel Fox calls the language of economizing (1990: 489). Examples include formula-driven rate-setting programs such as diagnosis-related groups, or DRGs (legislated in 1983 to reimburse hospitals under Medicare, Part A). A more recent effort, the resource-based relative value scale (RBRVS, which reimburses physicians under Medicare) was originally designed to be different: it would factor explicit social values (like the need for more primary care physicians) into reimbursement rates. As I shall show below, the effort to hold clear, visible value judgments up to the political light was soon buried by arcane budget rules and bureaucratic folkways. New government agencies (in both the executive branch and Congress), the growth in private sector bureaucrats (operating managed care plans), and federal sponsorship of medical outcomes research all extend the realm of bureaucratic politics.

The result is a deep change in our health policy process. Bureaucratic politics are obscure—an important advantage in a weak, fragmented polity suspicious of its own public officials. Formula-driven rate-setting programs can be legislated even during the stalemate over big issues like national health insurance. But the bureaucratic changes come at a price.

The entrance costs to the health policy dialogue grow very high and distinctly skewed. Without a social ideal to aim for, there is no concern when health policy drifts beyond the comprehension of the general public. Even legislative control becomes increasingly difficult to assert. The medical profession, too, loses authority over what was once its sphere. The health policy debate proceeds with different assumptions, methods, and rules— all biased to exclude the doctors, the Congress, and the people. Max Weber neatly summed the contest between democratic and bureaucratic politics: "The political 'master' always finds himself, vis-à-vis the trained official, in the position of a dilettante facing the expert. Under normal conditions . . . the power position of a . . . bureaucracy is . . . overtowering" (Weber 1978: 991).

The rise of bureaucratic politics puts American health policy (and American public administration) in distinctly uncharted waters. We are diverging from both our own past politics and from international experience. More important, the new bureaucratic politics sets the institutional infrastructure for future change. After all, successful political reforms are rarely invented entirely new. Rather, they draw on existing programs, organizations, and institutional memories (Skocpol 1992; Skocpol and Finegold 1982).

Contemporary programs—ranging from Medicare payment methodologies to corporate managed care plans—establish a framework for future changes. From a reform perspective, this is not a benign development; and from any angle, it is not a neutral one. The burgeoning American administrative apparatus can be expected to articulate and pursue its own interest. In any case, it will powerfully influence both the shape and the prospects of future health policies.

In the following section, I sketch the traditional American health economy, dominated by organized medicine. Next, I examine the challenges to the professional model; I suggest how and why Americans managed change amid the political gridlock. I then show how incremental adjustments sum into the new bureaucratic politics and suggest the consequences—both for the medical profession and for health care reformers.

Interest Group Liberalism

A clear pattern dominated American health care politics through most of the twentieth century: public authority over medicine was ceded to physicians, operating through associations (most famously, the American Medical Association, or AMA). Professional associations controlled licensure, proscribed unacceptable arrangements in health care organization (like prepaid practices), and dominated legislation on every level of government. In many ways, the medical profession's power constituted an exaggerated case of interest group liberalism—government authority wielded by an industry, generally for the benefit of its members (Morone 1990a; Starr 1982).

The doctors' power rested on two very different sources. First, they flexed the muscle of a well-organized, richly financed, highly prestigious interest group. By the 1920s, the AMA had developed a reputation for political influence that would grow for almost a half century. The American Medical Association, exaggerated the *New York Times* in 1954, "is the only organization that could marshall 140 votes in Congress between sundown Friday night and noon on Monday" (quoted by the editors, *Yale Law Journal* 1954). In political reality, liberal health reforms were generally sacrificed to maintain the shaky political coalition between northern and southern Democrats—a victim of the American system of checks and balances as much as the dread AMA. Even so, the medical association masterfully opposed threatening programs while offering politicians uncontroversial health care alternatives that reinforced both the prestige and the autonomy of the profession (Morone 1990a: 254–57).

Secondly, beneath the politics lay the deeper authority of professional knowledge. Physicians acted on the basis of technical expertise, acquired through prescribed training, guided by internalized norms, and accurately evaluated only by colleagues (rather than by patients, politicians, or anybody else) (Freidson 1972; Stone 1984).

While liberal reformers repeatedly wrangled with the AMA over financing national health insurance, they never challenged the underlying assumption of professional authority. Reformers would reduce the economic barriers to medicine, never meddle with the practice of medicine itself. Consequently, health providers were central to the implementation of all government health care programs. Public officials sought out professional advice, approval, and participation.

For example, the Hospital Construction Act of 1946 (popularly named Hill-Burton after Senators Joseph Lister Hill and Harold Burton) was a model of restrained public power, full of checks to governmental incursion into the health sphere. The program funded hospital construction; the state financed medicine's workshops and laboratories, while it studiously avoided meddling with professional decisions. The statute was only nine pages long, but there was room in it to forbid any federal regulation of hospital policy and to invite local administrators to appeal to the courts if the surgeon general rejected their project. Not that federal bureaucrats were permitted any discretion; local providers proposed projects, a formula allocated funds by state. Over the next thirty years, Hill-Burton funds contributed to almost a third of the hospital construction projects in America. (For descriptions, see Rosenblatt 1978; Thompson 1981.) The state provided funds while ceding authority over the program to the profession, which used the money to build up a sophisticated institutional infrastructure for the private practice of medicine.[1]

Even Medicare (1965), the first significant government challenge to providers in the twentieth century, continued to reflect the patterns of deference. The statute itself broke with all legislative tradition: Rather than promising all things to all citizens, this bill opened with promises to alter almost nothing at all: "Nothing in this title shall be construed to authorize any federal official or employee to exercise any supervision or control over the practice of medicine." The next five passages embellished the theme, forbidding state control over medical personnel or compensation or choice of provider or selection of insurer (title 18, sections 1801, 1802, and 1803 of the Social Security Act).

Implementors worked hard to secure the confidence and cooperation of providers who had long opposed the program. Medicare was lodged in the Social Security Administration, an agency structured around swift claims processing rather than meddlesome oversight (see Feder 1977).

---

1. The legislation's one intrusive stipulation was a requirement that grantee hospitals "provide a reasonable volume of . . . services to persons unable to pay." Congress immediately appended a loophole by adding "unless such a requirement is not feasible from a financial standpoint." The implementing bureaucracy simplified matters for the grantees by failing to write regulations for or monitor compliance of the indigent care provision. More than twenty-five years later, the courts denied standing to indigent consumers who sued for free care in Hill-Burton hospitals; the regulations were still unwritten. Government meddling in the medical business violated the spirit of the enterprise.

Shunning payment schedules or other controls, Medicare reimbursed providers their "reasonable costs"—essentially, whatever they charged. In order to avoid the stigma of governmental bureaucracy, private insurance companies would process the payments; hospitals were permitted to select their own fiscal intermediaries, a solid protection against overly zealous scrutiny of reimbursement claims. The general expectation was that medical professionals would guide Medicare, defining "reasonable" reimbursement levels, monitoring the quality of health care, and advising public officials on needed regulations.

The implementation of Medicare offers a cautionary tale for at least one important reason: it succeeded. The implementing bureaucracy was set a daunting task: sixteen million Americans would be eligible in a year, physicians were threatening mutiny, and there were few guides for how to organize such a program. The job was to get care to people over sixty-five without upsetting—indeed, without affecting—the medical system (Ball and Hess 1992; Johnson 1971).

In retrospect, of course, Medicare's implementation is often criticized for its generosity—it was virtually "captured" by the medical profession. But the criticism stands outside of the historical context. At the time, all officials—public and private, liberal and conservative—shared the same assumptions and biases. Their approach to medical policy, even the conceptual categories by which they perceived it, was shaped by six decades of deference to the medical profession. The task was to pay for the care of sixteen million people without affecting medicine itself. That is what the program's implementors set out to do.

The solution to one problem had unforeseen consequences, which revised the political agenda for health policy. Cost concerns rose, access worries faded. A new dilemma soon scrambled the traditional political economy of health care.

Small Changes beneath the Gridlock

The discovery of a cost crisis followed fast on the implementation of Medicare and Medicaid. President Richard Nixon declared "a massive crisis" in 1969. *Business Week* ran a cover story on the "sixty-billion-dollar crisis." *Fortune* judged American medicine "on the brink of chaos." Writing in the inaugural issue of the *Journal of Health Politics, Policy and Law*, Senator Jacob Javits (R-NY) summed up the political consensus: "It is . . . urgent that we . . . do better" (Javits 1976: 8; see Starr 1982: 381).

Corporations, labor unions, insurance companies and consumer groups joined the politicians in calling for solutions.

Almost a quarter century later, the "massive crisis" remains unsolved. A long string of cost control programs have come and, in some cases, gone—Lawrence Brown counted eleven major initiatives between 1972 and 1985 (Brown 1986: 569–571). In perhaps the most memorable summation, Robert Alford called it all "dynamics without change" (Alford 1975). In contrast, our industrial partners in the Organization for Economic Cooperation and Development reacted to the fast rising costs of the late 1970s with successful controls by the mid-1980s—some nations were more effective, others less, but (at least in raw statistical terms) they all have done better than the U.S. (see Schieber and Poullier 1991; U.S. General Accounting Office 1991). The obvious question is, why?

The answer lies in the design of the American political regime. The broad global budget reforms that other nations have wrestled into place are not easy to win in a polity that is suspicious of its own state (Morone 1990a). Perhaps more importantly, American political institutions are thick with checks and balances; it is difficult to win new forms of state authority, even for the extension of narrow benefits to broad constituencies. Proposals must run an awesome political gauntlet: first, the Office of the President; then, the competing, overlapping committees in each branch of Congress (five separate committees have major jurisdiction over health care bills); after that, the Washington bureaucracy; and, finally, the multiple layers of American federalism—all divided by function and bedeviled by an extensive (and much-called-upon) judiciary. It is not a policy-making apparatus designed for swift or concerted action. On the contrary, American government is designed to be maladroit at securing broad, coordinated policy changes—like national health care reform (Morone 1990a, 1992).

In this context, federal and state officials have faced rising health care budgets with few effective policy alternatives. They filled the cost control vacuum with narrowly focused, apparently haphazard programs. The first efforts remained within the old health care paradigm—they called on the professionals to solve the problem. The Physician Standard Review Organization of 1972, for example, forbade anybody but physicians from making regulatory judgments. By the 1980s, however, the efforts began to fall into a new, quite distinctive pattern. Public as well as private officials began to develop complex, highly technical, often formula-driven, cost control programs. Diagnosis-related groups offer a good example;

so do the resource-based relative value scales. Private payers developed preferred provider arrangements (PPOs, essentially bargaining with providers over price) and managed care protocols (that monitor, with wildly varying levels of managerial intensity, what providers actually do to their patients). In contrast to the weak programs of the 1970s, these efforts regulate important streams of money; in contrast to broad-gauged, global budget reforms, these narrow changes are well adapted to the American political process.

First, they appear (and in politics, appearance is crucial) to operate automatically, scientifically—without visible decisions by politicians or bureaucrats. The illusion of self-enforcing, automatic, scientific process is important in a nation that is suspicious of its own public officials (Morone 1990b). Second, formula-driven rate-setting programs are complex, difficult to describe, hard to understand, and—consequently, crucially—not easily transformed into explosive symbols like "socialized medicine." To the public and the major media, these appear to be obscure policy fiddles, redolent of green eyeshades and dusty accounting methods; to the politicians they are relatively safe. Third, the programs are narrow, each addressing only the regulators' own costs. When the Health Care Financing Administration tries to cut Medicare costs, it is acting as prudent purchaser, cutting back on government spending. A more global effort would challenge the boundaries of legitimate state action.

Of course, the multiple, narrow, competing cost control efforts exact a high price. As a voluminous literature now makes plain, multiple payers each pursuing their own cost control programs leave multiple cost-shifting safety valves, through which providers can recoup their income. Worse, it has fractured our employment pools into increasingly small groups, as private insurers have pursued less expensive (read: healthier) clientele (Marmor et al. 1990; Stone 1993; Altman and Cohen 1993).

The usual focus on the policy wreckage, however, obscures an important underlying consequence for the policy process. The buildup of technical programs sums to an emerging health policy infrastructure. In many ways, it offers a partial, hidden, less effective way to achieve the political bargaining that characterizes traditional national health insurance plans. However, the obscure operation of this process sharply contrasts the social democratic ideal.[2] Instead, Americans have been developing an entirely new model of authority over health care.

2. In this, the organization of American politics and the classic bureaucratic mind-set fit together well. Recall Weber's maxim: "Bureaucratic administration always tends to exclude the public, to hide its knowledge and action from criticism" (Weber 1978: 992).

Bureaucratic Politics

Traditional national health insurance bargaining turns on explicit acts of political representation. The negotiations (largely over prices and funding) are organized to permit speeches, symbols, gestures, negotiating tactics. In short, the process rewards political skills. Peak associations, professional groups, legislatures, and citizens can all play a significant role.

Contemporary American rate-setting programs are, of course, equally political. However, the costs of entering the negotiations are much higher and distinctly skewed. Participants must be ready to argue statistical models, assumptions, and formulae—indeed, I have suggested that the relative obscurity that results is precisely the political advantage of these programs. But the political benefit comes at a cost. There is a systematic bias at work. The American bargaining methods rest on the classic strengths of bureaucratic administration: the precise coordination of highly specialized information. This is a system for health policy experts; it cannot easily be entered by interest groups, politicians, physicians, or the public. As the systems develop, it becomes increasingly difficult to bring political pressures to bear on public officials. Traditional political accountability is sacrificed for the politically useful illusion of technical precision.

For example, hospitals in Newfoundland (or the members of parliament for their districts) can protest budget allocations; hospitals in New Jersey (or their representatives in Congress) must, somehow, challenge the total impact of hundreds of DRG prices that disadvantage them (even while they advantage competitors). Indeed, when the DRG reimbursement methodology was first introduced in New Jersey, the legislature— prodded by local providers—sought to delay implementation. However, lawmakers were uncertain about how to frame alternatives to a program that was partially in place. The Assembly was reduced to censuring the Department of Health in a resolution (that had no force of law). In this case, at least, control over health policy had passed from providers and legislators to the health bureaucracy (Dunham and Morone 1983).

Recent conflict over physician payment reform offers a more baroque example of the same pattern. Congress intricately balanced experts, physician groups, and Medicare constituents in designing the reform. The ideal was long-run cost control linked to a national dialogue over the relative social value of different procedures and services. Here, in short, was the social democratic ideal in the American institutional context. Congress designed the relative value scales to be budget-neutral—Medicare payments to physicians as a group would not be reduced. Yet, when the Health Care Financing Administration released its implementation plan (in proposed regulations), the first-year projection included a startling 16 percent drop ($7 billion) in the total payments to physicians. The simplest explanation (there are several complicated ones) points to a congressional drafting error in the frenzied last-moment negotiations over the bill (see Grey 1992). Naturally, a furor ensued. The traditional political solution would have been simple: Congress restores the money, perhaps slapping the bureaucrats on the wrist. (Of course, in the traditional health care economy, Congress would not have been manipulating medical incentives with innovative payment modes—physicians would get their "customary" and "usual" fees [Oliver 1993; Resneck 1992].)

In contemporary Washington it is not so easy. The 1990 budget agreement requires budget neutrality. Money added to one program must be cut from another. The Office of Management and Budget (OMB, then in Republican hands) keeps the fiscal score. The drafting error that "lost" the money had occurred in the previous year and accounts must be squared each year. The OMB could have (and rumors suggest some officials thought they should have) required Congress to cut $7 billion from other programs before it restored the $7 billion to Medicare.

On the surface, the outcome may look like old business as usual. The providers screamed, Congress mobilized, and after a bout of recrimination and confusion, the money reappeared. The case was complicated, of course, because the usual checks and balances were exacerbated by divided government—Democrats in Congress allocated funds that Republican administrations did not want to spend. However, these details should not obscure the broader trend: The rules of the Washington game made congressional intervention very difficult. Congress had to raise the political stakes quite high in order to accomplish that most standard of political operations—distributing benefits to a mobilized constituency. Restoring the funds required elaborate rounds of multiparty bargaining. But what is crucial were the terms of engagement.

The battle was fought on technical terrain amid a complex welter of rules. There were multiple layers of intricacy: the budget process, congressional–executive branch rivalry, the reimbursement methodology itself. This was pure bureaucratic politics; high-minded notions of social accountability were quickly thrown aside. Bradford Grey examined a related bill in the same budget package and "marvel[ed] that any legislation ever gets passed" (Grey 1992: 65). An HCFA official offered a more pungent epilogue: "We released the numbers [at a press conference] and those media guys just sat there. They didn't have a clue" (personal communication, 14 April 1992).

The increasingly bureaucratic process leads to the development of more bureaucratic capacity: in Congress (Brown 1992 32), on the state level (Hackey 1992), in private industry (HIAA 1991: 22); throughout the billing departments of the medical establishment (Rabkin and Wallace 1992), and, of course, in the federal bureaucracy itself—where the latest transformation involves the reconfiguration of the National Center for Health Services Research (NCHSR) into the Agency for Health Care Policy and Research (AHCPR. Apparently the agency was to be the Agency for Health Care Research and Policy till someone worked out the acronym, AHCRAP) (Grey 1992: 50). All this activity—indeed, the bureaucratic model itself—has broad political ramifications. Consider the implications, first for doctors, then for social democrats.

Implications for the Doctors

The upshot for physicians is more than a waning of political power. The dynamics described above challenge not just the political influence of organizations like the AMA but the professional claims on which they ultimately rest. Both the traditional political pattern in the United States and the social democratic model abroad leave medical judgments to medical professionals (though Europeans are watching the American experiments in professional regulation with considerable interest). Without the luxury of system cost control, American cost regulation has begun to penetrate the offices, clinics, and hospitals of the profession itself.

Many American cost control programs are designed to induce providers to behave differently (read: less expensively). Managed care plans reward physicians who are slower to put patients into hospitals; diagnosis-related groups reward the hospitals who are faster to get them out. The efforts contrast with global negotiations, which simply set the price and leave the practice patterns to the profession. And they offer an even more striking contrast to the old American pattern, codified in those first passages of Medicare, that insisted nothing would change except the source of the cash.

The Agency for Health Care Policy and Research presses the challenge to professional autonomy forward. Congress charged AHCPR with determining "how diseases, disorders and other health care conditions can most effectively be diagnosed and treated." John Wennberg laid out the logic of the enterprise in a series of influential articles: Large differences in hospitalization in Boston and New Haven did not appear to be guided by scientific factors. "Residents of Boston incurred about $300 million more in hospital expenditures (in 1982 dollars) and used 795 more hospital beds than would have been the case if the use rates of New Haven had applied" (Wennberg 1990: 1203–4).

The theory is that research teams can determine what is appropriate medicine under which conditions. The guidelines, it is often said, could help physicians practice better medicine. And yet, external arbiters meddling with the content of medicine (much less arbiters funded by the federal government) are a powerful, long-resisted challenge to the nature of professionalism itself.

The inroads into what was once exclusively professional turf is facilitated by the American faith in painless, automatic, nongovernmental cost savings. After all, *AHCPR* sounds nothing like "national health insurance" or "government rationing." And who could oppose research into what makes for good medicine? Researchers will spare Americans the hard budget choices by exposing the excesses in the extra $700 million of spending that John Wennberg found in Boston; RAND Corporation researcher Robert Brook speculated that "we could trim $50 billion from the nation's health bill" (Kosterlitz 1991: 575). And Secretary of Health and Human Services Otis Bowen raised the ante by suggesting that up to 25 percent of the health care delivered in America is not necessary (Grey 1992: 45–46).

The tender political point is, what happens to the data? Some of the research faithful trust that simply showing physicians the numbers will nudge them toward more efficient medicine—the apotheosis of a simple, automatic solution to a complex problem. The issue was exposed in the skirmish to keep the research out of HCFA. That agency, asserted the American Medical Association, cares mainly about cost control and would swiftly convert research findings into reimbursement formulae. But that is precisely what many parties are after.

As Fred Grandy (R-IA) put it, "Questions are being raised about the value of the outcome of . . . medical treatments" (quoted in Grey 1992: 60). If anybody missed the programmatic implications, the final vote on AHCPR came amid a flurry of deals on whether Medicare would set an expenditure target for their physician payments—a much-feared step down the slippery slope to global budgets. While Congress pondered the research program (and the uncontrolled spending for Medicare), a consortium of corporations in Cleveland, Ohio, quietly mandated outcome studies of their own (Freund 1994).

Skirmishes over which bureaucracies control outcomes research are part of a much larger conflict: the effort to reshape the practice of medicine from outside the profession. Already, a multitude of cost containment programs have that effect. Outcomes research makes the efforts more systematic. The managed care movement—among both private and public payers—judges medical practice in an extraordinary number of ways. In this new medical world, a Blue Cross (of Illinois) program sends monitoring teams into physician offices to judge everything "from appropriateness of primary and specialized care" to the "cleanliness of the office" (Cox 1992).

Till recently, medicine was the province of highly trained professionals, answering only to internalized norms and to colleagues who shared them. Now, AHCPR, Blue Cross of Illinois, and the business consortium in Cleveland, Ohio, all seek—essentially—ways to code and operationalize that once specialized knowledge. Once the protocols are developed, less expert (even nonprofessional) employees can judge medical practice and authorize or withhold funding. The classic professional model is evolving into the classic bureaucratic one.

Reacting to these developments, sociologists have recently opened a debate about whether medicine has become "deprofessionalized" and "proletarianized" (McKinlay 1988; Mechanic 1991; Light 1991). While the matter is hotly contested, what is startling is that the issue is plausible in the first place. The hard political reality that emerges from this profession's fall can be illustrated by the reactions that physicians got when they asked for the criteria that triggered HCFA investigations of unnecessary care. The responses (reported in Rich 1991) ranged from the doubtful (*Washington Post*: "Can Doctors Be Trusted?") to the hostile (Congressman Pete Stark: "That's like telling drug dealers when you're going to carry out a raid"); HCFA decided to settle the matter with a $400,000 study designed to evaluate the costs of informing the doctors.

Can the decline of professional autonomy—still in relatively early stages—be reversed? Some physician groups have begun to try. The boldest efforts have come from the American College of Physicians. Quoting Jefferson, Tocqueville, and the 1935 Committee on the Cost of Medical Care, they propose the European bargain: global budgetary controls in exchange for the restoration of physician autonomy and an end to the "intrusions . . . paper work, administrative time and . . . hassle factor" of "the current situation" (*Annals of Internal Medicine* 1990, 1992; Brown 1992).

Of course, many of their colleagues will think twice about trading away the lavish funding, even for professional autonomy. But their own preferences no longer count as much as they once did: Interest group liberalism operates on the expressed preferences of organized groups, but bureaucratized regimes balance those preferences with the interests of the regulators and *their* institutions. The administrative apparatus we have developed injects a new kind of interest (protected by new layers of inertia) into the discourse of health care reform.

Implications for Reform

Even great breakthrough reforms are rarely invented new. They rely on existing models, conceptions, and experiences. Medicaid, for example, revised and extended the Kerr-Mills program; Medicare had been on the drawing boards of the Social Security Administration for fifteen years (Stevens and Stevens 1974; Brown 1983).

The web of technical changes described above suggests a potential infrastructure for contemporary reform. Today, the innovations remain scattered across many programs (both public and private); they involve a wide variety of methods (some more effective than others). Taken together, however, recent bureaucratic reforms offer conceptions, precedents, and organizations for reformers to build on. The path of least organizational resistance is to emend the current patchwork of controls by pushing them forward—extending, combining, systematizing.

Nor are contemporary administrators merely onlookers, waiting for political change. Pluralist analysis—calculating the probabilities of action by touting up the interest groups—obscures the influence of the administrative apparatus itself. Health care bureaucrats play an increasingly active role in formulating health care legislation (Robinson 1991). They implement with far less deference (some would say, less attention) to the concerns of organized interests. (See Ball and Hess 1992 for a measure of the change.) The often-lamented administrative costs of American health care represent not just a policy problem or an employment machine but a powerful political force. Both experience and self-interest lead administrators to defend what is familiar to them. The future of American health policy is likely to involve a great deal more of the complex, bureaucratic same.

That prospect raises the forgotten matter of popular control. It is an issue that Americans have not yet begun to grapple with, one that their institutions are ill equipped to cope with.

I have argued that American bureaucratic reforms bury questions of democratic accountability. As the state pushes further into the details of medicine, the hard choices are hidden deeper in the technique. Political leaders find few opportunities and no rewards for publicly grappling with cost control trade-offs or the limits of medicine. Citizens have no sustained way of holding leaders to account for their administration of the health care system. Indeed, the American political reflex is precisely the reverse: Make choices untainted by politics in some organizational equivalent to the Federal Reserve Board. Search for a better algorithm. Develop a more effective technique.

The reformist question ought to press beyond financing schemes or bargaining arrangements or regulating physicians. The issue, in an increasingly state-centered health care system, is how to achieve a measure of accountability for choices made (or not made) in the citizens' name. This may seem a philosophic fillip compared to the hard problems of costs and coverage. However, Americans might find that forcing leaders to account for how they juggle costs, quality, and access is the key to significant and sustained reform. It is not a likely model of reform. But it offers the only way to confront the difficult social choices that Americans have been avoiding.

References

Abel-Smith, B. 1992. Cost Containment and New Priorities in the European Community. *Milbank Quarterly* 70:393–416.

Alford, R. 1975. *Health Care Politics*. Chicago, IL: University of Chicago Press.

Altman, S., and A. Cohen. 1993. The Need for a Global Budget. *Health Affairs* 12 (Suppl.): 194–203.

Annals of Internal Medicine. 1990. Universal Access to Health Care in America: A Moral and Medical Imperative. 112:637–39.

————. 1992. Universal Insurance for American Health Care. 114:511–19.

Ball, R., and A. Hess. 1992. The Early Implementation of the Medicare Program. Transcript of discussion with the Study Panel on Implementation Aspects of National Health Care Reform, National Academy of Science, Washington, DC, 31 January.

Brown, L. 1983. *New Policies, New Politics*. Washington, DC: Brookings Institution.

————. 1986. Introduction to a Decade of Transition. *Journal of Health Politics, Policy and Law* 11:569–83.

————. 1992. Political Evolution of Federal Health Care Regulation. *Health Affairs* 11:17–37.

Cox, B. 1992. Illinois Blues Begin Physician Evaluation Program. *National Underwriter*, 20 January, p. 13.

Dunham, A., and J. A. Morone. 1983. *The Politics of Innovation*. Princeton: Health Research and Education Trust of New Jersey.

Feder, J. 1977. Medicare Implementation and the Policy Process. *Journal of Health Politics, Policy and Law* 2:173–89.

Fox, D. M. Health Policy and the Politics of Research in the United States. *Journal of Health Politics, Policy and Law* 16:481–99.

Freidson, E. 1972. *Profession of Medicine: A Study of the Sociology of Applied Knowledge*. New York: Dodd, Mead.

Freund, D. 1994. Outcomes Assessment: Market Incentives or Regulatory Fiat. In *Competitive Approaches to Health Care Reform*, ed. R. Arnould, R. Rich, and W. D. White. Washington, DC: Urban Institute Press.

Grey, B. 1992. The Legislative Battle over Health Services Research. *Health Affairs* 11:38–66.

Hackey, R. 1992. Trapped between State and Market. *Medical Care* 49:355–88.

HIAA (Health Insurance Association of America). 1991. *Sourcebook of Health Insurance Data*. Washington, DC: HIAA.

Hsiao, W. 1992. Comparing Health Care Systems: What Nations Can Learn from One Another. *Journal of Health Politics, Policy and Law* 17:613–36.

Javits, J. 1976. National Health Policy for the Future. *Journal of Health Politics, Policy and Law* 1:5–8.

Johnson, L. 1971. *The Vantage Point*. New York: Holt, Rinehart and Winston.

Kosterlitz, J. 1991. Cookbook Medicine. *National Journal*, 9 March, pp. 572–76.

Light, D. 1991. Professionalism as a Countervailing Power. *Journal of Health Politics, Policy and Law* 16:499–506.

McKinlay, J. B., ed. 1988. The Changing Character of the Medical Profession. *Milbank Quarterly* 66 (Suppl. 2).

Marmor, T., J. Mashaw, and P. Harvey. 1990. *America's Misunderstood Welfare State*. New York: Basic.

Mechanic, D. 1991. Sources of Countervailing Power in Medicine. *Journal of Health Politics, Policy and Law* 16:485–98.

Morone, J. A. 1990a. *The Democratic Wish*. New York: Basic.

————. 1990b. American Political Culture and the Search for Lessons from Abroad. *Journal of Health Politics, Policy and Law* 15:129–43.

————. 1992. The Bias of American Politics: Rationing Health Care in a Weak State. *University of Pennsylvania Law Review* 140:1923–38.

Oliver, T. R. 1993. Analysis, Advice, and Congressional Leadership: The Physician Payment Review Commission and the Politics of Medicare. *Journal of Health Politics, Policy and Law* 18:113–74.

Pitkin, H. 1967. *The Concept of Representation*. Berkeley and Los Angeles: University of California Press.

Rabkin, M., and E. C. Wallace. 1992. Provider Concerns and the Implementation of

Health Care Reform. In *Implementation Issues and National Health Care Reform*, ed. C. Brecher. New York: Josiah Macy Foundation.

Resneck, J. 1992. Medicare Physician Payment Reform. B.A. thesis, Taubman Center of Public Policy and American Institutions, Brown University.

Rich, Spencer. 1991. Medicare: Can the Doctors Be Trusted? *Washington Post*, 18 February, p. A23.

Robinson, C. 1991. *The Bureaucracy and the Legislative Process*. New York: University Press of America.

Rosenblatt, R. 1978. Health Care Reform and Administrative Law. *Yale Law Journal* 88:243–336.

Schieber, G. J., and J.-P. Poullier. 1991. International Health Spending: Issues and Trends. *Health Affairs* 10:106–16.

Skocpol, T. 1992. *Protecting Soldiers and Mothers*. Cambridge, MA: Harvard University Press.

Skocpol, T., and K. Finegold. 1982. State Capacity and Economic Intervention in the Early New Deal. *Political Science Quarterly* 97:255–78.

Starr, P. 1982. *The Transformation of American Medicine*. New York: Basic.

Stevens, R., and R. Stevens. 1974. *Welfare Medicine in America*. New York: Free Press.

Stone, D. 1984. *The Limits of Professional Power*. Chicago: University of Chicago Press.

―――. 1993. When Patients Go to Market. *American Prospect* 13:109–14.

Thompson, D. 1988. Representatives in the Welfare State. In *Democracy and the Welfare State*, ed. Amy Gutmann. Princeton, NJ: Princeton University Press.

Thompson, F. 1981. *Health Policy and the Bureaucracy*. Cambridge, MA: MIT Press.

U.S. General Accounting Office. 1991. *Health Care Spending Control: The Experience of France, Germany and Japan*. GAO/HRD-92-9. Washington, DC: U.S. General Accounting Office.

Weber, M. 1978. *Economy and Society*. Vol. 2. Ed. G. Ross and C. Wittich. Berkeley and Los Angeles: University of California Press.

Wennberg, John. 1990. Sounding Board: Outcomes Research, Cost Containment and the Fear of Health Care Rationing. *New England Journal of Medicine* 323 (17): 1202–4.

Yale Law Journal. 1954. The American Medical Association: Power, Purpose, Politics. 63:933–1022.

The Courts and
the Reconstruction of American
Social Legislation

Rand E. Rosenblatt

Abstract Because of budgetary and other political pressures, American health care reform (and other social reform) legislation is often not enforced, or is implemented in ways that undermine its egalitarian goals. About 25 years ago the federal courts began to try to reduce this gap between statutory promise and policy reality by interpreting federal funding laws as creating rights for their ultimate beneficiaries, including low-income patients and the providers who serve them. This major innovation in the concept of legal rights was confirmed by hundreds of judicial decisions and accepted by Congress itself. Over the past few years, however, a new Supreme Court, led by Chief Justice William Rehnquist, has issued opinions denying that such rights exist and vastly increasing agency power to reduce important statutory provisions to virtually meaningless formalities. Thus, at the very moment that national health care reform is prominent on the political agenda, the federal courts are abandoning a rights-enforcing role that may be critical for the reform's success. This essay explains the struggle around the courts' rights-enforcing role, defends the role, and suggests ways that it can be maintained even if the courts themselves are not currently in a good position to fulfill it.

A fierce struggle is currently raging over the courts' role in interpreting federal statutes,[1] particularly laws about federal spending for health

---

1. There are two major ways in which the courts will interact with national health care reform. First, the courts will inevitably be involved in interpreting and enforcing the federal and state laws that establish the structures and methods of reform. Second, the courts will likely continue to perform their traditional role of defining and enforcing physician-based but ultimately judge-made standards of medical malpractice, perhaps as modified by federal and state statutes. This article deals with the first role, that of interpreting statutes.

I am assuming that federal legislation will play a major role in national health care reform. Federal legislation, in turn, is judicially interpreted and enforced largely by federal courts; hence, by "courts" I mean primarily federal courts. In addition to interpreting statutes, federal courts have the authority to enforce the federal Constitution, and can refuse to enforce statutes that the and other social programs. The intensity of this debate recalls the New Deal constitutional crisis of the 1930s and involves similarly fundamental issues: the norms of legal interpretation, the concept of the judge's role, and the sources and meaning of legal rights. On one side of this debate stands a vision of law that recognizes important rights implicit in the modern welfare state, and sees courts as the legitimate interpreters and enforcers of these rights. These rights include fair agency procedures for deciding individual cases, agency policies that reflect the choices and values embodied in legislation (or, on occasion, the Constitution), and, where appropriate, particular benefits or outcomes. On the other side stands a vision of law that denies the existence of these rights if they are only implicit or based on interpretation, and commands the federal courts to refuse their enforcement unless Congress has defined and required them in super-clear terms. The purpose of this essay is to explain and defend the first vision of the courts' limited but important rights-enforcing role, and to discuss that role's significance for national health care reform.[2]

It is important not to exaggerate or idealize what the courts can do. Because of their limited authority, resources, and remedial powers, the courts cannot be the primary actors in solving the large underlying problems of American health care, notably the fragmented tax and insurance pools, the inability to control costs, and the vast impact of racism, poverty, and drugs. What the courts can do is modest but nonetheless important: to provide a forum with some decisionmaking power where politically fragile commitments to egalitarian reform can be supported toward becoming reality.

It is likely that any national health care reform will contain egalitarian commitments, and that they will continue to be fragile. Egalitarian commitments will be made in an effort to respond to market dynamics that virtually no one can defend: 35 million citizens uninsured because

---

courts find to be unconstitutional. However, the Supreme Court has largely abdicated its constitutional role with respect to what it has termed "social and economic legislation." See, e.g., Dandridge v. Williams, 397 U.S. 471 (1970); Rosenblatt 1990. The primary focus of this essay is therefore on the courts' role in interpreting statutes.

To the extent that national health care reform relies on state initiatives and legislation, state governments, including state courts, may also play a significant role. It is also worth noting that a number of state supreme courts, unlike the United States Supreme Court, have been willing to articulate state constitutional principles with large implications for educational financing, zoning, and other social issues. See, e.g., Neuborne 1989.

2. The phrase "rights-enforcing role" is not entirely satisfactory. The difficulties lie in the words "rights" and "enforcing." As will appear, my position is that the federal courts have over 25 years expanded the term "right" to include a right to a certain kind of allocation or decision process. This relatively new meaning of "rights" inevitably collides with the vision of negative, individualistic rights associated with the American and French revolutions. See Hobsbawm

of low incomes, unemployment, and health status; employers and insurers scrambling to deny or limit benefits to those who make—or who are at risk of making—significant claims;[3] and medical education and hospitals organized to support lucrative subspecialties and high technology while basic primary and preventive care is shortchanged. Egalitarian commitments to alter these market dynamics and others, however strongly supported by general public opinion and however sincerely intended by Congress and the new Administration, will remain fragile for at least four reasons. First, money and political influence are grossly unequally distributed in favor of interests that are likely to resist egalitarian change. Second, and relatedly, American political culture has been so dominated by fragmented, self-regarding politics for so long—what Robert Kuttner (1993) describes as our polity's "decayed avenues of participation [and] corrupted institutions of representation"—that it is difficult to conceive of, and organize, a political consensus for equality and mutual care. See also Lerner 1993. Third, the economic incentives for health care payors and providers to exclude "undesirable" patients because of their health status, race, occupation, etc., will remain a strong countercurrent to efforts to restructure markets in an egalitarian, or, to use the currently fashionable (but not entirely equivalent) phrase, "managed" direction.[4]

These three factors will interact to amplify a fourth: Congress's unavoidable effort to implement its value choices through mechanisms of "structured discretion." Although Congress typically makes some clear choices in health care financing legislation, notably about the source of funding, many important issues are delegated for resolution, under more or less clear guidelines, to federal and state agencies and nongovernmental entities. There are many reasons for this pattern: the inevitable imprecision of legislative language, the limited time and political resources

---

1984. Second, the term "enforcing" may imply that the right is clearly "there" in the statutory text, and that "all" a court is doing is "enforcing" it. As will become evident, the relationship of the courts to American social reform legislation is much more complex than this. Elsewhere I have characterized this kind of judicial role, with somewhat varying emphases, as a "structural due process approach" (Rosenblatt 1978), an "entitlement model" (Rosenblatt 1982, 1990), and a "model of social duties" (Rosenblatt 1990). The term "norm-realizing" might best capture what I mean by "rights-enforcing."

3. See, e.g., McGann v. H. & H. Music, 946 F.2d 401 (5th Cir. 1991), *cert. den. sub nom.* Greenberg v. H. & H. Music, 113 S.Ct. 482 (1992) (self-insured employer's reduction of lifetime maximum medical benefits from $1 million to $5,000 for AIDS-related claims only, after employee had filed AIDS-related claim, upheld as legal under the federal Employment Retirement Income Security Act [ERISA]).

4. "Managed competition" means structuring competition through regulation and financial incentives to achieve the policy goals of equality (universal, affordable coverage), cost containment, and quality of care. See, e.g., Starr 1993.

that Congress can spend on any one area, lack of clear political consensus (aggravated by the maldistribution of money and influence), the fragmented structure of American government (both among the federal branches and between the federal government and the states), and the long American tradition of anti-government beliefs and assumptions. See, e.g., Morone 1990.

Against this background, we can expect Congress and the new Administration to make commitments, in the form of law, in the direction of universal coverage, cost containment, and quality of care. Federal and state agencies and nongovernmental entities (e.g., employers, insurance companies, "health insurance purchasing cooperatives," and health maintenance organizations) will then be expected to implement a list of countervailing values, such as efficiency versus quality of care, or cost containment versus equality.[5] But these institutions will themselves be subject to similar budgetary, market, and political pressures as shaped the original congressional compromises and evasions.[6] Given these pressures, and the general political culture in which they operate (e.g., the absence of a strong labor movement or other well-organized forces in favor of egalitarian change), it is likely, as in the past, that serious gaps will develop between the Congress's egalitarian promises and the realities of health care delivery. Frustrated health care beneficiaries and/or providers may well then claim, as in the past, that these gaps result not simply from market dynamics or good faith judgment calls by government agencies, but rather from the agencies' failure to take Congress's egalitarian commitments into account at all, or in any defensible fashion. Should a court be able to investigate that claim?

Part 1 of this essay explores the nature and roots of the courts' rights-enforcing role. This role rests on the idea that funding laws for the ultimate benefit of individuals, or of the providers who serve them, are presumed to create legal rights (unless explicitly foreclosed by the statute) that members of those groups can enforce through the courts. This does not mean that the claims of beneficiaries or providers will or should always prevail; in any particular case, the arguments for and against recognition of a right and granting relief will vary in their persuasiveness. Moreover, the courts may not have the technical authority

5. See, for example, the proposed Russo/Wellstone Universal Health Care Act of 1991, 1991 H.R. 1300 Sec. 2121(a)(1)(a), 9/15/92. For a comprehensive analysis of various national health care reform proposals, see Marmor and Barr 1992.

6. For analysis of how these dynamics have functioned in many previous contexts, see, e.g., Edelman 1964; Morone 1992, 1990; Rosenblatt 1978.

or political or public support to provide full and effective remedies for legislative ambiguity and agency neglect regarding egalitarian reform. But at the very least the courts can perform and have performed three important (and usually interconnected) functions: (1) a "blocking function," blocking illegal, often grossly illegal agency actions or refusals to act;[7] (2) an "unmasking function," forcing into political daylight the gap between statutory standards and agency structure and performance;[8] and (3) a "rationality function," requiring agencies to articulate their policies and explain them in relation to statutory goals.[9]

Section (A) of Part 1 discusses the roots of the rights-enforcing role in the welfare rights litigation of the 1960s and early 1970s, and the contrary legal traditions that had to be (and were) overcome. Section (B) then focuses on how the lower federal courts have developed this role in the 1980s and early 1990s in the context of Medicaid reimbursement of institutional providers, a topic likely to figure prominently in national health care reform.

Although thoughtful and courageous judges pursuing a rights-enforcing role have made major contributions in many institutional and policy settings (see Rosenblatt 1990, 1978; Neuborne 1989), the legitimacy of this judicial role has always been under attack. Part Two of this article explores that attack and its increasing judicial triumph. The judicial attack is grounded in a laissez-faire legal consciousness that holds that citizens in general, and beneficiaries of government spending in particular, have no statutory "rights" against government or its agents, unless those rights are very explicitly declared in laws enacted by Congress and signed by the President.[10] The long tenure of the Reagan and Bush administrations has filled the federal courts, including the Supreme Court, with judges who

---

7. See, e.g., the *AMISUB* case discussed below; Cook v. Ochsner Foundation Hosp., 61 F.R.D. 354 (E.D.La. 1972) (finding that Health, Education and Welfare (HEW) Secretary's failure to issue regulations protecting low-income patients from exclusion from Hill-Burton grantee hospitals, and failure to require such hospitals to accept Medicaid patients, violates the Hill-Burton Act), discussed in Rosenblatt 1978: 276–82.

8. See, e.g., the *Rosado* case discussed below; Estate of Smith v. Heckler, 747 F.2d 583 (10th Cir. 1984) (holding that the Health and Human Services (HHS) Secretary has a duty to inform herself of nursing home conditions relevant to the Medicaid statutory standard of quality care, and that HHS certification of nursing homes under an inspection system that does not gather relevant information violates that duty).

9. See, e.g., *AMISUB*, *Temple University*, *Multicare*, and other Boren Amendment cases discussed below.

10. The point of the phrase "enacted by Congress and signed by the President" is to exclude or downgrade the use of legislative history (committee reports, patterns of amendments and substitute bills, etc.) in interpreting statutes. See Rosenblatt 1991: 807–12.

This perspective also denies constitutional rights in the same way, that is, the constitution creates no rights unless "explicitly" set forth in the text or "original intent" of the framers.

hold this view. The political momentum for national health care reform has thus gained strength at the very moment that the federal courts are abandoning a role that may be critical for the reform's success.

The vulnerability of the courts' modestly egalitarian role is not only due, however, to attacks by conservative politicians and judges. Part Three of this article explores the limits of liberals' conception of social reform, and the need for what the article's title refers to as "the reconstruction of American social legislation." I shall argue that liberals often create reforms with serious built-in weaknesses, by failing to attend to the politics of administration and implementation that take place after the politics of legislation are seemingly over. The question of "the role of the courts in national health care reform" is actually a variation on the most central question: will the forces that favor national health care reform be able to mobilize enough vision and energy to begin creating the kind of society and political culture which, in my view, is the indispensable basis for humane and egalitarian national health care reform itself.

Part 1   The Role of the Courts in Social Welfare Legislation: Structured Discretion as a Legal Right

(A) The Roots of the Right to Structured Agency Discretion

When government promises in the form of law to act, particularly to meet basic human needs, do the people who will benefit from that promise have a "right" to enforce it in the courts? Prior to the 1960s, the answer given by most American courts was "no." At one level, this answer was said to be based on the way the laws were written; the statutes' explicit language and structure generally conferred structured discretion on decision-makers as a condition of receiving federal funds, and did not explicitly confer rights on individual beneficiaries. Indeed, for many judges, the idea of agency discretion, however "structured," was inconsistent with the notion of rights. Traditionally, rights were conceived as clear, mandatory rules that gave the right-holder possession of a definite "thing," such as money or property, or of a zone of autonomy in which the right-holder could act without government interference (e.g., "liberty of contract"). To say that someone had a "right" to have a decisionmaker exercise discretion by taking into account certain factors was thought by many to be a contradiction in terms.

In addition, the courts' negative response reflected a more general judicial doctrine known as the "right-privilege distinction." According to this concept, "rights" were generated primarily by contractual relationships. Most government benefits—even employment—were conceived of as something else, a "privilege," as to which the beneficiary had few if any rights, and which could be diminished or withdrawn at any time, for any reason—even in retaliation for the beneficiary's exercise of a constitutional right such as freedom of speech. See Van Alstyne 1968. The major justification advanced for the right-privilege distinction was (and remains) the "greater power/lesser power" argument. If the government has no constitutional duty to maintain a Medicaid program, a welfare system, or a child protection agency, then it can terminate the service or benefit at any time. The power of complete termination is said to "include," as a matter of "logic," the "lesser" power to place conditions on access to the benefit, even conditions that might seem "harsh," such as refusal to pay for a constitutionally protected therapeutic abortion, or to provide effective protection against child abuse. See Harris v. McCrae, 448 U.S. 297 (1980); DeShaney v. Winnebago County Dept. of Social Services, 109 S.Ct. 998 (1989); Sullivan 1989; Kreimer 1984; Rosenblatt 1982; Hale 1935.

The New Deal, the Civil Rights Movement, and other social developments interacted with, and helped to form, new patterns of legal thought that rejected the right-privilege distinction and its underlying image of society as a set of disconnected individuals bound together only by explicit laws and agreements. See, e.g., Rosenblatt 1970, 1990; Mensch 1990. By the mid-1960s, the impact of unreviewable government discretion on welfare recipients and other government beneficiaries had been subjected to powerful critical analysis by legal scholars such as Jacobus TenBroek, Charles Reich, and Edward Sparer (TenBroek 1954; Reich 1964, 1965; Sparer 1965). The combination of social movements, critical legal scholarship, and other cultural changes helped persuade lower federal courts in the middle 1960s to recognize for the first time that welfare recipients had a legal entitlement to their benefits if they satisfied the eligibility standards set out in the federal law. The United States Supreme Court adopted this entitlement approach, and rejected the right-privilege distinction, in four landmark rulings decided between 1968 and 1970.[11]

11. See King v. Smith, 392 U.S. 309 (1968) (state cannot define mother's sexual partner as a "parent," thereby depriving child of welfare eligibility, because the Court interpreted the term "parent" in the federal Social Security Act to mean an adult with a legal obligation of support, 392 U.S. at 329); Shapiro v. Thompson, 394 U.S. 618 (1969) (state cannot impose, and federal

The Court's opinion in one of these cases, Rosado v. Wyman, 397 U.S. 397 (1970), embodied a broad judicial coalition in favor of a new conception of federal statutory rights. The opinion was authored by Justice John Marshall Harlan, a what-was-then-thought-of-as-conservative Republican, and was joined by justices across the political spectrum: his fellow Republican Stewart, liberal Democrats Douglas, Brennan, and Marshall, and conservative Democrat White.[12] Justice Harlan's opinion stood for several important principles, all of which contradicted the right-privilege distinction and related concepts about the limited, bright-line nature of legal rights. First, even obscure statutory provisions, dealing with complex issues of social policy (in *Rosado*, about cost-of-living adjustments to welfare eligibility standards), should be interpreted if at all possible as sources of meaningful law. In particular, courts (and agencies) should avoid reading statutes in ways that make them "a futile, hollow, even deceptive gesture," 397 U.S. at 415—laws that seem to promise something for the poor, but "really" mean nothing more than formal assurances and empty bureaucratic labels.

Second, courts should not shrink from a full inquiry into complex statutes and legislative history. "Congress," wrote Justice Harlan, "as it frequently does, has voiced its wishes in muted strains and left it to the courts to discern the theme in the cacophony of political understanding." 397 U.S. at 412. Third, congressional compromise may result in a statute that contemplates not a clear rule or benefit, but a process of structured discretion, in which a federal or state agency may make a policy choice, but also is supposed to take certain information and values into account. Even though such a provision confers discretion, it also creates an obligation to take certain factors into account in exercising it, and a corollary "right" on behalf of the ultimate beneficiaries to have that consideration

---

law cannot authorize, a one-year residency requirement prior to welfare eligibility, because such a requirement penalizes the constitutional right of interstate travel); Goldberg v. Kelly, 397 U.S. 254 (1970) (state cannot impose, and federal law cannot authorize, termination of welfare benefits without a hearing consistent with the constitutional right to due process, because erroneous termination of benefits might imperil a recipient's health or even life); Rosado v. Wyman, 397 U.S. 397 (1970) (state cannot reduce standard of need used to determine eligibility in violation of federal statute; federal statute judicially enforceable by recipients against state without waiting for federal agency to rule on the question). For a discussion of similar developments taking place at the same time in administrative law generally, see Stewart 1975; Rosenblatt 1978: 253–64.

12. Justice Black, joined by Chief Justice Burger, dissented, for reasons discussed in note 14 below. (There were eight justices, rather than the usual nine, on the Court when *Rosado* was decided.) Justice Harlan's opinion built on (but did not entirely affirm) federal District Judge Jack B. Weinstein's pathbreaking trial court opinion, 304 F.Supp. 1356 (E.D.N.Y. 1969).

take place.[13] Fourth, statutes such as these, even when framed as conditions on federal funding to the states, can be treated as individual (and, through class actions, group) rights, enforceable in court directly against the relevant decisionmakers. The fact that Congress has also delegated to a federal agency authority to define and enforce these statutory conditions does not preclude judicial action, unless Congress has clearly indicated such preclusion. This is particularly so where neither Congress nor the agency has given beneficiaries access to the administrative process or effective administrative remedies. "We are most reluctant," wrote Justice Harlan, "to assume that Congress has closed the avenue of effective judicial review to those individuals most directly affected by the administration of the program." 397 U.S. at 420.[14]

Between 1970 and 1990, the *Rosado* principles achieved remarkable acceptance by Congress, the lower federal courts, and the Supreme Court itself. First, in contrast to Justice Black's suggestion in his *Rosado* dissent (see footnote 14 above), Congress did not appear committed to HEW's primary enforcement responsibility, because it never amended the Social Security Act to require it, although it was aware of *Rosado* and other rulings and amended the law on other matters many times thereafter. On the contrary, Congress explicitly recognized and approved prospective judicial remedies (that is, court orders requiring states to change policies prospectively, as distinct from money damages for past violations) in the legislative history to a 1976 Medicaid amendment. Wilder v. Virginia Hospital Association, 110 S.Ct. 2510, 2521–22 (1990). Moreover, in 1980 Congress explicitly endorsed beneficiary litigation against state officials to enforce federal funding requirements when it removed the $10,000 amount in controversy provision for federal court jurisdiction over cases involving federal statutes (Rosenblatt 1991: 832).

13. *Rosado* can be viewed from a technical perspective as not being about structured discretion, because the Court interpreted the particular provision at issue as a mandate to the states to adjust their standards of need, leaving them no, or virtually no, discretion as to that matter. However, the opinion places this interpretation in a broader context: the states still have discretion to set grant levels at less than the standard of need, and the requirement of updating that standard is understood as part of a process of structuring (through an information requirement) the discretionary process. 397 U.S. at 413–414.

14. In contrast, Justice Black's dissent focused on the statutory sections providing for HEW review of state plans, found an "unmistakable [legislative] intent" to give HEW primary jurisdiction," 397 U.S. at 431 (Black, J., dissenting), and therefore concluded that all judicial consideration of issues subject to HEW review should be precluded until HEW had reached its decision, although judicial review might be available thereafter. 397 U.S. at 435. Interestingly, HEW itself, through its *amicus* brief, chose not to discuss the jurisdictional or administrative process issues, and focused solely on its interpretation on the merits of the statute.

From the mid-1960s to the present, the lower federal courts have decided hundreds, perhaps thousands of cases brought by beneficiaries and providers involving federal funding requirements in the cash assistance, Medicaid, housing assistance, and other federal programs. The Supreme Court itself has decided many of these cases on the merits, and has further clarified the statutory basis of the *Rosado* principles. In Maine v. Thiboutot, 448 U.S. 1 (1980), a cash assistance case, the Court held that any federal statute, including those imposing conditions on federal funding, could create a right enforceable in federal court under the general federal cause of action statute, 42 U.S.C. § 1983.[15] Moreover, in a case involving environmental restrictions on federal funding of highways, the Supreme Court stated again that courts could review, albeit deferentially, the way agencies exercised their structured or bounded discretion. The court's task is not to substitute its judgment for that of the agency, but rather to determine if the agency action was based upon "a consideration of the relevant factors and whether there has been a clear error of judgment." Citizens to Preserve Overton Park v. Volpe, 401 U.S. 402, 416 (1971).

The rights-enforcing role that American courts developed from the late 1960s to the present can be seen as a matter of some pride. In human and political terms, it represents at least in part an effort to protect vulnerable individuals and groups (e.g., the poor, the chronically ill, nursing home residents, abused children, institutionalized mental patients, and the retarded) from powerful pressures to de-fund their programs and ignore laws designed to meet their needs. In intellectual terms, it represents a major effort to articulate a theory of law for the modern welfare state, one that recognizes and seeks to reconcile the tensions among the fundamental interests of individuals, the needs of groups, and the competing claims on and complex processes of the polity at large. See Rosenblatt 1991, 1990. At the same time, one can feel a certain despair about the whole enterprise. A nation that repeatedly articulates humane intentions in its laws, then often fails miserably at translating those goals into practical reality, and then spends large human and financial resources litigating whether the goal was really adopted and who has authority to decide its practical

15. This statute, first enacted in 1871, provides a federal cause of action (that is, a right to seek federal judicial relief) to any person who has been deprived under color of state law of "any rights, privileges, or immunities, secured by the Constitution and laws. . . ." 42 U.S.C. § 1983. Although originally enacted in the context of assuring equal legal rights for the newly emancipated slaves, the law has long referred to rights secured "by the Constitution and laws," without specific reference to the issue of racial discrimination. The Court's opinion in *Thiboutot* confirmed the implicit position of many precedents that the Social Security Act and other federal laws could be judicially enforced on the basis of this general statute.

consequences, is, to put it kindly, wasteful and politically paralyzed, as well as failing to meet important human needs.[16]

(B) Judicial Review of Agencies' Structured Discretion: The Example of Medicaid Reimbursement of Institutional Providers

Against this background, how have the federal courts developed the concept of rights in the context of health care financing agencies' structured discretion? Useful illustrations can be found in the many cases brought by institutional providers concerning the Boren Amendment. Enacted in 1980 and 1981 as part of the Omnibus Budget Reconciliation Acts (OBRA), the Boren Amendment repealed the prior requirement of retrospective "reasonable cost" reimbursement and granted states much more discretion in paying hospitals and nursing homes. At the same time, the states' discretion was structured or limited in three ways that were supposed to protect providers and Medicaid beneficiaries. The Boren Amendment requires the states, as a condition of federal funding of their Medicaid programs, to pay hospitals and nursing homes

> through the use of rates (determined in accordance with methods and standards developed by the State . . . and which, in the case of hospitals, take into account the situation of hospitals which serve a disproportionate number of low income patients with special needs . . .) which the State finds, and makes assurances satisfactory to the Secretary [of Health and Human Services] are reasonable and adequate to meet the costs that must be incurred by efficiently and economically operated facilities [in order to provide services consistent with applicable laws and quality standards] . . . and to assure that individuals eligible for [Medicaid] have reasonable access (taking into account geographic location and reasonable travel time) to inpatient hospital services of adequate quality.

42 U.S.C. § 1396a(a) (13) (A) (1982 ed., Supp. V), quoted in Temple University v. White, 941 F.2d 201, 207 (3d Cir. 1991). In more accessible English, the Boren Amendment requires the states, in setting reimburse-

16. In contrast, see Whitney 1993 (newspaper report on German health care system, noting 88 percent of the population covered by government-mandated sickness funds; 1990 health spending of 8.1 percent of Gross National Product [GNP], compared with 12.1 percent of GNP in the United States; recent soaring increases in health care costs; and a "draconian" new cost control law supported by "all the major political parties").

ment rates for institutional providers, to take into account three values or factors: (1) the needs of hospitals that serve a disproportionate number of low-income patients with special needs; and (2) the costs incurred by efficiently and economically operated facilities in order to (a) meet applicable laws and quality standards and (b) assure reasonable access to hospital services for Medicaid patients.

As in the *Rosado* case, the exact signal that Congress was trying to send to federal and state agencies and providers was far from clear. On the one hand, the 1981 Senate Report stated that "[t]he Committee expects that the Secretary will keep regulatory and other requirements to a minimum to assure proper accountability. . . . It is expected that the assurances made by the States will be considered satisfactory in the absence of a formal finding to the contrary by the Secretary." S. Rep. No. 139, 97th Cong., 1st Sess. at 478. On the other hand, the same Senate Report stated that the "flexibility given the States is not intended to encourage arbitrary reductions in payment that would adversely affect the quality of care," and the 1980 Conference Committee Report noted the conferees' "intent that a State not develop rates . . . solely on the basis of budgetary appropriations." S. Rep. No. 139, 97th Cong., 1st Sess. at 478; H.R. Conf. Rep. No. 1479, 96th Cong., 2d Sess. at 154.

To compound this lack of clarity, neither the Boren Amendment nor the legislative history defined any of the key terms, such as "disproportionate share," "reasonable and adequate," "efficiently and economically operated facility," or "reasonable access to inpatient hospital services." Moreover, in its regulations implementing the statute, the federal Department of Health and Human Services (HHS) expressly declined to provide federal definitions; any such attempt "would unnecessarily intrude upon the legislatively mandated flexibility provided to States . . . ." 48 *Federal Register* 56049 (Dec. 19, 1983). Going even further, HHS declined to require each state to provide its own definition of an efficiently and economically operated facility. "The reason for this is that the State's methods and standards implicitly act as the State's definition of an efficiently and economically operated facility, and no explicit definition is necessary." *Federal Register* at 56049. While HHS requires the states to make the "findings" specified in the statute, it does not give guidance as to the form and basis of those findings, nor does it require the states to submit the findings themselves or any underlying data. *Wilder*, 110 S.Ct. at 2516. The state must submit only "assurances" that the required findings have been made, plus general information about estimated average payments to types of providers (e.g., hospitals, nursing homes), changes in such payments since the previous year, and estimated consequences of the changes.[17]

Anyone familiar with the history of the free care and community service requirements of the Hill-Burton hospital construction program,[18] or with previous state efforts to evade federal Medicaid coverage, quality, and reimbursement requirements,[19] is likely to view the above administrative scheme with skepticism and, perhaps, as an open invitation to the states to disregard the Boren Amendment's protective provisions. The lack of definition of key terms, the absence of any operational standards by which to measure compliance, the failure even to ask the states to develop their own criteria and collect information, the lack of a national pool of data—all of this eerily recalls the Hill-Burton experience and suggests that the designers of this plan are practicing what Murray Edelman terms "symbolic politics": the appearance of serving an important public value, while hiding the reality of subverting it (Edelman 1964; Rosenblatt 1978). As in earlier struggles over Hill-Burton and Medicaid, the federal courts have been virtually the only forum in which the political-legal debate could take place about whether the Boren Amendment's protective provisions should be treated as window-dressing, or whether they should have real impact on state policy.

Given Congress's lack of clarity, it is not surprising that the federal

17. In addition to the information noted in the text, states are supposed to include estimates of the short-term and (if feasible) long-term effects of the changes in average payments on availability of services, type of care furnished, extent of provider participation, and the degree to which costs are covered in hospitals that serve a disproportionate share of low-income patients with special needs. 42 C.F.R. § 447.255 (1991). While these requirements could in theory provide a basis for scrutiny (although the apparent focus on statewide averages and estimates might well miss important local problems), it appears from the *AMISUB* and *Temple University* cases discussed below that at least in some cases, HHS accepts assurances with little inquiry into their underlying basis.

18. See, e.g., Cook v. Ochsner Foundation Hosp., 61 F.R.D. 354 (E.D.La. 1972) (finding HEW Secretary's failure to issue regulations protecting low-income patients from exclusion from Hill-Burton grantee hospitals, and failure to require such hospitals to accept Medicaid patients, violates the Hill-Burton Act), and other Hill-Burton developments discussed in Rosenblatt 1978: 264–86.

19. See, e.g., Mitchell v. Johnson, 701 F.2d 337 (5th Cir. 1983) (striking down repeated state attempts to drastically cut dental benefits to children, as violating federal statutory coverage requirements); Smith v. Vowell, 379 F.Supp. 139 (W.D. Tex.), *aff'd* 504 F.2d 759 (5th Cir. 1974) (requiring state to provide safe transportation to seriously disabled Medicaid beneficiaries so they could obtain needed care from available providers). Cf.Estate of Smith v. Heckler, 747 F.2d 583 (10th Cir. 1984) (holding that the HHS Secretary has a duty to inform herself of nursing home conditions relevant to the Medicaid statutory standard of quality care, and that HHS certification of nursing homes under an inspection system that does not gather relevant information violates that duty).

courts have responded to this question in different ways. Four broad patterns are evident in the opinions. Some courts focus on the state discretion theme in the statute and regulations and uphold virtually *any* state reimbursement plan, no matter how inconsistent with the Boren Amendment protections.[20] A second approach is not to require the state to make written findings or studies of hospital efficiency and reasonable access, but to look for some process in which it can plausibly be said the Boren protections were taken into account, and to guard against rate reductions so severe "that a dangerous number of hospitals, or single medically important hospitals, might withdraw from the program." Mary Washington Hospital v. Fisher, 635 F.Supp. 891, 902 (E.D. Va. 1985). A process in which the state considers a number of budget reduction options, evaluates their impact on each hospital, and chooses an option which does not cause severe financial hardship to any provider or group of providers is regarded as falling "within range of what could be considered reasonable and adequate." *Mary Washington*, 635 F.Supp. at 901.[21]

A third approach is to take the HHS administrative system seriously—more seriously, apparently, than HHS does itself. Thus in 1982, Nebraska, pursuant to a new reimbursement plan, refused to accept updated cost reports from nursing homes and imposed a 3.75 percent cap on increased costs. The plan was filed with HHS with the requisite Boren Amendment assurances and approved. Yet when providers challenged the 3.75 percent cap in federal court, the state conceded that it "did not conduct any objective analysis or studies to determine the effects [of the new reimbursement system] on the level of care Medicaid patients would receive or the extent to which facilities would continue to participate in Medicaid." Citing the HHS regulation requiring (at that time) that the states submit a "quantified estimate" of the short-term and (to the extent feasible) long-term

20. See, for example, *AMISUB (PSL) Inc. v. State of Colorado Dept. of Social Services*, 698 F.Supp. 217 (D.Colo. 1988) (upholding DRG-based reimbursement system that reduced allowable costs by 46 percent to limit hospital reimbursement to the sums "historically appropriated by the State legislature," even though the payments thus arrived at had "no relation to the actual costs of hospital services"), 698 F.Supp. at 219, *reversed*, 879 F.2d 789 (10th Cir. 1989).

21. See also Colorado Health Care Assoc. v. Colorado Dept. of Social Services, 842 F.2d 1158, 1168 (10th Cir. 1988). Notably, in this approach the burden of proving severe financial impact and its effect on "reasonable access" is on the providers; if no particular provider comes forward with such evidence, the plan is presumed to be adequate. *Mary Washington*, 635 F.Supp. at 902 (upholding plan); Kansas Health Care Assoc. v. Kansas Dept. of Social & Rehabilitation Services, 958 F.2d 1018, 1022–23 (10th Cir. 1992) (vacating injunction on grounds that industry associations do not have standing; whether reimbursement policy is illegal depends on facts specific to each nursing home). Cf. Anderson and Hall 1992: 213, 234 (predicting that few hospitals would or could prove that reduced Medicaid reimbursement would lower access or quality of care).

effects of the rate change on availability, type of care, and provider participation,[22] the court concluded that the state's assurances violated HHS's own regulation, because they were not supported by the type of information HHS itself required. HHS's own approval was therefore invalid, and the state could be prohibited from implementing the new reimbursement plan. Nebraska Health Care Assoc. v. Dunning, 778 F.2d 1291, 1294 (8th Cir. 1985).

A fourth approach takes, in a sense, the opposite tack from the third. Where *Nebraska Health Care* focuses on what the state has not reported to HHS, other courts look at what decisionmaking process and studies the state has undertaken itself. Noting that HHS does not even look at the state's findings and exercises virtually no independent review, these courts conclude that the requirement of findings in the statute and regulations is largely independent of the administrative process, and therefore if it is to mean anything at all, it must be a serious duty imposed on the states and reviewable by the courts.

> While it is true that a state is free to create its own method for arriving at the required findings, this does not absolve the state from making the required findings. . . . Mere recitation of the wording of the federal statute is not sufficient for procedural compliance. There is a presumption that a state will engage in a bona fide finding process before it makes assurances to HCFA [the relevant sub-agency within HHS]. . . . To rule otherwise would completely eviscerate the federal requirements so long as the magic words are submitted to HCFA.

AMISUB (PSL) Inc. v. State of Colorado Dept. of Social Services, 879 F.2d 789, 797 (10th Cir. 1989). Under this approach, in contrast to cases such as *Mary Washington*, the efficiency and economy provisions of the Boren Amendment are understood as imposing an obligation on the state agencies

> to make "findings" which identify and determine (1) efficiently and economically operated hospitals; (2) the costs that must be incurred by such hospitals; and (3) payment rates which are reasonable and adequate to meet the reasonable costs of the state's efficiently and economically operated hospitals.

22. The requirement of a "quantified estimate" was contained in HHS's interim regulations. In the final regulations, issued December 19, 1983, HHS dropped the term "quantified," in response to state concerns that "quantified data may not always be available or may be burdensome to gather. . . ." 48 *Federal Register* 56056 (Dec. 19, 1983).

AMISUB at 796. Since in the *AMISUB* litigation the relevant state official "readily admitted the State did not determine which hospitals are efficiently and economically run, and made no efforts to do so. . . . [nor did the State] determine the costs that must be incurred by the efficiently and economically operated hospitals," *AMISUB* at 796, the Tenth Circuit Court of Appeals had little difficulty concluding that the state reimbursement plan violated the procedural requirements of the Boren Amendment regarding the necessary findings. *AMISUB* at 797. The court also held the Colorado plan in violation of the Boren Amendment's substantive efficiency and economy requirements, finding that under the plan no Colorado hospital was reasonably or adequately compensated, including those that qualified as efficiently and economically operated under one of several methodologies. *AMISUB* at 797–99.

The *AMISUB* opinion demonstrates the considerable significance of the courts' rights-enforcing role. Once a court concludes that a statutory provision creates a "right," there is inevitable pressure to give that right some operational or coherent meaning. The Boren Amendment requires states to pay health care institutions on the basis of rates "which the State *finds* . . . are reasonable and adequate to meet the costs that must be incurred by efficiently and economically operated facilities [in order to achieve quality and access goals]" (emphasis supplied). What must the states actually do to comply with this provision? The position taken by HHS and many states was that the state rate-setting methodology itself operates implicitly "as the State's definition of an efficiently and economically operated facility, and no explicit definition is necessary." 48 *Federal Register* 56049 (Dec. 19, 1983). In particular, both HHS and the states focus on the extent of dollar changes in the new rates; if a state's new rates are the same as last year's budget, perhaps with a small inflation factor, they are said to be "adequate" for an "efficient" hospital, regardless of the actual increased costs that the hospitals may have experienced, and the degree of shortfall between Medicaid rates and any accepted cost methodology. See *AMISUB*, 879 F.2d at 796, 799, 800–01. Here is the critical issue: do the states have discretion to define adequacy and efficiency solely in terms of their own rate-setting methodologies, or must they use, however "implicitly," concepts of efficiency, adequacy (and the other Boren factors) that have some grounding outside the state's own rate-setting methods and, as is almost always the case, budgetary pressures? See Multicare Medical Center v. State of Washington, 768 F.Supp. 1349 (W.D. Wash. 1991) (rejecting as circular the state's argument that rate-setting methods define efficiency).

The real-world impact of these questions is apparent. Thus federal District Judge John Fullam found that Temple University Hospital, located in a "North Philadelphia community that is principally black, hispanic, and indigent," would lose about $7.8 million in 1988–89 by treating Medicaid patients, about 55 percent of its caseload. Temple University v. White, 729 F.Supp. 1093, 1095–96 (E.D.Pa. 1990). The hospital presented "a mass of evidence, which stands unrebutted, to the effect that it has cut costs in every conceivable way, and that, as a practical matter, no further 'efficiency' or 'economy' is possible," *Temple University* at 1096. The state's reimbursement system paid the hospital on the basis of a peer group median, added 2.5 percent for Temple's disproportionate share of low-income patients, and cut 14 percent from all hospitals in order to hold total hospital payments within a pre-set budgetary appropriation. In establishing this system, Judge Fullam found, and the Third Circuit Court of Appeals agreed, that Pennsylvania "had conducted no analysis and made no findings" as to the reasonableness and adequacy of its rates in relation to economy and efficiency and reasonable access. *Temple University* at 1100; 941 F.2d 201, 210 (3d Cir. 1991), *cert. denied*, 112 S.Ct. 873 (1992). Both courts held the state's reimbursement system in violation of the Boren Amendment and secured significant additional funding for Temple and other hospitals.

Temple University stands as an unusual case in which litigators and judges were able to get additional resources to institutions that were actually serving the poor.[23] In the majority of Boren Amendment cases, courts have used the first or second approaches discussed above and have denied relief, either on the merits or on procedural and jurisdictional grounds. Are the opinions in *AMISUB* and *Temple University* correct in interpreting the law so as to require the states to make findings based on studies that focus on economy, efficiency, and reasonable access to services?[24] Litigation over this question has not, for the most part, reached this issue

23. See Strickler 1991. However, the fragility of this relief is striking. The hospitals and the state of Pennsylvania eventually settled the *Temple University* case by funding additional Medicaid hospital reimbursement through "hospital contributions" to the Medicaid program (letter from Matthew M. Strickler, Esq., to author, January 4, 1993). This in effect operates as a temporary contribution by hospitals, which is then leveraged by matching federal Medicaid payments. In response to use of this device by an increasing number of states, Congress "narrowly restricted the types and amounts of such taxes and donations that may qualify for federal matching funds. Pub. L. No. 102-234 (signed into law Dec. 12, 1991)." Anderson and Hall 1992: 230 n.101. See also Spivey 1992. As a result, when the *Temple University* settlement expires on June 30, 1993, "Pennsylvania anticipates a substantial deficit in the Medicaid program and intends to cut payments. . . . Anticipate further litigation on July 1" (letter from Matthew M. Strickler to author, January 4, 1993).

24. For an analysis critical of these cases, see Anderson and Hall 1992. Anderson and Hall do not rely primarily on the textual formalism advanced by Chief Justice Rehnquist, see Part Two of this article, but rather on utilitarian and institutional competence arguments.

squarely, but rather has focused on more primitive or preliminary disagreement about the proper *methods of thought* to be used in interpreting statutes and, more broadly, identifying sources of law. Advocates and judges have been drawn back to the questions raised in Section (A) and in the Introduction: What are "rights" and their sources? Must they be clear, "bright lines" explicitly set out in procedurally correct texts? Or may they be opaque compromises that signal an (unclear) political "context" or "direction"? Is the courts' only legitimate role to "implement" the clear value choices made by the political branches, or do the courts have a legitimate, albeit specialized, role in helping to construct and clarify policy choices and direction? These questions have been made highly visible by the first (and thus far only) Boren Amendment case to generate a full Supreme Court opinion, in which the justices re-opened the question seemingly answered by *Rosado* twenty years before: *Could* the courts, at the request of providers, consider the Boren Amendment at all?

Part II The Contemporary Judicial Challenge to the Courts' Rights-Enforcing Role

Despite the broad acceptance by Congress and the courts of the rights-enforcing judicial role embodied in *Rosado* and other cases, it is not surprising that this role has always generated significant opposition. This is because the "problem" that generates the *need* for the role is rooted in strong political forces. On the one hand, the government and politically dominant interests wish to present themselves as responsive to important human needs and political movements, and indeed as presiding over a reasonably humane, civilized, and bonded-together society. On the other hand, these decisionmakers often have a simultaneous desire not to pay the costs in money and power that really achieving such a society would entail. The result is the familiar and depressing gap between statutory promise and administrative/political reality that we have observed with respect to the Boren Amendment and other social legislation.

There are three possible judicial responses to litigation challenging the gap as illegal. The first is to confirm that the statute creates rights and legitimate expectations, take those rights seriously in operational terms, acknowledge the existence of an illegal gap between those rights and agency practice, and order the gap to be closed or at least reduced. See *AMISUB* and *Temple University*, discussed above. A second approach purports to confirm that the statute creates rights and legitimate expectations, and then declares that there is no gap—for example, that "normal"

state methods of reducing hospital reimbursement are deemed to constitute the required Boren Amendment findings. See *Mary Washington*, 635
F.Supp. 891, discussed above. The first approach will obviously be opposed by all the forces (including bureaucratic) in whose interests the gap
was created in the first place. The second approach, if managed properly
from the perspective of the gap-maintainers, can serve the useful function
of taking the statutory promises just seriously enough to support the belief
that the promises are real, but not so seriously that any money has to be
spent or power shared, i.e., to maintain simultaneously the gap and the
belief that it does not exist. This approach is inherently risky, however, because once a right has been recognized and a judicial forum provided for
its elaboration and enforcement, there is a danger that some litigators and
judges may persuade themselves and others to move to the first approach.

Chief Justice Rehnquist and his like-minded colleagues on the United
States Supreme Court have recently promoted a third approach: to close
the gap by denying that the statute creates any rights at all, except under
very stringent conditions. The gap is said to disappear because if the
statute creates no rights, then it consigns all policy issues to the unbounded
or unstructured discretion of the government agencies. Whatever they do
is adequate, because the statute delegates to them the authority to define
what is adequate. Of course, from the perspective of the managers of this
system, this approach largely forgoes the benefits of even the appearance
of caring about the values purportedly protected by the statute—such as
the Boren Amendment's reasonable access and economy and efficiency
provisions. On the other hand, this approach more clearly and decisively
allocates power to the Executive Branch and (where relevant) the states,
and makes it much more difficult for Congress to "structure" federal and
state agency discretion.

Chief Justice Rehnquist's approach was prominently articulated in his
dissent in Wilder v. Virginia Hospital Association, 110 S.Ct. 2510 (1990).
A five-justice majority of the Court, in an opinion by Justice William
Brennan,[25] rejected the state's argument that the Boren Amendment created no rights for hospitals, and explicitly re-affirmed the rights-enforcing
role established by *Rosado*, *Thiboutot*, and many other cases. See Rosenblatt 1991. In particular, Justice Brennan held that the mere existence of
HHS authority to receive the states' "assurances" was not a clear indication of congressional preclusion; nor was the very limited HHS process,

25. Justice Brennan's opinion was joined by Justices White and Marshall (who had been,
with Brennan, members of the *Rosado* majority), and by Justices Blackmun and Stevens.

which contained no opportunity for provider or beneficiary input, a "comprehensive administrative scheme" that would be disturbed by judicial intervention. 110 S.Ct. at 2523–25.

The remarkable aspect of *Wilder* was not the majority opinion, which defended a long line of precedents, but the slim size of the majority (five justices out of nine), and the sweeping nature of Chief Justice Rehnquist's dissent on behalf of himself and Justices O'Connor, Scalia, and Kennedy. Chief Justice Rehnquist advanced three arguments. First, he noted that the literal words of the Boren Amendment do not create explicit rights on behalf of providers; rather, the words are addressed to the states and establish conditions for receiving federal funding. 110 S.Ct. at 2526–27. This alone, he argued, is enough to defeat the hospitals' claim, because

> the first step in our exposition of a statute always is to look to the statute's text and *to stop there if the text fully reveals its meaning*. . . .
> " '[O]ur starting point must be the language employed by Congress' and we assume 'that the legislative purpose is expressed by the ordinary meaning of the words used' . . . ."

110 S.Ct. at 2526 (citations omitted) (emphasis added).

Second, Chief Justice Rehnquist took the position that even if the Boren Amendment is interpreted as creating a right to "reasonable and adequate rates," the statute immediately qualifies that right by defining the "procedures" by which those rates are to be determined, namely, that the state must make certain "findings" and submit certain "assurances" satisfactory to the Secretary of HHS. Thus the hospitals' only federal right is to have the state "make findings" and submit assurances satisfactory to the Secretary. Once the state has done that, as a formal matter, hospitals have no right to challenge the basis of those findings or whether the state has actually considered any of the statutory factors; the statute assigns such review solely to the Secretary. 110 S.Ct. at 2527. Third, Chief Justice Rehnquist buttressed this position by reference to the "basic purpose" of the Boren Amendment, which, according to him, is "to allow the States more latitude in establishing Medicaid reimbursement rates," 110 S.Ct. at 2527. This purpose would be frustrated by allowing courts to order the states to adopt rates other than ones they wished to use and which were acceptable to HHS. 110 S.Ct. at 2527, 2525.

Justice Brennan's response to these arguments echoed *Rosado* and other cases in the rights-enforcing tradition. First, he disputed Chief Justice Rehnquist's method of interpreting texts. Relying on detailed precedent, Brennan argued that the proper method is not to search for magic words such as "right" or "cause of action," but rather to inquire whether the statute creates a "binding obligation" on a government agency to do something. If so, and if that obligation was intended to benefit the party seeking to enforce it, then that party (in this case, hospitals) has a federal right under the statute and a federal cause of action (again, a right to seek judicial relief) under 42 U.S.C. § 1983. Since the language of the Boren Amendment clearly states a mandatory condition of federal funding ("a State [Medicaid] plan . . . must . . . provide . . . for payment . . . of hospital [and nursing home] services . . . [according to the Boren Amendment factors]"), it creates a binding obligation for the benefit of hospitals and nursing homes. 110 S.Ct. at 2517–19.

Second, Brennan rejected Rehnquist's argument that if the Boren Amendment creates a right, it is only a right to have certain "procedures" adhered to as a matter of form.

> Any argument that the requirements of findings and assurances are procedural requirements only and do not require the State to adopt rates that are actually reasonable and adequate is nothing more than an argument that the State's findings and assurances need not be correct.
>
> We reject that argument because it would render the statutory requirements of findings and assurances, and thus the entire reimbursement provision, essentially meaningless. . . . We decline to adopt an interpretation of the Boren Amendment that would render it a dead letter. See *Rosado v. Wyman* (citation omitted), ...

110 S.Ct. at 2519–20. Justice Brennan conceded that the statute granted the states discretion to make choices, and that there might well be a range of rates that would qualify as reasonable. But "there certainly are *some* rates outside that range that no State could ever find to be reasonable and adequate under the Act." 110 S.Ct. at 2523.[26]

Given that the statute *can* be given operational, judicially enforceable meaning, Brennan believed that it *should* be given such meaning, especially because there are strong arguments that that is what Congress intended. Rather than being too "vague and amorphous" to be judicially

26. As examples of such impermissible findings, Justice Brennan cited *AMISUB* and *West Virginia University Hospitals v. Casey*, 885 F.2d 11 (3d Cir. 1989), a case successfully attacking on behalf of out-of-state hospitals the Pennsylvania reimbursement system that was also struck down on behalf of in-state hospitals in *Temple University*. Justice Brennan further supported his position by reference to the 1976 legislative history of another Medicaid provision expressing approval of judicially enforceable provider rights, and the Boren Amendment committee reports noting that the states were not supposed to make arbitrary payment reductions. 110 S.Ct. at 2520–22.

enforceable, Justice Brennan read the statute as requiring the state, "in making its findings, to judge the reasonableness of its rates against the objective benchmark of an 'efficiently and economically operated facility' providing care in compliance with federal and state standards while at the same time ensuring 'reasonable access' to eligible participants." 110 S.Ct. at 2523. While not deciding the exact degree of deference that courts should give to state agencies, Brennan did suggest that the state's findings regarding the costs of efficient facilities had to refer to some "objective benchmark" other than the state's rate-setting methodology itself.

Both Justice Brennan and Chief Justice Rehnquist focus their debate on "what is Congress' true intent?" But as to that issue, it seems to me that Justice Brennan clearly has the better arguments. He is correct that there are more than twenty years of judicial precedents recognizing and enforcing rights derived from federal funding conditions. He is correct that Congress is aware of, and has approved of, those judicial decisions. Justice Brennan does not say this, but it seems quite likely that a Congress with a Democratic majority, locked in constant, long-term conflict over social legislation and spending with a series of Republican Administrations, would value highly the additional pressure that litigants could exert through the courts in support of congressional goals. Whatever the exact weight of that value, and conceding that the Democratic Party is split on many issues and undergoing change, it seems inconceivable that the Democratic majority would overturn twenty years of judicial precedents that generally operate to its political and policy advantage without any discussion or explicit statutory language. Yet that is the conclusion that Chief Justice Rehnquist purports to derive from what he calls "the ordinary meaning of the words used."

A more plausible reading of Rehnquist's dissent is that while he claims to be talking about what congressional intent "is," he is actually talking about how *courts* should "determine" that intent. From a political perspective this makes much more sense. While Congress has been controlled by the Democrats for many years (with a brief exception for the Senate), the political complexion of the *courts* has changed dramatically, as Presidents Reagan and Bush have appointed the majority of the federal judiciary. Ironically, while Chief Justice Rehnquist makes elaborate obeisance to congressional intent, he is actually instructing the increasingly Republican judiciary to disregard the most likely meaning of that intent, and instead to interpret statutes as granting unreviewable, plenary discretion to the (hitherto Republican) federal Executive and to state agencies forced by budget pressures to disregard congressional safeguards for the poor and other politically weak groups.

This is not to say that Rehnquist's approach is "political" and Brennan's is not, or that Rehnquist's is a "narrower" form of politics than Brennan's. Both Rehnquist's and Brennan's approaches can be discussed in terms of their impact on short- and medium-term partisan struggles, and both can also be linked to long-standing debates about political and legal theory. I do believe, however, that Brennan's is a more defensible kind of politics, in the broad sense of the term. While Brennan's approach is consistent with the interests of the Democratic congressional majority, it is also consistent with a more general norm that judges should interpret statutes in the light of *congressional* intent. A president whose party is a congressional minority certainly has an opportunity for input, through legislators of his own party, through persuasion and favor-trading generally, and through the veto power.[27] But if, after all this, the congressional majority can secure enactment (and presidential signature or veto override) of provisions that the President may not favor, are not those provisions law? Should not their interpretation be guided by the most likely intent of Congress itself, given the text, statutory structure, legislative history, context of other statutes and judicial precedents, and the statute's political context or direction?

There is a second basis for arguing that Brennan's political-legal choices, in the broad sense, are more defensible than Rehnquist's. By maximizing the opportunity for unreviewable agency discretion, Chief Justice Rehnquist increases the chances of low-visibility, even secret agency nullification of the statutory text. Rehnquist's approach to statutory interpretation, while claiming fidelity to the "ordinary meaning" of the text, in effect adds a secret clause so that the statute reads as follows: "the states must pay provider institutions reasonable and adequate rates to meet the specified statutory goals, *unless budget pressures make it politically convenient not to do so.*" Rehnquist's approach has this effect because it permits the federal agency to approve any assurance, no matter how formal, implausible or false, without the possibility of judicial

---

27. A president can also have post-enactment influence over statutory interpretation through regulations and policy decisions made by executive agencies under his control. However, courts have long held that agency interpretations and policies, while deserving some degree of deference, should not be upheld if they are inconsistent with the statute or represent an arbitrary exercise of discretion in relation to the statute. In *Wilder*, Justice Brennan explicitly declined to decide which of the several different lower court approaches to reviewing state agency action was correct. 110 S.Ct. at 2523 n.18.

review,[28] in a program where this kind of nullification is a known danger. Moreover, this effect is secret because (i) it is not in the text of the statute, and (ii) it would not likely occur to anyone reading the statute as the meaning, ordinary or not, of the words used. The reason it would not likely occur to anyone is that the statute goes to the trouble of speaking of findings and assurances about reasonable access, etc., suggesting that the authors of the statute intended to have some actual effect on policy. Such an interpretive methodology violates not only the most likely meaning of congressional intent, but also the basic premises of our political system. Both Congress and the Executive are supposed to be accountable to the people, but how can they be accountable if they claim the power to act on the basis of secret, or nearly invisible, choices?

Despite these criticisms, it may not surprise readers to learn that Chief Justice Rehnquist's approach now has the support of a majority of the Supreme Court. Justice Brennan retired from the Court in 1990, and Justice Marshall retired in 1991. They were replaced by Justices David Souter and Clarence Thomas, respectively. Having control over which cases it will hear, the newly constituted Court wasted little time in choosing to re-open the question addressed in *Wilder*. In Suter v. Artist M., 112 S.Ct. 1360 (1992), the plaintiffs were children claiming that the Illinois Department of Child and Family Services (DCFS), charged with protecting children from neglect and abuse, had failed to make reasonable efforts to supply appropriate services so as to prevent the removal of children from their homes, or to facilitate reunification of families once removal had occurred. Specifically, after extensive evidentiary hearings, federal District Judge Milton Shadur found that appointment of a caseworker was the essential first step toward providing any services; without a caseworker, no services can be provided. Despite the importance of this step, DCFS often failed to appoint a caseworker for two to six weeks after assuming jurisdiction over a child. Moreover, even after a caseworker was assigned, there was no system for re-assigning the case promptly if, as often happened, the caseworker resigned, was fired, or was absent for an extended

28. In addition to judicial review of state action under 42 U.S.C. § 1983, the federal Administrative Procedure Act (APA), 5 U.S.C. §§ 701–706, authorizes judicial review of federal agency actions to determine if the agency violated a statute or made an arbitrary and capricious decision. However, the APA also exempts from judicial review decisions committed to the agency's discretion, and the Solicitor General argued in *Wilder* that the Secretary of HHS's decision to accept a state's Boren Amendment assurances would be exempt on that ground. 110 S.Ct. at 2520 n.12. Justice Brennan did not resolve this issue, but requiring hospitals to frame their claims not against the agency that made the substantive rate decision (the state agency), but against a federal agency that exercises little oversight for "abuse of discretion," would be to make the hospital's case much more difficult, if it were allowed to be litigated at all.

period. As a result of these problems, hundreds of children had no case-worker assigned to them, and/or were without a caseworker for a month or more. The impact of not having a caseworker is very serious; Judge Shadur found, inter alia, that abused children continue to be abused, hungry children remain hungry, and children in shelters cannot be placed elsewhere, even with relatives willing to care for them.[29] After making these findings, Judge Shadur ordered DCFS to assign or re-assign case-workers within three days of the need to do so, a time frame that DCFS itself had suggested was feasible.

The children's request for federal judicial relief was based on a statute similar in content and structure to the Boren Amendment. The federal Adoption Assistance and Child Welfare Act of 1980 (AACWA), (like the Medicaid law, codified as part of the Social Security Act), 42 U.S.C. §§ 620–628, 670–679a, requires, as a condition of federal funding, that the states submit to the Secretary of HHS for approval a plan that provides, among other requirements,

> that in each case, reasonable efforts will be made (A) prior to the place-ment of a child in foster care, to prevent or eliminate the need for removal of the child from his home, and (B) to make it possible for the child to return to his home. . . .

42 U.S.C. § 671(a)(15). It is worth noting that in developing this statute, Congress had before it massive evidence of harm to children caused by existing state agency foster placement and other child protection prac-tices. Unlike the Boren Amendment, one of whose purposes was to grant the states greater discretion, the AACWA was designed to give the states additional federal funds in return for less discretion and badly needed reforms.[30]

The importance of federal *judicial* enforcement of this provision was made clear in the brief of the American Bar Association, which had made child protection issues a high organizational priority for many years:

> Federal enforcement of the AACWA through administrative moni-toring does not attempt to address states' systemic failures to make reasonable efforts. The Federal Government requires only that there be present in individual case files agency and court documents which re-

29. See Respondents' Brief to the United States Supreme Court, Suter v. Artist M., Docket No. 90-1488, at 4–9, citing to Judge Shadur's unpublished findings of fact.

30. See Artist M. v. Johnson, 917 F.2d 980, 985 (7th Cir. 1990), *rev'd sub nom.* Suter v. Artist M., 112 S.Ct. 1360 (1992); Respondents' Brief to the United States Supreme Court, Suter v. Artist M., Docket No. 90-1488, at 15–17 (citing legislative history).

cite that reasonable efforts were made. As a result, states can ensure that they meet federal requirements simply by amending their child welfare agency and court forms.

Accordingly, without a private cause of action to enforce reasonable efforts on a system-wide basis, there is no effective remedy for grave systemic failures to provide reasonable efforts.

Amicus Brief of the American Bar Association to the United States Supreme Court, Suter v. Artist M., Docket No. 90-1488, at 5.

Chief Justice Rehnquist's opinion for the Court[31] in *Suter* shows strikingly little interest in the facts about agency inaction and its consequences for children. After dryly noting that the District Court made factual findings (without giving any details), the Chief Justice focuses on his real concern: that states, in accepting federal funds, might not have detailed enough notice of all the obligations they were undertaking. Treating the state and the federal governments as arms-length, almost hostile participants in a bargaining process, Rehnquist argues that

"The legitimacy of Congress' power to legislate under the spending power thus rests on whether the State voluntarily and knowingly accepts the terms of the 'contract.' There can, of course, be no knowing acceptance if a State is unaware of the conditions or is unable to ascertain what is expected of it. Accordingly, if Congress intends to impose a condition on the grant of federal moneys, it must do so unambiguously."

Suter, 112 S.Ct. at 1366 (quoting Pennhurst State School and Hospital v. Halderman, 451 U.S. 1, 17 (1981)).

This passage in itself represents a major attack on the rights-enforcing model. As we have seen, the *Rosado* opinion, the Boren Amendment litigation, and many other cases stand for the principle that even though congressional intent may be complex and ambiguous, the role of the courts is, if at all possible, to give a federal funding statute some operational meaning so as to advance its intended goals. Chief Justice Rehnquist stands this principle on its head: in order to protect the states from alleged surprises, congressional ambiguity should be interpreted as an intent *not* to have any operational effect, and the statutory text should therefore be understood either as merely "hortatory" (Rehnquist's conclusion in the *Pennhurst*

31. The opinion was joined by Justices O'Connor, Scalia, Kennedy, Souter, Thomas, and, mysteriously, White, who had voted with the *Wilder* majority. For why I consider Justice White's silent joinder of Rehnquist's opinion "mysterious," see footnote 33 below.

case),[32] or, as in *Suter*, limited "exactly" to its express words. Since the AACWA's reasonable effort provision is framed as a mandatory condition on federal funding, Rehnquist concedes that it places a "requirement" on the states, but that "requirement," according to the statute's "exact" words, is only to submit an assurance to the Secretary of HHS. Illinois had submitted such an assurance, and the statute, according to Rehnquist, delegated to the Secretary the decision as to whether it was adequate. Thus the statute created no rights that individuals could enforce.

This, of course, is exactly the approach to statutory interpretation that Chief Justice Rehnquist unsuccessfully advanced in *Wilder*. In his *Suter* opinion, Rehnquist does not literally overrule *Wilder*; rather, he purports to distinguish it by arguing that the Boren Amendment contains more detailed requirements than the AACWA's reasonable effort provision and, therefore, that the former can be properly interpreted as creating enforceable rights, while the latter cannot. 112 S.Ct. at 1368. (Of course, Rehnquist had argued in his *Wilder* dissent that the Boren Amendment created no such rights and required only the filing of assurances.) In an interesting turn of phrase, the Chief Justice states that in *Wilder* "we held that the Boren Amendment actually required the States to adopt reasonable and adequate rates. . . ." 112 S.Ct. at 1368. The clear implication is that in his *Suter* opinion, the federal statute is being interpreted *not* to require the states to actually make reasonable efforts to prevent family breakup and to reunite families once broken.

Although *Wilder* has not been overruled, and thus hospitals still have an enforceable right under the Boren Amendment, the methodology of

---

32. *Pennhurst* involved a claim by institutionalized mentally retarded persons under a section of the Developmentally Disabled Assistance and Bill of Rights Act of 1975, 42 U.S.C. § 6000 et seq., titled "Bill of Rights," that provided, inter alia, that persons with developmental disabilities have "a right to appropriate treatment, services, and habilitation," and that the federal and state governments have "an obligation" not to fund institutions that do not provide such services. 42 U.S.C. § 6010. Justice Rehnquist's opinion for the Court held that because this section was not explicitly framed as a mandatory condition of federal funding, it did not create any obligations on the states or enforceable rights on behalf of individuals, 451 U.S. at 13–27, and was instead simply "encouraging" the states through "hortatory" language. 451 U.S. at 24, 27. In an ominous preview of the *Wilder* and *Suter* cases 15 years later, Justice Rehnquist also questioned whether another provision of the Act requiring states to submit assurances to the Secretary of HHS created any enforceable rights under 42 U.S.C. § 1983. 451 U.S. at 28.

Justice Blackmun, concurring in the judgment and in part of Justice Rehnquist's reasoning, disagreed with what he took to be Rehnquist's view that Congress had intended to enact "politically self-serving but essentially meaningless language. . . ." We should avoid, wrote Justice Blackmun, "the odd and perhaps dangerous precedent of ascribing no meaning to a congressional enactment. . . ." 451 U.S. at 32. Justice White, joined by Justices Brennan and Marshall, also disagreed with Justice Rehnquist's statutory interpretation.

Wilder and more than 20 years of precedents has been, without discussion, dramatically ignored.[33] Justice Harry Blackmun's dissent, joined by Justice Stevens, makes the point very clearly:

> In sum, the Court has failed, without explanation, to apply the [doctrinal] framework our precedents have consistently deemed applicable; it has sought to support its conclusion by resurrecting arguments decisively rejected less than two years ago in *Wilder*; and it has contravened 22 years of precedent by suggesting that the existence of other "enforcement mechanisms" precludes sec. 1983 enforcement. At least for this case, it has changed the rules of the game without offering even minimal justification, and it has failed to acknowledge that it is doing anything more extraordinary than "interpret[ing]" the Adoption Act "by its own terms." (citation omitted). Readers of the Court's opinion will not be misled by this hollow assurance. And, after all, we are dealing here with children. . . . I dissent.

Suter, 112 S.Ct. at 1377 (Blackmun, J., dissenting).

Justice Blackmun is correct: Chief Justice Rehnquist is far too modest. While purporting to be simply "following the text," Rehnquist has sought consistently for many years, and has substantially achieved, a counterrevolution in Supreme Court doctrine, indeed, his own "reconstruction" of American social legislation. It is properly called a "counterrevolution" because it draws upon, and to a large extent reinstates, the methodology, premises and doctrines of the pre–rights enforcement era. Thus Rehnquist's *Suter* opinion helps to revive the "right-privilege distinction." As in the past, government spending and benefits do not create rights but are merely privileges, to be granted or withheld according to bureaucratic discretion or, as suggested by the facts in *Suter*, bureaucratic incompetence or indifference. See also Deshaney v. Winnebago County Dept. of Social Services, 109 S.Ct. 998 (1989) (opinion by Rehnquist, C. J.) (four-year-old boy severely injured by father's abuse has no constitutional right to

33. It is for this reason that I characterize Justice Byron White's support of Chief Justice Rehnquist's *Suter* opinion as "mysterious." It may be that Justice White sees a difference between the Boren Amendment and the AACWA reasonable effort requirement, and that difference might justify, in his view, different votes in the two cases. But it is very hard to understand how a justice who agreed with Justice Brennan's methodology in *Wilder* less than two years before *Suter*, who was a member of the original *Rosado* majority, and who wrote a strong dissent from Rehnquist's methodology and conclusion in *Pennhurst*, could support without explanation Rehnquist's radical break in methods of interpreting federal funding statutes. A minimal concern for consistency and craftsmanship would counsel a separate concurring opinion, in which Justice White could have explained why he voted the way he did, the extent to which he agreed with the Chief Justice's new approach, and why.

any level of protection from child protection agency who had assumed jurisdiction over him). Indeed, echoing the late nineteenth century, Chief Justice Rehnquist has held that government benefits can be conditioned on the relinquishing of constitutional rights; thus if they wish to accept federal funds, family planning centers may not exercise professional judgment and freedom of speech by engaging in counseling about abortion. Rust v. Sullivan, 111 S.Ct. 1759 (1991) (opinion by Rehnquist, C. J.).

In addition to the points made above in connection with *Wilder* and *Suter*, Chief Justice Rehnquist's general approach can be usefully understood as "managerial formalism." (See Rosenblatt 1990.) It is formalistic both in its methods of interpretation and in its results. In interpretation, Rehnquist's approach denies its own value-laden premises, ignores the most relevant parts of interpretive context, and purports to be "simply" following "neutral legal principles" and the "obvious" meaning of statutory words.[34] This methodology breaks with the great twentieth-century Supreme Court tradition of contextual interpretation championed by such diverse justices as Holmes, Brandeis, Stone, Frankfurter, and Harlan, and returns to almost a parody of late-nineteenth-century legal formalism. In results, as we have seen, Rehnquist consistently proclaims that the meaning of statutory provisions is to create formalities; if the state files the right piece of paper with the Secretary, containing the proper formal phrases, then the law has been satisfied and courts cannot inquire into what is actually happening to endangered children or to hospitals serving the poor. Rehnquist's approach is "managerial" because its deepest commitment is to enhancing the discretionary power of executive agencies, and limiting the power of what have been to date the two most active federal sources of rights for those at a disadvantage in political, economic and bureaucratic competition: Congress and the federal courts. Whether and to what extent this vision triumphs as the model of American social legislation depends on the values, energies, and skills of those who might oppose it, and whether those values can establish themselves firmly in the political branches of government.

Part III The Need for Reconstruction of American Social Legislation

Those who favor national health care reform that will provide universal coverage, real access to adequate care, and cost control consistent with

34. On the meaning of "formalism" in legal thought, see, e.g., Unger 1975; Kennedy 1973; Mensch 1990; Rosenblatt 1970, 1990.

defensible priorities, perhaps owe Chief Justice Rehnquist some thanks, for making it abundantly clear that the New Deal era model of social legislation is no longer viable. Indeed, if congressional Democrats (assuming they remain in the majority) continue to enact laws on the model of the Social Security Act's welfare and Medicaid provisions—without explicit enforcement rights for providers and beneficiaries, and relying on HHS to monitor complex policy discretion by the states—they can properly be charged with responsibility for the program's likely failure. The challenge is to come up with a much broader and more active concept of what it means to undertake "reform."

A broader vision is needed because the obstacles to change are so deep and so well known. Government agencies put in charge of programs to help the disadvantaged are often hostile to their purported clients, and see their real constituency as the taxpayers and budget directors who have "power to cripple, scuttle, or change an agency that fails to meet [their] expectations" (Edelman 1977: 87). Murray Edelman provides a small but telling example. In 1972, an advocacy group for the poor, the Food Research and Action Center, informed a congressional committee that the Agriculture Department had "knowingly misled" Congress by reporting that only 1,100 schools had asked to participate in a breakfast program for needy children, when actually 4,900 schools had applied. The assistant secretary responsible for the program acknowledged that these figures "would not be that far from being accurate," but still denounced the criticism as "immature, unfair, and intemperate." In Edelman's view, the assistant secretary did not view his job as helping needy children, but as satisfying his real clients (perhaps the budget director and/or the appropriations committee chairman) who did not want a large program. From this perspective, telling the truth about the number of needy children was "unfair" (Edelman 1977: 87–88).

To be sure, many who staff and administer agencies and institutions who serve the disadvantaged are not personally hostile to their clients, and even strive heroically to meet their needs. But the limited resources of welfare and Medicaid agencies, schools and child protection agencies, family courts and public health clinics, often require "street-level bureaucrats" to behave in uncaring ways. The elaborate functions of these programs envisioned by federal funding laws are usually totally unmatched by adequate federal (or any other) funding, generating despair and cynicism among the workers placed in this institutional bind (Lipsky 1980: 29–39).

In addition, American legislators have often conceived of reform as simply supplying additional resources so that people who cannot afford market prices can buy into a functioning market for services. Medicare and Medicaid are in essence designed around this model. For many it may appear to be an adequate model, as long as government reimbursement is sufficient to attract providers and there are no other barriers such as racism, rural residence, and lack of primary care providers.[35] But for many others the subsidized market model is not adequate. It is refreshing, but also shocking in the amount of delay, that after more than 25 years of serious access problems for Medicaid recipients, New York City is beginning to try something more active than just issuing Medicaid cards, by actually contracting with organized providers to supply managed primary care to Medicaid patients (see Belkin 1992). Not surprisingly, this initiative has a double-edged quality: on the one hand, to provide Medicaid patients with a better source of primary care than hospital emergency rooms and, on the other, to control costs and change patterns of both physician and patient behavior. These latter goals are certainly legitimate, but the meaning of the system for patients and doctors depends on the details of how the "management" process is administered and implemented. See Rosenblatt 1986; Annas, Law, Rosenblatt, and Wing 1990: 537–60.

The great lesson of the role of the courts in American social legislation over the past 25 years is that the political process does not end when legislation is enacted. Indeed, one could apply Winston Churchill's World War II comment about the Battle of Egypt and say that enactment of legislation is not the end, or even the beginning of the end, but perhaps the end of the beginning.[36] Theodore Marmor and Michael Barr, in their detailed analysis of competing national health care reform proposals (1992), concur on this point: "[T]he traditional policy analyst's checklist—enumeration of a reform proposal's benefit package, beneficiaries, administration, and financing—gives the appearance of comprehensive analysis without explaining how (or how well) a plan would actually work" (p. 230). One of their five "key questions" about any reform proposal is: "How do we ensure accountability, good quality, and acceptable administration?" (p. 230). As we have seen, these questions are acutely important about any government spending program regarding politically vulnerable social groups, such as minorities and the poor. But they are also important with respect to middle- and higher-income citizens, whose health care interests have also been vitally affected by government policies and by "private"

35. For discussion of some of the deficiencies of market competition models of health care delivery even for middle-income patients, see Rosenblatt 1981.

36. See Winston Churchill's speech at the Mansion House, London, on November 10, 1942, reproduced in his book *The End of the Beginning* (1943) and cited in *The Oxford Dictionary of Quotations* (1992), p. 202, no. 17.

administration by corporations and insurance companies. Moreover, all citizens have been seriously put at risk, and some harmed, by governmental administrative failures to regulate adequately the quality of health care. See, e.g., Annas, Law, Rosenblatt, and Wing 1990: 506–25; Bogdanitch 1991; Estate of Smith v. Heckler, 747 F.2d 583 (10th Cir. 1984) (Secretary of HHS ordered by courts to implement patient-oriented standards to protect nursing home patients from substandard and dangerous care).[37]

I do not claim to have a blueprint for the administration of national health care reform or for the reconstruction of American social legislation. Such topics are surely daunting, in a society afflicted by massive inequalities in income and political influence, severe distrust of government, pervasive focus on one's immediate self-interest, and widespread fraud, corruption, and legalized plunder. See, e.g., Schneider 1992; Barlett and Steele 1992; Phillips 1990; Edsall 1984.[38] At the same time, there remains a substantial reservoir of good will, civic mindedness, and desire to build a better society. Even conceding the large, complex, and unknowable nature of the enterprise, some lessons from our experience of health care (and other social) legislation can be at least tentatively posed as a series of questions or criteria for guiding and evaluating proposals for national health care reform.[39]

1. Does the proposal take account of the large political, bureaucratic, judicial, cultural, and other barriers to change, particularly change designed to moderate inequalities of resources, influence, or access to services? What barriers are identified, and how does the proposal undertake to deal with them?

---

37. It is worth noting that middle-income citizens, in ways somewhat analogous to the poor, have suffered significantly from governmental administrative disregard of their interests in the regulation of savings and loan institutions, banks, corporations, and other sectors of the economy. See generally Barlett and Steele 1992. Barlett and Steele also make clear that while some of these harmful effects have come from administrative failures, most have come from congressional and presidential choices "to favor the privileged, the powerful, and the influential. At the expense of everyone else" (Barlett and Steele 1992: 2). See also note 38 below.

38. If the statement in the text seems too extreme, consider this quotation: " 'To say these guys [the leveraged buy-out tycoons] are entrepreneurs is like saying Jesse James was an entrepreneur,' observed Electronic Data Systems founder Ross Perot. 'In my day, you could make a lot of money creating a new product or backing a new company. But now, if you're an investment banker, you can make many times that amount of money in three or four weeks—and through the miracle of junk bonds leave all the risk with pension funds, S&Ls and banks, all of which are insured by the government. . . . Now it's the taxpayer, the average citizen, who's become the entrepreneur in fact, with all the risk and very little of the reward' " (Phillips 1990: 72).

39. These criteria were influenced and informed by a presentation by Louise Trubek at the 1992 Conference on Critical Legal Networks. See Louise Trubek, "Critical Perspectives on Universal Health Care Plans" (unpublished paper, April 1992).

2. In particular, does the proposal acknowledge the long history of "gaps" between statutory promises and agency performance? How does the proposal undertake to deal with them? Specifically, does the proposal:

   a. create explicit, clear enforcement mechanisms for egalitarian statutory provisions, including the right of beneficiaries to seek judicial relief, and attorneys' fees provisions to finance the litigation?

   b. create clear rules and standards by which higher administrators and courts should review the performance of line decisionmakers?

   c. create positive incentives (e.g., promotions, bonuses, awards) for administrators who effectively and creatively implement egalitarian commitments? penalties for those who disregard and sabotage those commitments?

   d. open the administrative process by requiring consultation with affected interests and groups, with a prominent place for beneficiaries and other traditionally unheard perspectives?

3. Does the proposal take steps to empower beneficiaries and other traditionally unheard perspectives, so they can participate in the administrative, judicial, and political process? Empowerment might include attorneys' fees provisions, and by analogy, advocates' and experts' fees, and subsidies of various kinds (training, travel expenses, staff support, and mandatory job leave with pay) to enable "ordinary citizens" to make their voices heard through "citizen juries."

4. Is the proposal sufficiently flexible in its benefits and reimbursement to fund innovative programs to meet needs most effectively and perhaps also efficiently? An effective program to expand prenatal care, reduce the number of low birthweight babies, and reduce unwed pregnancy might look quite different in a big city housing project than in a rural area, and both might be quite different than a traditional medical model. Even if all health-related services are not included in the national health plan, the plan should take care to coordinate with other approaches, and not privilege a medical model and stifle innovation.

5. Does the proposal attend to meanings and relationships, and not

only to the distribution of authority and material resources? One gets the definite impression, in reading cases like *Suter*, that the point of child protection services—to protect children and help families—has been lost in turf wars, patronage, agency litigation strategy, case processing, and the forms of administration. What does it take to connect the human beings who work for government with the substance of their programs?

These are the kinds of questions that the federal courts began to address, or opened up space for addressing, when they developed the rights-enforcement model in the late 1960s and early 1970s. To be sure, courts and litigation are not the optimum forum for addressing most of these issues, and in most instances, progress in answering them was not spectacular. On the other hand—and this is a sad commentary on American politics and administration—there were not many other forums in which these types of questions were being addressed.[40]

40. An alternative perspective and vocabulary in which some of these questions have been recently addressed is that of "entrepreneurialism" in government. See Osborne and Gaebler 1992. From this perspective, people in government agencies should identify their objectives and "customers," and attempt to supply energetic, creative, and high-quality management and performance said to be characteristic of entrepreneurialism at its best. Osborne and Gaebler are shocked that this approach has not been applied to welfare and public housing programs. They see both programs, first established in the 1930s, as working relatively well as long as their clientele was primarily white. But after World War II, when whites were replaced by "uneducated black sharecroppers from the South, both programs faced an entirely different clientele. Yet both kept operating exactly as they had before. Not surprisingly then, they soon found themselves in deep crisis. Had each program defined its intended outcomes and measured whether they were being achieved, policymakers would have known by 1960 that they had a massive failure brewing. Had their funding been tied to outcomes—how many welfare recipients left the rolls for jobs, how long each family stayed in public housing, the crime rate at each public housing development—the funding would have shifted gradually to those innovators who devised new strategies to deal with the new clientele. But by 1990—*30 years later*—that process had barely begun" (Osborne and Gaebler 1992: 153–54).

The entrepreneurial and rights-enforcing approaches can operate either harmoniously or in tension, depending on how both are conceived. If "rights" are conceived as rigid rules that limit goal-oriented creativity, then the approaches will often be at odds. But if "rights" are conceived as goal-oriented principles, then the two approaches can be mutually supporting. The *Suter* litigation is a good example of rights-enforcement as an effort to induce an agency to achieve minimally adequate management.

Having noted some of the similarities between entrepreneurialism and the questions raised in the text (e.g., systematic identification of goals, barriers, and resources required; strategic planning; positive incentives to reward desired action; measurement and accountability; flexibility and pervasive goal-oriented administration), I also want to note that I do not agree with all of the premises or tone of Osborne and Gaebler. While goal-oriented government management may well contribute to solving the problems of poverty, racism, capital flight, the isolation of the better-off in the suburbs, etc., other factors, forces, and perspectives will be needed as well. For a more realistic and complex view of the phenomena that Osborne and Gaebler treat in two paragraphs—and one that includes the voices of African Americans themselves—see Lemann 1991.

Chief Justice Rehnquist and his like-minded colleagues in the federal judiciary have announced that the federal courts are no longer interested—at least for now—in these sorts of issues. Of course, if reform-minded Democrats continue to control the White House and Congress, and maintain control for a long time, they could eventually change the orientation of the courts through judicial appointments. Even in the short and medium term, it is conceivable that a reformist President and Congress, enacting clear legislation with strong public support, might persuade the more moderate conservative justices to form a new coalition with the remaining liberal justices and revive, at least to some extent, the courts' rights-enforcing role.[41] In addition, many lower federal court judges may remain committed to the rights-enforcing tradition, and resist the new direction to the extent possible in a hierarchical system mitigated by lower court discretion and the flexibility of legal reasoning. Nevertheless, it is at least equally likely that Chief Justice Rehnquist's approach will come to dominate the federal judiciary for a considerable period of time.

This possibility, and its political background, highlight the need for proponents of national health care reform to create alternative forces and mechanisms to support long-term, meaningful change. If they wish to prevail against strong countervailing forces, the Clinton Administration and Congress should seriously consider new forms of citizen participation and structures to support change: citizen juries and commissions, expert advocates, entrepreneurial management, and specialized entities designed to deal with the inevitable blockages and gaps in performance. In short, the rights-enforcing *role* of the federal courts needs to be defended and actualized, even if the federal courts themselves are not in a good position to fulfill that role at the current time.

Conclusion

We are a society in which millions of people are without health insurance and have great difficulty obtaining needed care. Unprecedented millions are in poverty, homeless, unemployed, and otherwise in severe need. In such a situation, it may seem like utopian frivolity to recommend spend-

41. An argument that three members of the current Supreme Court—Justices Sandra Day O'Connor, Anthony Kennedy, and David Souter—are more likely to use open-ended "standards" instead of the rigid rules favored by Chief Justice Rehnquist and Justice Scalia, can be found in Sullivan 1992. However, Professor Sullivan's analysis focuses on constitutional law rather than statutory interpretation, and there is no indication in the *Suter* case that these three justices have begun to take a different view of statutory rights than that advanced by Chief Justice Rehnquist.

ing material and human resources on "empowerment," "participation," and "innovation." It is also true that efforts of this sort in the past—for example, in the War on Poverty, or in the movement for community control of schools—led at times to narrow self-interest and corruption in community-based agencies and boards. But that is only to say that these efforts occur in our society, in which narrow self-interest and corruption appear to be widespread, even (or perhaps especially) among the political and corporate elite (Barlett and Steele 1992; Phillips 1990). If every instance of corruption and maladministration were an argument against the possibility of something different, we would have long ago lost any hope for positive change.

My response is this: given the history of frustration of egalitarian social legislation, particularly in the area of health care delivery, it is "utopian" (in the sense of highly unrealistic) *not* to try new methods to achieve reform. If we set up a maze in which one path leads nowhere, while a second leads to food, and we watch a rat repeatedly go down the first path, we say: that rat cannot learn. How many times can the proponents of health care (and other social) reform set up a system for change and assume rather than struggle for the political consensus and technical expertise necessary for its success? How many times can the proponents for change ignore the near certainty of a continuous struggle over the premises and details of that system? Once that struggle is recognized, will the proponents for change bring as much confidence, energy, and long-term commitment to their values as Chief Justice Rehnquist evidently brings to his?

References

Anderson, Gerard F., and Mark A. Hall. 1992. The Adequacy of Hospital Reimbursement under Medicaid's Boren Amendment. *Journal of Legal Medicine* 13:205–36.

Annas, George J., Sylvia A. Law, Rand E. Rosenblatt, and Kenneth R. Wing. 1990. *American Health Law*. Boston: Little, Brown.

Barlett, Donald L., and James B. Steele. 1992. *America: What Went Wrong?* Kansas City: Andrews and McMeel.

Belkin, Lisa. 1992. Brooklyn Beginning a City Plan to Link All Poor with a Doctor, *New York Times*, October 1, p. A1.

Bogdanitch, Walter. 1991. *The Great White Lie*. New York: Simon and Schuster.

Edelman, Murray. 1964. *The Symbolic Uses of Politics*. Urbana: University of Illinois Press.

————. 1977. *Political Language: Words That Succeed and Policies That Fail*. New York: Academic.

Edsall, Thomas. 1984. *The New Politics of Inequality*. New York: Basic.

Hale, Robert. 1935. Unconstitutional Conditions and Constitutional Rights. *Columbia Law Review* 35:321–59.

Hobsbawm, Eric. 1984. Labour and Human Rights. In *Workers: Worlds of Labour*, ed. Eric Hobsbawm. New York: Pantheon.

Kennedy, Duncan. 1973. Legal Formality. *Journal of Legal Studies* 2:351–98.

Kreimer, Seth. 1984. Allocational Sanctions: The Problem of Negative Rights in a Positive State. *University of Pennsylvania Law Review* 132:1293–1397.

Kuttner, Robert. 1993. Unsparing Change. *The American Prospect* (Winter, no. 12): 8–10.

Lemann, Nicholas. 1991. *The Promised Land: The Great Black Migration and How It Changed America*. New York: Knopf.

Lerner, Michael. 1993. Memo to Clinton: Our First Hundred Days. *TIKKUN* (January/February): 8–10, 81.

Lipsky, Michael. 1980. *Street-Level Bureaucracy*. New York: Russell Sage.

Marmor, Theodore R., and Michael S. Barr. 1992. Making Sense of the National Health Insurance Reform Debate. *Yale Law and Policy Review* 10:228–82.

Mensch, Elizabeth. 1990. The History of Mainstream Legal Thought. In *The Politics of Law*, rev. ed., ed. David Kairys. New York: Pantheon.

Morone, James A. 1990. *The Democratic Wish*. New York: Basic.

————. 1992. The Bias of American Politics: Rationing Health Care in a Weak State. *University of Pennsylvania Law Review* 140:1923–38.

Neuborne, Burt. 1989. Foreword: State Constitutions and the Evolution of Positive Rights. *Rutgers Law Journal* 20:877–901.

Osborne, David, and Ted Gaebler. 1992. *Reinventing Government: How the Entrepreneurial Spirit is Transforming the Public Sector*. Reading, MA: Addison-Wesley.

Phillips, Kevin. 1990. *The Politics of Rich and Poor*. New York: Random House.

Reich, Charles. 1964. The New Property. *Yale Law Journal* 73:733–87.

————. 1965. Individual Rights and Social Welfare: The Emerging Legal Issues. *Yale Law Journal* 74:1245–57.

Rosenblatt, Rand E. 1970. Note: Legal Theory and Legal Education. *Yale Law Journal* 79:1153–78.

————. 1975. Book Comment: Dual Track Medicine and the Decline of the Medicaid Cure. *University of Cincinnati Law Review* 44:643–61.

————. 1978. Health Care Reform and Administrative Law: A Structural Approach. *Yale Law Journal* 88:243–336.

————. 1981. Health Care, Markets, and Democratic Values. *Vanderbilt Law Review* 34:1067–1115.

————. 1982. Legal Entitlement and Welfare Benefits. In *The Politics of Law*, ed. David Kairys. New York: Pantheon.

————. 1986. Medicaid Primary Care Case Management, the Doctor-Patient Relationship, and the Politics of Privatization. *Case Western Reserve Law Review* 36:915–68.

────── . 1990. Social Duties and the Problem of Rights in the American Welfare State. In *The Politics of Law*, rev. ed., ed. David Kairys. New York: Pantheon.

────── . 1991. Statutory Interpretation and Distributive Justice: Medicaid Hospital Reimbursement and the Debate over Public Choice. *St. Louis University Law Journal* 35:793–835.

Schneider, William. 1992. The Dawn of the Suburban Era in American Politics. *The Atlantic* (June):33–44.

Sparer, Edward V. 1965. The Role of the Welfare Client's Lawyer. *U.C.L.A. Law Review* 12:361–80.

Spivey, Michael O. 1992. Patching the Patchwork Quilt: "Reforming" the Medicaid Program—The Medicaid Voluntary Contribution and Provider-Specific Tax Amendments of 1991. *Annals of Health Law* 1:37–51.

Starr, Paul. 1993. Healthy Compromise: Universal Coverage and Managed Competition under a Cap. *The American Prospect* (Winter, no. 12): 44–52.

Stewart, Richard. 1975. The Reformation of American Administrative Law. *Harvard Law Review* 88:1667–1813.

Strickler, Matthew M. 1991. Practical Issues in Representing Providers in Legal Actions under the Boren Amendment. *St. Louis University Law Journal* 35:893–901.

Sullivan, Kathleen M. 1989. Unconstitutional Conditions. *Harvard Law Review* 102:1415–1506.

────── . 1992. Foreword: The Justices of Rules and Standards. *Harvard Law Review* 106:22–123.

TenBroek, Jacobus, and Richard Wilson. 1954. Public Assistance and Social Insurance: A Normative Evaluation. *U.C.L.A. Law Review* 1:237–302.

Unger, Roberto. 1975. *Knowledge and Politics*. New York: Basic.

Van Alstyne, William. 1968. The Demise of the Right-Privilege Distinction in Constitutional Law. *Harvard Law Review* 81:1439–64.

Whitney, Craig R. 1993. Medical Care in Germany: With Choices, and for All. *New York Times* January 23, pp. 1, 4.

In the summer of 1969, as a law student, I assisted Lee Albert, Sylvia Law, and other attorneys at the Columbia University Center on Social Welfare Law who were representing the welfare recipient plaintiffs in Rosado v. Wyman, 397 U.S. 397 (1970), one of the cases discussed in this essay. Early in my work, Sylvia Law asked. "What is this statutory entitlement theory?" and asked me to write a memorandum on it. Although I submitted something at the time, this essay can be regarded as the latest phase in more than 20 years of thinking about an answer. See Rosenblatt 1970, 1978, 1982, 1986, 1990, 1991.

I wish to thank Ann Freedman for thoughtful comments and wonderful personal support. I also wish to thank Perry Dane, David Frankford, and Mark Hall for helpful comments on this and earlier work. I dedicate this essay to the memory of my teacher, Thomas Emerson, Lines Professor of Law Emeritus at the Yale Law School, who died in 1991. A great scholar about, and advocate of rights in the areas of freedom of speech, privacy, and gender equality, and a participant in and supporter of the social welfare tradition of the New Deal, his calm, forceful, unswerving commitment to human rights and social justice is a needed inspiration in the light of the developments discussed in this essay.

Part 3
Business

Dogmatic Slumbers: American Business and Health Policy

Lawrence D. Brown

Abstract For more than a decade students of health policy have predicted a revolution waged by corporate purchasers of health care who would rise in demand of public policy cures for increasing and burdensome health care costs. This forecast has been largely disappointed, however, as the business sector has remained oddly diffident in its demands for health policy reform. There are three reasons for business's reticence—the economic stakes of the corporate sector in health reform are uncertain, organizational encumbrances hamper business activism in this arena, and ideological convictions make business wary of governmental solutions. Although business is sometimes said to manipulate the policy process for its own material ends, in the health sphere the most likely road to reform may reverse this image: a newly activist federal government may have to mobilize business support for reforms that advance both corporate interests and larger social goals.

Once upon a time a band of sociologists and political scientists called "elitists" taught that big business in the United States comprised a power elite or ruling class, effectively controlled public policy, and shaped and steered it to its own material ends. Pluralist critics battered this model severely, and today few policy analysts contend that corporate power determines policy outcomes across a range of arenas. Fewer still, however, doubt that business (like other interest groups, only more so) weighs into policy struggles when it has strong economic motives to do so, or that the more salient the economic spur to action, the greater the resources business will wield, and the more formidable a political force it will be.

Against this backdrop the reluctance of U.S. corporate efforts to enter the lists in the battle to reform the health care system is surely a tantalizing political mystery. If political engagement follows the dollar, business should be very much in evidence in the corridors and power centers of health care policy. Employment-based coverage is the centerpiece of the U.S. health insurance system. By tradition, and in many quarters by strong continuing preference, employers are the main shoppers and buyers in the private health insurance market. In 1990, 57.3 percent of the non-aged population (some 141 million people) had employer coverage and business's share of total U.S. health care spending was 29 percent (U.S. CBO 1992: 38; Levit and Cowan 1991: 85). Moreover, business contributions to health care spending have been rising rapidly for some time. Between 1970 and 1989 employer spending (in constant 1989 dollars) rose 1 percent for wages and salaries, 32 percent for retirement benefits, but 163 percent for health benefits (Biacentini and Anzick 1990, cited in Alliance for Health Reform 1992: 15). Health expenses rose from 19.8 percent to 55.1 percent as a share of pretax profits and nearly equaled profits after tax (98.3 percent) (Levit and Cowan 1991: 88). Between 1985 and 1990 health spending by business rose at an average of 13 percent per year (MEDSTAT 1992: 5).

Nor are these hidden costs; business executives complain of them loudly and often. Because the expenditures afflict individual firms and business "as a sector," one might expect them to stimulate a potent political response. After all, business tends to be most formidable when it is both mobilized and unified (Vogel 1989: 291). Furthermore, political activism by business in other arenas has increased "partly as a response to public policy initiatives perceived as placing new and unwarranted constraints on firm behavior" (Plotke 1992: 190), which presumably include the sizable shifting of costs by public sector purchasers who use payment shortfalls in Medicare and Medicaid to relieve their own health care budgets. But neither individual firms nor peak associations that represent the business sector have been notably energetic in proposing and pursuing major policy initiatives in a system that apparently wreaks serious damage on their economic interests and prospects.

Arguably, the mystery is becoming old news. For a decade political observers have forecast the imminent awakening of these sleeping giants, who would launch a corporate revolution to instill fiscal discipline into a health care system that had too long dared to defy the iron laws of economics. In 1981 these predictions looked highly persuasive: amidst a recession, sharp foreign competition, and constrained profits, corporate

America faced soaring health care costs that it declared insupportable.[1] But a decade later it was déjà vu all over again: a recessionary economy, foreign competition, and eroding profits plagued many corporations, health care costs continued to rise unacceptably, everyone deplored the situation, and no one knew exactly what to do. Contrary to expectation, economic stimulus had not triggered an effective political response; a decade of reform opportunity had been lost.

It is important to be clear about what is mysterious and needs explanation. The premise here is not that business has done nothing to counter health care costs but rather that it has largely failed to exert itself vigorously in the public policy arena. Business power in health affairs can be viewed as a continuum spanning several forms of engagement, chief among them being (1) nondecisions (nothing happens because the unshakable legitimacy of a status quo that business favors makes change unthinkable); (2) intraorganizational reform (companies experiment with cost sharing, utilization review, selective contracting, and more—measures that lie in their individual hands and lack overt community connotations); (3) self-education (firms band together to explore the workings of the health system and perhaps the ways and means of reform); (4) position taking (they analyze their common problems and seek formal agreement in white papers and task force reports on broad directions for change); (5) communication (firms and perhaps associations and coalitions disseminate their views to their peers and the public); (6) lobbying (firms and associations try to persuade policymakers to act as they suggest); (7) coalition building (they work to enlist broad support both within their own ranks and among policymakers); and (8) public-private partnerships (business cements alliances between its own cohesive elements and public purchasers to enhance leverage and concert political influence that advances the sectors' shared reform agenda).

What needs explaining is that, nondecisions aside, business responses to the health cost "crisis" have mainly settled along points 2–5 of the continuum—internal "reforms" supplemented by self-educational endeavors and modest efforts to adopt and advertise policy positions that are often nebulous. Those strategic options (6–8) that carry business into the political arena have not gone unexercised (Bergthold 1990) but have seen far less action than a straight economic reading of political motivation would predict. Business, after all, is not congenitally shy of politics. On

---

1. For a skeptical contemporary view, see Sapolsky 1981.

tax policy, tariffs, labor law, consumer protection, environmental regulation, and many more such issues it has been politically aggressive and (at times) effective (Vogel 1989; Martin 1991). And the modest health strategy interventions have failed to deliver relief, so why not onward? There lies the mystery: One need not be a Marxian to wonder why these most capitalist of interests in this most capitalist of societies have been so slow to press policy levers that might counter the economic carnage of health care costs.

This paper argues that business's political diffidence (and, perhaps, exceptionalism) in the health sphere derives from sectoral fragmentation that anesthetizes three key potential motives for political action: economics, organization, and ideology. Limits of space and of detailed information about business and health politics preclude any claim to a comprehensive canvass of the topic. Indeed, the very term *business community* conveys a specious homogeneity that masks marked variations among firms by profit picture, labor market, managerial philosophy, organizational culture, and other variables that shape attitudes toward health costs and preferred policy remedies for what ails the health care system. The argument here is that these exceptions prove the "rule": sectoral fragmentation is a barrier not only to confident generalization in these pages but also to coherent policy initiatives by business itself.

Economics: Where's the Beef?

In 1976 Victor Zink, a benefits official in General Motors, told the national Council on Wage and Price Stability that Blue Cross/Blue Shield had become a far larger supplier to G.M. than U.S. Steel (Council on Wage and Price Stability 1976: 23). Since then this and kindred shocking data have been widely cited to prove that uncontrolled health spending is ruining the profits and international competitive standing of U.S. business.

It is not entirely clear, however, that CEOs in general share the alarm that the cost-of-care/cost-of-car example is meant to generate. For example, a poll conducted by the Robert Wood Johnson Foundation in 1989 found that, of the 38 percent of corporate chiefs who responded, 60 percent labeled health care costs a major concern, but only 35 percent called them a "top" concern (Cantor et al. 1991). More recent polls suggest wider, deeper agitation among top corporate personnel, but these too should be handled with care. Surveys discovering sizable, rising support for "fundamental" changes in the system rarely probe deeply into what respondents mean by "fundamental." Obviously business leaders would prefer to bump health care costs elsewhere if they could; that understandable longing does not prove the familiar contention that health costs constitute a terminal illness for corporate America. Several factors intrude between economic perception, on one side, and public policy, on the other.

First, as Uwe Reinhardt (1989) cogently argues, costs ascribed to corporations are not necessarily "corporate" costs. Reinhardt notes that the business sector's ability to compete in international markets turns not on health spending per se but rather on the total compensation package firms offer (among other variables). Depending on market conditions, business may pass health costs along to consumers, meet them by reducing shareholders' returns, or—most important—trade them off for slower wage growth. It is not "business" that swallows rising health care prices, says Reinhardt; rather, "almost always, it is employees who pay the bulk of that price in the form of lower real cash income, at least in the longer run" (Reinhardt 1989: 20). Presumably the 163 percent rise in health benefits between 1970 and 1989 has something to do with the measly 1 percent growth in real wages over those years. Wasted health dollars, argues Reinhardt, are a legitimate ground for corporate and social concern, but competitiveness is largely a specious issue.

Even if one granted that health costs are the competitive disaster they are often said to be (and Reinhardt's contentions have indeed been challenged: see *Health Affairs* 1990) business still might not rise to the political occasion for pressing change. One reason is that, to a degree not always recognized, health care is not merely a cost of doing business but rather (or also) a prominent, powerful member of the top corporate club itself. Health care is very big business. In city after city—New York, Boston, Cleveland, Atlanta, Houston, Birmingham, and other places, small as well as large—health services are, if not the largest local industry, close to the top. This lofty and relatively recession-proof economic status doubtless triggers ambivalence about cost containment and recalls Samuel Goldwyn's alleged warning not to bite the hand of the goose that lays the golden egg. For example, in the 1980s health care accounted for one-fourth of the net job growth in New York State. Health services in New York State are the state's top source of employment; the 630,000 health jobs exceed the runner-up, business services, by nearly 200,000 jobs. The national pattern is more dramatic still. Now the fourth largest nonagricultural source of employment, health care accounts for more than one in six new jobs projected in the United States and has become "the leading growth sector of the economy." Nationally, health jobs are expected to increase 34 percent by the year 2000, 2.5 times the rate for all other jobs (Ehrenhalt 1991: 1–2, 9, 11).

These numbers imply that health cost containment can be a mixed economic blessing. Lower spending on health services might reduce income growth and economic activity in some communities and thereby depress demand for corporate products, health-related and other. The auto industry itself knows the score. Asked in an interview why Ford Motors, once fairly active in cost containment politics in Michigan, had not sustained and enlarged its leadership role, a benefits specialist smiled wryly and replied with three little words: "Doctors buy Lincolns." He meant of course that it would be poor corporate strategy to weaken this "market's" willingness or ability to stay in the Ford family. Communities and companies differ in these respects, to be sure, but the variations do not rebut the basic point: economically, health cost containment is something of a double-edged sword.

Even if business "as a sector" were resolved in principle to promote cost containment policies, its corporate components might have second thoughts because policies do not present uniform gains and losses to all firms, which often have trouble assessing how they would fare under various proposals. In the early 1980s, for example, the American Medical Association tried to parlay the antiregulatory sentiments of the Reagan administration into curbs on the power of the Federal Trade Commission to regulate physicians. Business groups split: some, including the Chamber of Commerce, stayed neutral, while the Washington Business Group on Health opposed the plan, fearing that deregulation would push costs higher (Vogel 1989: 263–64). Lee Iacocca, representing a Rust Belt industry facing tough foreign competition and a strong union, the United Auto Workers, with broad health benefits it is determined to defend, has every reason to seek a national health plan that would confer on the taxpayer more of Chrysler's health care tab. Heads of service sector firms with strong market niches and nonunionized workers are not so sure that what is good for Detroit is also good for them. Big firms that insure their employees and pay premiums that include the costs of uncompensated care for workers whose employers fail to do likewise may favor employer mandates or a "play-or-pay" plan. Small companies that do not now extend coverage (or fear that mandates will drive their costs too high) demur. Some companies want government to lead the way toward cost containment—but not if that means ending ERISA preemptions that permit them to self-insure and escape state regulations, including mandated benefits.

Business "as a sector" may not have a clear-cut economic stake in health care reform.

Even if corporate leaders agreed in detail on what they wanted from health policy reform, they might not fight for their convictions, because they have deeper economic stakes in other legislative projects and choose to save their political capital for battles that count more heavily. Mizruchi (1992) counted the cases in which two or more of a sample of fifty-seven manufacturing firms in the Fortune 500 testified before congressional committees on various issues between 1980 and 1987. Energy was the subject in forty-three hearings; automobile and transportation issues in thirty-five; government regulation and taxes, thirty-one; environmental protection issues, thirty; industrial health and structure, twenty-two; public works and government budget concerns, twenty-two; science, technology, and education, twenty-two; foreign trade, eighteen—and health care, just one (pp. 160–61). Apparently, health costs, however annoying, took a back seat politically to arenas that spoke more directly to the heart of business profits and autonomy. Perhaps rising costs since 1987 are forcing new policy priorities and political patterns. Be this as it may, the dollars do not speak for themselves. As Plotke observes (1992: 175), business tends to exert itself politically "when economic phenomena are interpreted in the light of normative and cultural commitments," which remain problematic in the health field.

Organization

Even if the economic case for close corporate attention to health costs were clear-cut, business would still often fail to exert itself effectively in the policy process, because organizational obstacles impede action. Those who exhort business to form buyer coalitions to concert economic power and to build political coalitions that wield legislative clout too seldom ponder the organizational prisms through which economic interests are beamed and refracted.

It is widely agreed that if firms, individually or in concert, are to play a decisive role in health affairs at the community (or national) levels, strong leadership at the top is essential. Such commitment can be difficult to secure, however. Corporate CEOs generally view health care as territory alien to their expertise. They rose through the ranks and command a large salary, because they know how to build cars, invest money, write advertising copy, or whatever, not because they can fix the health care system. Busy people, they have only so much time to explore the mechanics of health care and the pros and cons of strategies for change. Their personal involvement in community-regarding endeavors can go only so far: the CEO who heads the cost containment coalition this year may let it languish when persuaded to chair the United Way fund drive next year. They get annoyed that health care departs so pervasively (and self-righteously) from the sound market principles to which they suppose the larger U.S. economy conforms and listen with rising indignation to insider accounts of why market-based panaceas, so obviously right and true, do not or cannot work in health matters. They have little taste for sustained public conflict with health professionals (inevitable if they are to lead a charge for change) and grow livid at the patronizing responses of providers, who rise to correct the misconceived critiques of business colleagues who doubtless mean well but, alas, overlook vital points they would (doubtless) have grasped were they more expert in the arcane topics at hand. They have equally little taste for battling with employees and their union representatives—or with each other, when, for example, seeking a united front in a "buy-right" strategy that limits individual firms' freedom of action. If [the firm] is not an important local employer headquartered in the community (and sometimes even if it is), CEOs may be reluctant to meddle in local health care arrangements (including, of course, payment and income flows). And frequently they identify with local health care institutions, especially the hospitals on whose boards they sit and whose aspirations to be the biggest and best they endorse and defend.

For all these reasons, CEOs are rarely prepared to commit much time and effort to struggles to reform some piece of the health care system and readily delegate these problems to the benefit manager, who is, after all, trained for, good at, and paid to address such challenges. But the training, inclination, and perceived mission of most benefit managers discourage them from donning the mantle of corporate agent on controversial community questions and encourage them to keep their innovations within the precincts of the corporation itself. Not surprisingly, corporate cost containment by benefit managers focuses on managing benefits—devising new cost-sharing schemes, installing utilization review programs, developing managed care options. These stratagems can be pursued with more or less acumen and energy, but even at their best their organizational virtues remain their main policy vice: they are narrow approaches that deliberately decline to tackle the big systematic issues intrinsic to true cost containment.

For most benefit managers, leadership stops at the organization's edge. In consequence, corporations tend to exhibit a cycle of expectation and disillusion. Annoyed at rising health costs and apprised of the latest glowing trade and consultant accounts of benefit redesign, utilization review, and managed care, CEOs give their benefit managers a hearty mandate to innovate. The intraorganizational departures are implemented, time passes, and it grows clear that they have saved little or nothing, or that such savings as were realized were swamped by cost shifting from public programs (or other private purchasers) and by other powerful external forces. Intermittent postmortems reveal uncertainty within the decision hierarchy on just who should be doing what. Benefit managers lack both the reach and the grasp to seize levers that lie beyond the sphere of corporate policy. The CEO has neither the time nor the taste to play health reform crusader on the community stage, which might in any case be too small to produce the desired results (Brown and McLaughlin 1990). And the two levels often coordinate poorly. As Joseph Duva notes, "A typical benefit manager rarely sees the CEO, and when he does, 'he has to talk in sound bites' " (Faltermayer 1992: 58). These elusive divisions of labor reflect a deeper organizational reality: health care costs are not unimportant to the corporate financial picture, but the hard work of controlling them is too peripheral to most business missions and mind-sets to elicit a heavy commitment of scarce managerial time and talent.

Although the organizational politics that shape position taking on health affairs within business peak associations have been little studied, these ambiguities around roles and responsibilities probably produce a comparable paralysis in these venues, too. Without clear marching orders from a solid phalanx of prominent CEOs, the development of association positions falls largely to staff. But staffers, like benefit managers, are loath to improvise aggressively without clear directives from CEO cadres and so settle for sober studies portraying the intolerable rise of costs accompanied by platitudinous antidotes ("greater cost consciousness among consumers, payers, and providers"). The National Leadership Coalition on Health Care is a star-studded body that has generated an unusually detailed and refined set of policy recommendations, but as Cathie Jo Martin observes in her paper in this issue, one price of concreteness was the defection of important constituents who begged to differ with one or more items on the list. Specificity of the reform agenda may relate inversely to breadth of corporate support.

Ideology

Even if the economic motives for corporate leadership in containing health costs were clearly compelling and organizational structures were conducive, business might still not fashion coherent policy positions because ideology inhibits them. Despite the manifold oddities of the health care market and the lateness of the hour in the quest to slow costs, many business leaders retain a faith in private, market, voluntary, and communitarian correctives and remain chary of regulatory interventions. A few CEOs would hand the health cost mess to government, and good riddance. More than a few obdurately oppose a larger governmental presence and might even repeal existing regulations if they could. The modal position is probably the "moderate antistatism" that has gained ground in corporate councils on public policy in recent years (Plotke 1992: 186).

This worldview largely explains why a decade of cost containment opportunity was lost in the 1980s. Having stirred early in the decade, the corporate revolutionaries marched bravely forth to do what came naturally: augment cost sharing in employee benefit plans, celebrate the virtues of competition and managed care, and join community coalitions (some employer-only, some multiparty) to bring important people together to devise strategies to constrain costs. As the decade wore on, cost sharing brought at best short-term relief from larger forces that soon overwhelmed it. Competition mainly meant cost shifting, cream skimming, and shadow pricing, which left most competitors in an incomprehensible bog. Coalitions, with few exceptions, produced information, pamphlets, data, seminars on how to encourage wellness and discourage drugs in the workplace, and the like—strategies as unavailing against costs as they were uncontroversial (McLaughlin et al. 1989). Their legacy was (again, with a few exceptions) epitomized by the head of the big-city coalition who recently declared that the main achievement of his group in 1992 was "survival."

These outcomes were not inevitable. Had the awakening corporate activists cast a critical eye on their ideological instincts and the limits of their worldview, their policies might have been less apolitical. Instead of competition, voluntarism, and community they might have reconsidered the case for regulation, global budgets, public-private purchaser coalitions, and state- and nation-based reform. Had they done so, the United States might have entered the 1990s in better shape to address health care costs.

However this may be, some observers contend that business ideology in health affairs is now changing rapidly. The Chrysler Corporation's ardent—albeit atypical—appeals for a national health plan are often cited as evidence of this supposed shift. Polls do indeed suggest that corporate leaders are increasingly troubled by the system's costs, receptive (at least in principle) to major changes, and ready to entertain a larger government role. But surveys inquiring what employers want government to do find

highest on the list such comparatively unintrusive steps as malpractice reform, more spending on prevention, less duplication of equipment, and
price controls on hospitals and doctors. Tougher measures, such as global
budgets for hospitals and doctors, closing underused hospitals, and tight
public control on capital spending by hospitals, fare less well (Harris and
Associates 1992).

This stubborn strategic lag suggests that the power of nondecisions may
be the most telling type of all. Having convinced itself that a laissez-
faire, employer-based health insurance system is a precious expression of
the American way of life and of the need to keep government small and
weak, business cannot easily appeal for government relief from duties it
is ever less suited to discharge. Torn between the cultural legitimacy of
private-dominated purchasing and the growing practical implausibility of
that inheritance, business cannot live contentedly with the status quo or
without it.

Hesitation over whether the current hodgepodge of public and private
functions should continue or cease is not the only durable ideological
barrier to business activism. If this were all, an agonizing reappraisal
might have emerged by now from economic anxieties and organizational
frustrations. A more tenacious, because more dynamic, ideological variable is the eternal promise that some optimal, competitive, market-based
scheme can be invented to discipline the system without surrendering
to the regulatory intrusions business instinctively deplores. For two decades, corporate leaders, like other policy observers, have watched with
fascination as policy entrepreneurs unveil one new line after another of
market-based fashions—enhanced consumer cost consciousness, HMOs,
buy-right plans, managed care very broadly defined, managed competition rather strictly defined, and more. The very richness of the market
menu at once increases the abstract appeals of competition and lessens
the prospects of realizing it.

The market-based plans differ widely in their premises and presupposi-
tions—in how they work, why they are supposed to work, and how much
public regulation one needs to make them work. Worlds of difference
divide plans that, for example, modestly rig the market to make consumers shop harder among providers and those that build a broad framework of "procompetitive regulation" to tilt the system toward HMOs.
Economists disagree on which scheme is preferable and what it would
take to make competition realize its promise. If theoreticians cannot sort
out these weighty matters, what is a practical businessman to do? Like
many policymakers, corporate leaders may therefore withhold support for

new regulatory interventions in hopes that a better market-centered approach can be found, but watch with exasperation as devotees of diverse competitive camps—some of which propose an extensive framework of policy rules that would constrain business's health purchasing options or require it to assume new roles (for instance, to become or join "sophisticated sponsors")—hawk their wares, insisting all the while that critiques of their plans are a priori invalid because their version of competition has never been tried. Corporate leaders, in short, pledge allegiance to the idea of competition (or at any rate to the idea that anything is better than bigger government) but do not know what to make of it. Understandably, in health matters, "there's no CEO spokesperson for business and no consensus among business people" (Paul Ellwood, quoted in Faltermayer 1992: 58). Ideologically inhibited, business is unable to lead, uncertain whom to follow, and unwilling to get out of the way.

Exceptions and the Rule

Occasionally, business has played a major role in shaping health policy innovations at the state and local levels. In 1982, for example, the Massachusetts Business Roundtable (MBRT), headed by Nelson Gifford, CEO of Dennison Manufacturers, led a broad coalition of interests—Blue Cross, commercial insurers, hospitals, physicians, and the state bureaucracy—to broker legislative changes in the state's rate-setting program. Several converging factors promoted this corporate activism—concern over the state's high health costs, annoyance at cost shifting, encouragement from the administration of Governor Ed King and the Rate Setting Commission, and, not least important, Gifford's unusual commitment and connections. (Aside from his CEO status, he was "vice chairman of the MBRT, chairman of its Health Care Task Force, and political friend of Margaret Heckler [then secretary of HHS], Governor King, and other influential Massachusetts politicians" [Bergthold 1990: 86]). Nor were these business exertions a flash in the pan. Bergthold concludes that the Roundtable was an "effective and relatively united spokesman for large corporate interests throughout the 1980s," one that conferred on business "a permanent and often dominant policy role" in health affairs (Bergthold 1990: 107, 101).

By the end of the decade, however, that policy role was strained severely. Costs continued to rise unacceptably, some segments of business flirted with competition and deregulation, and consumers and other groups were pressing for universal access—the level playing field without which, some (including Gifford) argued, competition made little sense. Gifford found his constituents more committed to capping their own costs than to fighting for broader coverage. With Gifford caught in an "increasingly untenable position" and "unable to act as an effective broker," policy leadership shifted to state government, especially to Senate Ways and Means Chair Patricia McGovern (Goldberger 1990: 867–69). The Health Care Task Force of the Business Roundtable disbanded, the Roundtable itself withdrew from health care issues, and its successor, the Associated Industries of Massachusetts, has been much less active than the Roundtable (Kronick 1990: 906). Drawn by their political involvement down a slippery slope toward policy measures they could not embrace, employers, writes Kronick (1990: 912), "stopped sliding down the slope by getting off the hill."

Surely the most remarkable and durable example of business leadership in health affairs is found at the community level, in Rochester, New York. There an Industrial Management Council led by Kodak (and, to a lesser degree, Xerox) has long insisted that they, the dominant health insurance purchasers, should have the courage to call the tune. The pattern was established nearly forty years ago, when Marion Folsom, a Kodak executive who had served as secretary of Health, Education, and Welfare under Eisenhower, took the then eccentric position that no one had proved that in health care more meant better, and that (therefore) business should discipline the expansion of health resources in the community. Blue Cross, the dominant payer, contentedly played "handmaiden to industry" (as a former plan executive put it), refusing to cover costs of services and facilities the corporate purchasers had not endorsed. Constrained by this united front of purchasers and payers, the hospitals adapted by forming the Rochester Area Hospital Council (later Rochester Area Hospital Corporation), a planning group that discussed the proposals of each hospital in light of the community's needs. Hospitals that acted unilaterally risked the purchasers' wrath and refusal of payment for unauthorized services. The community likewise supported planning on a broad scale, first in a voluntary areawide body, then in the comprehensive health planning program, and later in a health systems agency.

This regulatory discipline allows Rochesterians to enjoy comparatively broad benefits at comparatively moderate costs. And maintaining the system remains a priority with Kodak and its industrial colleagues. To a degree unusual elsewhere, corporate executives concur that preserving their achievement is an important part of their community service mission. Kodak vice presidents sit on the boards of all area hospitals and note proudly that they do not check their brains at the hospital door. They ask hard questions, insist on sound answers, and refuse to be intimidated by the technical medical issues that come before them. Impressing rising managers with the importance of the cost containment mission, they do their homework and dutifully attend breakfasts and luncheons at which they articulate the purchaser's perspective, ponder the community's interests, and prepare themselves to hold the line. Shaping the health care system is, in short, part of Kodak's corporate culture, which (given Kodak's dominance and headquarter status in Rochester) is a prominent element in the larger community culture.[2]

Rochester hosts a stream of admiring visitors seeking to learn how to do it. Most depart, admiration enhanced, but despairing of duplicating this feat of organizational will in sites that lack a headquarters firm that is both committed to the community and willing to enter local frays, or in firms where CEOs decline to force hospitals to temper the progressive medical innovations that boosterish chamber of commerce pamphlets routinely celebrate in their quest to attract executive talent to their homeland. Every community knows why Rochester works, but apparently none (other) knows how to do it.

A Rude Awakening?

The heart of business's enigmatic role in health policy is its wish to have its costs contained without much growth in the role of government. Each passing day makes this preference less plausible; whether and when business wakes up to reality may influence importantly the content of changes that may now be inevitable.

Business-government dealings in health reform will likely evolve into one of three political patterns. First, the long-expected awakening and mobilization of corporate America might finally arrive. Business leaders may clarify their options, resolve their differences, work through a few cohesive organizations, and make common cause with public purchasers. This dramatic rallying cannot be ruled out, but it is doubtful, because the corporate slumbers of past and present are not accidental but rather the product of economic differences, organizational uncertainties, and ideological devotions that impose powerful political inhibitions. And even if economic interests were more cohesive and organizational dynamics more

---

2. This account of Rochester comes from Brandon 1986 and from this author's interviews with a small sample of participants in that system.

coherent, business's abiding commitment to competition, coupled to its continuing confusion about what it means, could tie corporate position taking in conceptual knots indefinitely.

Second, the forces of change may gain enough momentum to carry the day, passing business by and neither seeking nor offering occasions for constructive corporate participation in policy-making. Arguably, however, change will proceed faster and better if large private purchasers become part of the solution, not the problem.

The 1990s have opened with growing agreement in most social quarters that sizable change in the financing (and perhaps the delivery) of health care is in some sense imperative. This growing agreement, however, falls well short of practical consensus on what changes to adopt. Public opinion registers deep discontent with the status quo but gives little clue about the trade-offs and sacrifices it would accept in a new regime. Interest groups clamor to thrust into the public eye their proactive, constructive plans for "comprehensive" change, but most plans assign the costs of change to other players, which suggests that when policy deliberations focus and the range of legislative options narrows, groups threatened by change will mount a strident counterattack (which will of course include extensive, expensive efforts to scare the public). Politicians see that they can no longer go abroad in their districts without a health plan that honors universal access and cost containment, but the dozens of legislative entrees cover a wide spectrum from insurance reform to Canada, with play-or-pay, Medicaid expansion, and more in between, and no consensus has emerged (Brown 1992a, 1992b).

In this unsettled political climate, pressure for change could dissipate, as it has so often in the past. On the other hand, there are good grounds to suspect that policy has finally turned a corner and can no longer retreat down the road to indecision. Simply put, the health care system seems to have superimposed on the cost crisis a price crisis. The cost crisis, long familiar, evokes lamentations over percentages of GDP and per capita costs that everyone knows are excessive, but in which no one feels a strong enough personal stake to compel action. (This crisis mimics the federal budget deficit, "insupportable" at $100 billion in 1981, at $350 billion in 1992, and perhaps ad infinitum.) The price crisis, by contrast, turns on anxiety about the affordability and availability of health insurance for millions of people long accustomed to coverage but increasingly doubtful that they can retain it on reasonable terms for themselves and their dependents. These vexations are politically analogous not to the size of the federal deficit but rather to the rates of inflation, unemployment, and consumer credit, which have real electoral resonance. Added to other elements of the loose coalition for change—the 37 million uninsured (whose plight has not been sufficient in itself to promote political action), top officials in fifty states incessantly aggravated by Medicaid costs, influential interests such as organized teachers who resent the diversion of money from them to health spending, and the usual liberal suspects in labor and elsewhere—these millions of uneasily insured middle-class voting types may supply the hitherto missing ingredient for change. Their concerns are unlikely to evaporate because they derive from twenty years of failed cost containment policies. Policymakers may therefore soon find it no longer possible to sit there, do nothing, and await a social consensus that they then rush in to ratify.

The future probably holds repeated ventures in "mere" incrementalism that accumulate to something like fundamental change. Reformers will take that first incremental bite (insurance reform or employer mandates, for example), find that these measures do not work without others on the reform agenda, and thence proceed at irregular but inescapable intervals to descend the slippery slope toward something like a German or Canadian system (Brown 1992c). What one does, how far one goes, and how long it all takes, however, are by no means determined but rather are contingent on the political balance of forces—a balance in which the presence and preferences of business may be pivotal.

The reason for this imposing corporate potential lies in the impending group struggle over reform. As reform advocates try to clarify their various preference schedules and reach common ground, they will face strong, skillful interest groups of providers and insurers who will fight to protect their incomes and autonomy. The heavyweight interests—especially organized labor and the elderly, who led the charge for Medicare in 1965—will be unable (and perhaps unwilling) to supply sufficient countervailing power this time. In this odd political constellation, interest mediation and legitimation will be at a premium, and the large private sector purchasers—American business—will be the best, perhaps only, adequate suppliers. Business, in short, might tip the balance of power and energize both the contents and the pace of incrementalism.

If business sides with the interests that fight above all to limit the role of the federal government and its power over them, the path to reform will be long and each step along it modest. If the corporate world concerts action with the emerging reform coalition and aggressively pursues a united front with public purchasers, reform may move more quickly and with fewer, bolder steps. Arguably, the latter course makes sense for society and business alike: the longer and slower the reform process, the more protracted the work of exposing and confronting the hard choices required to curb the growth of costs and the higher the base (percentage of GDP and per capita spending) that may be held harmless when budget caps arrive.

Moreover, in a nation with a deeply ingrained antigovernmental ethos that in the 1980s was exploited and inflamed for short-term electoral gain, political leadership in health reform requires large, concentrated doses of legitimation. Sustained business engagement in reform politics might well supply that invaluable resource more effectively than any other means. Persuading business to play that role, not to mention successfully organizing and orchestrating its expression in the political process, would not be easy, for the history of corporate (non-) involvement shows that a group's perception of a problem by no means guarantees a coherent policy response. The economics of corporate interest are ambiguous and the organizational challenges are daunting, but the toughest obstacles to constructive corporate participation in health policy-making are ideological. As often happens in the politics of material interests, the crucial variables lie mainly in the mind.

The constructive engagement of business in health policy reform is at once desirable and unlikely to emerge easily, a dilemma that highlights a third pattern, one that embraces neither the implicit pluralism of the first pattern (corporate awakening and mobilization) nor the explicit statism of the second (reform leaves business on the sidelines of politics). This third image blends these two in a kind of state-initiated pluralism in which government works to mobilize the consent of business leaders for the reforms it favors and tries to mediate and legitimate change by means of conspicuous public-private cooperation. As noted earlier, Massachusetts tried something similar in the 1980s, with mixed results. To date, the federal government has not pursued this avenue for several reasons, including the disinclination of the Reagan-Bush administrations to launch health policy reforms of any consequence, the antipathy of these regimes to regulation (procompetitive included), and their readiness to practice public sector cost shifting that a public-private partnership would presumably end.

In 1993 or 1997, however, an administration of more activist bent might acknowledge the need for broad-gauged reforms; recognize that cooperation between private and public purchasers could do much to advance it; work to identify and court those prominent business leaders who are open to new directions; and encourage them to sell the new public-private agenda to as many of their corporate peers as will listen. A federal government resolved to lead and in assiduous search of compatible corporate partners might win over a critical mass of business statesmen and thereby tip toward "real change" an otherwise precarious pattern of power.

The effective mobilization of business power in health affairs may, in short, require standing the old elitist image on its head. The government that business supposedly manipulates for corporate ends may have to mobilize hesitant corporate leaders by convincing them to invest political capital to advance their own material interests and a larger social good.

References

Alliance for Health Reform. 1992. *Chartbook: Health Care in America*. Washington, DC: Alliance for Health Reform.

Bergthold, L. A. 1990. *Purchasing Power in Health: Business, the State, and Health Care Politics*. New Brunswick, NJ: Rutgers University Press.

Biacentini, J. S., and M. A. Anzick. 1990. Employee Benefits in Total Compensation. *EBRI Issue Brief* 111:4.

Brandon, W. P. 1986. Rochester: Flower City and Flexnerian Seedling. In *The Training of Primary Physicians*, ed. Stephen J. Kunitz. Lanham, MD: University Press of America.

Brown, L. D. 1992a. The Politics of Health Care Reform. *Current History* 91:173–75.

———. 1992b. Getting There: The Political Context for Implementing Health Care Reform. In *Implementation Issues and National Health Reform*, ed. Charles Brecher. New York: Josiah Macy, Jr., Foundation.

———. 1992c. Policy Reform as Creative Destruction. *Inquiry* 29:188–202.

Brown, L. D., and C. McLaughlin. 1990. Constraining Costs at the Community Level. *Health Affairs* 9:5–28.

Cantor, J. C., N. L. Barrand, R. A. Desonia, A. B. Cohen, and J. C. Merrill. 1991. Data Watch: Business Leaders' Views on American Health Care. *Health Affairs* 10:98–105.

Council on Wage and Price Stability. 1976. *The Complex Puzzle of Rising Health Care Costs: Can the Private Sector Fit It Together?* Washington, DC: Executive Office for the President, Council on Wage and Price Stability.

Ehrenhalt, S. M. 1991. *Health Services in New York State: A Human Resources Perspective for the '90s*. Albany, NY: Nelson A. Rockefeller Institute of Government.

Faltermayer, E. 1992. Let's Really Cure the Health System. *Fortune* 125 (23 March): 46–50, 54, 58.

Goldberger, S. A. 1990. The Politics of Universal Access: The Massachusetts Health Security Act of 1988. *Journal of Health Politics, Policy and Law* 15:857–85.

Harris, Louis, and Associates. 1992. Unpublished survey of employers.

Health Affairs. 1990. Perspectives. Responses to an essay by U. Reinhardt on health care spending and American competitiveness. Vol. 9, pp. 162–77.

Kronick, R. 1990. The Slippery Slope of Health Care Finance: Business Interests and Hospital Reimbursement in Massachusetts. *Journal of Health Politics, Policy and Law* 15:887–913.

Levit, K. R., and C. A. Cowan. 1991. Business, Households, and Governments: Health Care Costs, 1990. *Health Care Financing Review* 13 (2): 83–93.

McLaughlin, C., W. K. Zellers, and L. D. Brown. 1989. Health Care Coalitions: Characteristics, Activities, and Prospects. *Inquiry* 26:72–83.

Martin, C. J. 1991. *Shifting the Burden: The Struggle over Growth and Corporate Taxation*. Chicago: University of Chicago Press.

MEDSTAT. 1992. *MEDSTAT Report*. 1:1–16. Ann Arbor, MI: MEDSTAT Systems, Inc.

Mizruchi, M. S. 1992. *The Structure of Corporate Political Action: Interfirm Relations and Their Consequences*. Cambridge, MA: Harvard University Press.

Plotke, D. 1992. The Political Mobilization of Business. In *The Politics of Interests: Interest Groups Transformed*, ed. Mark P. Petracca. Boulder, CO: Westview.

Reinhardt, U. E. 1989. Health Care Spending and American Competitiveness. *Health Affairs* 8:5–21.

Sapolsky, H. M. 1981. Corporate Attitudes toward Health Care Costs. *Milbank Memorial Fund Quarterly/Health and Society* 59:561–85.

U.S. CBO (U.S. Congress, Congressional Budget Office). 1992. *Projections of National Health Expenditures*. Washington, DC: CBO.

Vogel, D. 1989. *Fluctuating Fortunes: The Political Power of Business in America*. New York: Basic.

Together Again: Business, Government, and the Quest for Cost Control

Cathie Jo Martin

Abstract Corporate America leads the pack in the collective anxiety attack over health care costs. But will the business community add its considerable political power to the movement for national health reform? Conventional wisdom suggests not: businessmen seldom rally for collective concerns, have traditionally been biased against government action, and have diverse interests. This article guardedly offers grounds for greater optimism about corporate participation, arguing that the proper institutional context can help businessmen to see their preferences as consistent with health reform. Business groups have already proven critical to the issue development stage, where a dedicated group of corporate health reformists were key to getting reform on the national agenda. Business may also respond to strong leadership from President Clinton and assist in the legislation of national health reform. Yet the price of this corporate support is a decidedly conservative slant to the proposed legislation.

Health care cost containment and the Holy Grail have a lot in common: elusive but ever-inspiring, they capture our imagination but escape our grasp. Past cost containment efforts faltered under the attack of providers, who used their political power and administrative expertise to weaken cost control legislation and evade its implementation. Confined to the domain of incremental adjustment, these interventions lacked the scope and power necessary to effect real change. Providers, insurers, and businessmen all rejected more comprehensive national reforms as costly, invasive of physician power, and ideologically incorrect.

Of late, however, the escalating costs of health care have triggered a collective anxiety attack, intensifying the crusade for containment. Joined to the concerns about costs are worries about the 34 million uninsured Americans, many of whom are working poor (Fuchs 1988: 9). For the first time in fifteen years a fundamental national overhaul of our health financing system is on the public agenda. In a remarkable reversal of fortune, national health reform has become associated with keeping costs down rather than driving them up. As a result, although corporate America has in the past rejected national health insurance as one step short of Moscow, some businessmen are at the forefront of the latest national reform effort.[1] Worried about international competition and budget deficits, these businessmen fear that Americans now face a choice: between tightening the belt or tightening the noose. The gluttonous health sector, expected to consume 15 percent of the annual GNP by the year 2000, seems a prime candidate for fiscal dieting (Polzer 1990: 30).

Even providers no longer present a unified front against national health reform, with some groups now recognizing the great impetus toward national health reform and offering their own proposals (Peterson 1992). The American College of Physicians and the Catholic Health Association go so far as to support global budgets (Pear 1992a; Catholic Health Association 1992: 18). But the most powerful provider organizations (the American Medical Association and the American Hospital Association) seem inspired by a desire for damage control. They support assorted incremental reforms but continue to oppose the more threatening cost containment proposals (Kosterlitz 1992).

A strong business showing for national reform could counteract the traditional dominance of providers and insurers in health policy. Bringing businessmen to define their interests as consistent with the collective goals of controlled costs and expanded access would create the political openings for genuine cost containment. The essential problem is whether a critical mass of the business community can be mobilized, either alone or in consort with other reformist forces, to offset producer power.

The conventional view of business participation in policy-making is skeptical about mobilizing corporate support for health reform. Corporate activism happens when a firm's interests are concentrated, but corporations tend to be complacent about collective matters or about issues outside the fundamental concerns of companies (Olson 1965). For example, Sapolsky et al. (1981) found in health what Bauer et al. (1972) found in

---

1. National health reform is not necessarily the same as national health insurance, as will be made clear below; however, both entail a national plan for regulating the health care financing of all Americans.

trade two decades earlier: a quiescent corporate crowd largely oblivious to the burgeoning medical claims on their financial statements.

The conventional view is that nonincremental policy changes only transpire either when a dominant business sector's primary interests coincide with those changes or when government bureaucrats are sufficiently insulated from narrow sectarian demands to create policy designed to meet the collective interest (Ferguson 1984; Skocpol 1985; Morone and Dunham 1985). In the latter case, business is a hindrance rather than a help to the process. The former case offers some potential for business participation in reform processes. But this involvement is unlikely in health reform, since corporate consumers of health services do not have concentrated interests in reforming the system. Although health costs have greatly increased in magnitude since Sapolsky et al.'s seminal study (1981), they remain only one of many factors in production.

In addition, despite the considerable incentives for business as a whole to engage in the health reform crusade, three other constraints impede corporate action. First, businessmen are ideologically predisposed to distrust the state: a national plan that increases federal control over health financing decisions will elicit an automatic "no" from many corporate quarters. Second, although business as a whole has impressive reasons for wanting cost containment, individual interests vary widely. Large, unionized, export-oriented firms now subsidize the costs of the uninsured, many of whom work at minimum-wage jobs without benefits. A health system that seeks to distribute the costs more equally among employers obviously creates new winners and losers. Third, corporate executives may choose to join the political struggle for aggregate cost containment or may opt instead for short-term, self-interested solutions, such as cost shifting, that do little to halt the overall growth of the health burden.

In this paper, I break with the conventional view by offering a scenario in which corporate consumers of health care (with less concentrated interests than producers) can aid in the reform process. Business mobilization around this collective reform is possible but depends on two important developments in the political, institutional realm.

First, for business to contribute to the development of the issue, a core group of corporate reformers must organize. Some part of the business community must decide that health reform is a top political issue and that greater government direction is appropriate and necessary. This requires changes in corporate preferences. Whether these preferences change depends on specific developments in the institutions that mediate shared business interests. Thus, the particular characteristics and strategies of business associations will greatly influence the prospects for reform.

Second, at the legislative stage, business must be organized to support a given proposal and to lend resources and energy to the legislative battle. For a wide spectrum of business to take an active positive role at the legislative stage usually requires top-down mobilization by sympathetic political entrepreneurs, often strategically placed within the administration. Business groups alone have difficulties mustering the leadership and organizational scope necessary to focus on a chosen option and to coordinate the warlike campaign for legislation.

This sanguine view of business participation in the political process leaves us, however, with certain ironies. First, business seems to be critical to the policy-making process, but it is incapable of taking action on its own. Business activism depends on top-down mobilization by government. It seems, then, that government cannot act without business participation, but that business cannot mobilize until government acts.

Second, corporate involvement in the reform process greatly improves the chances of its political success. But recruiting business to overcome provider intransigence does not guarantee a happy ending. As soon as business is brought into the process, the dynamics change. Business mobilization has its own set of costs. Corporate reformers may have relaxed their ideological opposition to government coordination of health financing, but they have nonetheless pulled the debate to the right. Whatever we consider the merits of a single-payer system to be, corporate opposition has diminished the chances that it will be passed into law. Although President Clinton may be able partially to reconcile conflicting interests, it is by no means certain that this consensus position represents the best possible solution to the health care crisis. Even if the business community chooses to engage in collective political solutions, the many details, exclusions, and transition rules of the legislation will certainly favor its political supporters.[2]

Options for Health Care Reform

Four major reform proposals for restructuring the health financing system organize the national debate: the single-payer system, the play-or-pay

---

2. An alternative to mobilizing business is to use the disarray of the business community to increase the relative power of the state. This strategy works quite well when different producer groups lobby for their own narrowly concentrated interests; the state gets leverage to pursue a middle way. In the case of health, however, businesspeople enter as consumers, have more collective concerns, and can act as counterweights to providers.

plan, the Heritage Foundation's tax credit proposal, and the managed competition approach.

The single-payer approach creates a single pool into which all pay; this pool negotiates with hospitals and doctors. It is a tax-based rather than a premium-based system. Some plans abolish private insurance and depend entirely on government administration. Other plans allow for private insurance or at least allow these insurers to administer the public plan. Representative Marty Russo and Senators Bob Kerry (D-NE), Tom Daschle (D-SD), Howard Metzenbaum (D-OH), and Paul Simon (D-IL) have all sponsored single-payer bills.

Woolhandler and Himmelstein, in an unpublished manuscript (undated) argue that a Canadian-style system would save $69 to $83.2 billion in administrative costs. Critics retort that the Canadian national debt is twice as high as ours per capita and that the Canadian federal government is shifting costs to the provinces (Brown 1989: 29). Others worry that the national government is not competent to administer the plan and that quality will decrease without competitive market pressures. There is also concern that increasing taxes is not politically feasible; however, Blendon (1988) finds that 66 percent of Americans would tolerate a small tax increase targeted for health care.

The "play-or-pay" system is a mixed public-private system that imposes global budgets to limit costs, regulated rates to reduce inequities, and mandates on employers to expand coverage. The play-or-pay feature means that employers either play and offer health insurance, or pay a new payroll tax of 5 to 8 percent, used to expand the public program. Play-or-pay has been the Senate leadership's approach of choice since the HealthAmerica bill (S. 1277) was proposed in June 1991.[3]

Critics of the initial Democratic proposal charged that it had no cost containment mechanism (Knox 1991). This may be attributed in part to Senator Kennedy's close relationship with providers. But during markup, the committee strengthened the powers of the health expenditure board to contain costs.[4] Critics worry that the rate regulation of play-or-pay will generate some of the same market problems as price controls. The mandate has also been widely debated. Swartz (1990) argues that mandates

3. The bill was proposed by Majority Leader George Mitchell (D-ME), Edward Kennedy (D-MA), John D. Rockefeller IV (D-WV), and Donald Riegle (D-MI). It requires a payroll tax of 7 percent. Funds from this tax would be used to create a new public insurance plan called AmeriCare, which would also absorb Medicaid (Kennedy 1991).

4. In the leadership's original bill the board would provide a forum for the negotiation of rates between purchasers and providers. But in the marked-up version, the board would have the power to set the rates in the event of a stalemate (Rovner 1992b).

will fracture the insurance market and reduce the risk pool. Wilensky (1989: 32) asserts that mandated benefits will create a new burden on business, increase the hourly cost for workers receiving the minimum wage by up to 80 cents, and precipitate a loss of jobs. But Brown (1990) responds that the alternative to mandating benefits is to increase general revenues to cover access: mandates may not be an ideal option, but they are better than the alternatives. Finally, play-or-pay has been criticized as a first step toward a single-payer system. This view gained credence with the proposed setting of the "pay" rate at 7 percent of payroll. Many large employers' health costs are as much as 14 percent of payroll. Thus, skeptics conclude that the system was designed to give individuals an incentive to opt into the public plan (Zedlewski et al. 1992).

The Heritage Foundation tax credit or voucher system seeks to reintroduce competition into the health care market.[5] This plan changes all employment-related benefits into direct wages: workers pay for premiums directly. Individuals and families get tax credits from the government, adjusted for income, so that all sources of insurance (and out-of-pocket expenditures) are treated equally. All heads of households are required to buy at least catastrophic insurance, but state mandating of specific benefits is illegal. The plan limits malpractice suits and "experience rating" by insurers and encourages the use of a single, universal insurance claim form.[6] In its pure form, the Heritage plan entails almost as much government monitoring as play-or-pay (Kinsley 1992). It differs in leaving the reform process to the private market, rather than to government regulation and administration.

The plan presented by President Bush adopted pieces of the Heritage approach but fell far short of comprehensive reform. Also, Bush's plan included no realistic funding strategies.[7] While the Heritage proposal ended the tax deduction for employer-funded health benefits, Bush avoided antagonizing business with this politically difficult move. The maximum tax credits stipulated by the plan ($1,250 for individuals and $3,750 for families) are unlikely to be enough to cover the costs of health care for poor

5. In health financing, third-party payers (insurance companies and government purchasers) upset the supply-and-demand relationship because neither patients nor providers experience price constraints. Thus one way of keeping costs down is to reintroduce market incentives.

6. Routine care would be cheaper if purchased out-of-pocket. The current system directs government assistance to those employed workers who need the assistance the least. There is no reward in the system for providers who offer services efficiently, since consumers hardly notice the cost of health care (Haislmaier 1992).

7. The traditional Republican culprit—waste, fraud, and abuse in Medicare and Medicaid, plus a corresponding slack in the commercial insurance industry—was idealistically expected to produce much of the necessary funds (Rovner 1992c).

families. All states would be required to guarantee basic plans that could be purchased with the vouchers. But would these plans meet the needs of the very ill? Governors worried that the plan would pass the problem along to the states.[8]

A final option is the managed competition proposal. This approach, based on the work of Alain Enthoven, seeks to change the market incentives for both providers and consumers, primarily by aggregating consumers into large purchasing cooperatives. The Democratic Leadership Council's version of these groups, called regional health insurance purchasing corporations (HIPCs), would evaluate plans, negotiate rates, and offer their members a choice of the best plans. States would be responsible for regulating HIPCs, but the entities could take various forms (Rosner 1993).

The health plans themselves would also be regulated in order to ensure quality and minimize costs. A national board would determine a standardized benefit package; only plans that provided the package would be certified as "accountable health plans." Consumers would only receive a tax credit for their health care costs if they bought a certified plan. The proposal also restricts employers' deductions of their contributions: employers must offer their workers a choice of at least two certified plans, and deductions would be limited to the cost of the cheapest accountable plan in the region. The rationale for this is to redirect consumers toward less costly managed care plans (such as HMOs) or catastrophic plans if the consumer feels that he or she does not need the extra coverage. By limiting the tax deductibility to lower-cost options, it is argued, health decisions will become more cost effective (Rosner 1993).

According to its advocates, managed competition would move all consumers to the managed care market and would accomplish dramatic changes in the health care landscape without excessive government intervention (Faltermayer 1992). But since the plan stipulates both mandates and regulatory boards, the government would remain very involved (Abramowitz 1992).

One reason for the popularity of managed competition is its political

8. Nelson Rockefeller pointed out the case of a family who, after losing its job-related coverage, would be required to pay $9,000 for individual coverage but would only be eligible for a voucher of $560 under the president's plan. The states would be required to run the tax credit system and to ensure that basic coverage would be available. Also, the plan changed the way in which Medicaid reimbursements are given to the state. These reimbursements are now awarded retrospectively, based on the amount spent by the state. Bush's plan would change this, giving the states an annual amount prospectively based on the number of Medicaid recipients (Rovner 1992c).

feasibility. First, market approaches tend to be more acceptable ideologically. Second, the plan builds on the employer coalition movement of the 1980s. Throughout the eighties, firms in many regions tried to restrain costs through purchaser coalitions, a smaller-scale type of consumer cooperative that shares much with the managed competition idea. Although these efforts had varied success, an institutional legacy was established (Jaeger 1983; Cronin 1988).

Third, managed competition has been helped politically by the recent rage in corporate cost controls—managed care networks. These networks, administered by the large insurers, use their strength in numbers to secure advantageous rates for their customers. In a Foster Higgins sample, 45 percent of the employees are enrolled in a managed care plan; nearly three-fourths of the companies offer a managed care option (Foster Higgins 1992: 5). Companies using managed care in a Tower Perrin study reported that their growth rate decreased from 18 percent to 12 percent (Tower Perrin 1992: 2). The cognitive step from managed care to managed competition is a small one: businessmen are instinctively drawn to a national solution that is close to what they are already doing at the micro level. Finally, the move of big insurers into managed care offers another reason for the political feasibility of managed competition: these giants hope to administer the purchaser cooperatives (interview by author, September 1992).[9]

Managed competition has its share of detractors; criticism will undoubtedly increase as the details of the proposal emerge. Some worry that managed competition will increase administrative costs, as managed care networks have done at the micro level. We may find a way to pay doctors less, but do we want to pay insurers more? Others wonder if the competitive strategy will really work. Although managed care has worked at a micro level, this success may be partially due to cost shifting. Although competition generally drives prices down, in the past in health care it has driven them up. The Congressional Budget Office, for example, predicts very limited savings from this approach, at least in the short term (Pear 1992c). Another issue is what to do about Medicare (Marmor 1993). Do we push the elderly into purchaser cooperatives that are likely to move them away from fee-for-service arrangements with their long-time doctors? As a trade association representative remarked, "I don't want to have to tell my mother. Do you want to tell yours?" (interview by author, December 1992).

---

9. The interviews with industry representatives and others in this article were granted to the author on condition of anonymity.

All of these approaches are national in scope and profess to expand access to all Americans. The single-payer and play-or-pay plans entail government regulation of prices and aggregate limits to health spending. The tax credit and managed competition approaches use improved market incentives to contain costs, albeit with considerable government oversight. The play-or-pay and managed competition proposals preserve employer provision of health benefits; the single-payer and Heritage plans end the employer-based system. The single-payer system occupies the left flank; the Heritage Foundation tax credit approach, the right. The play-or-pay and managed competition approaches fall in the political center.

To date President Clinton gives signs of offering a blend of the play-or-pay and managed competition proposals, similar to the plan developed by John Garimendi, California's insurance commissioner. In keeping with the spirit of play-or-pay, Clinton has proposed that all employers be mandated to provide health benefits to their employees. To contain costs, Clinton has proposed that a national board would set spending targets for the amount to be spent on health care. Combined with these regulatory efforts to contain costs is the market-oriented managed competition proposal. Employer-paid premiums would be aggregated into nongovernment purchasing cooperatives that would coordinate coverage and restrain costs. This policy has attracted considerable support from Paul Starr (1992, 1993) and other health policy experts.

Clinton's appointment of Judith Feder as head of the transition team on health issues signaled his commitment to the global budgets and mandates found in the play-or-pay approach (Feder served on the staff of the Pepper Commission, which developed play-or-pay). Clinton's appointment of Ira Magaziner to coordinate the development of health policy within the administration suggested an interest in Garimendi-style managed competition. Most importantly, the president's appointment of Hillary Rodham Clinton to head a special health panel indicated a serious commitment to action (Friedman 1993). The form of this action, however, remains to be seen.

The transition team report created a flap in predicting a $150 billion shortfall between what it would cost to provide universal coverage and what would be saved by the proposed price controls. At this point, the special commission led by Hillary Clinton was organized, signaling to some a decline in the fortunes of play-or-pay advocates and a rise in the status of managed competition (Gosselin 1993: 10). Yet the pressures of the budget deficit may inspire a return to rate regulation as the easiest way to cap rising costs immediately. Many important decisions will have to be made concerning the details of the plan. The administration must decide whether to make employee-funded benefits above the cost of the minimum plan taxable to the employee. The number of health insurance purchasing corporations (HIPCs) in a region must be determined. Important to employers is whether companies will be allowed to have their own HIPCs or forced to join one regional HIPC and, thus, be lumped into the regional risk pool. If price controls are joined with the managed competition approach, will the accountable health plans also be subject to these price controls, or will they be free to organize their own internal prices in negotiating services with the HIPCs? If caps are developed for overall spending, will they be adjusted to reflect the different costs of health care in different regions?

Business and Cost Containment

American business as a whole has good material reasons for desiring health care cost containment. Health care costs have risen dramatically in the past forty years, increasing from 5.3 percent of the GNP in 1960 to 11.6 percent in 1989. A large proportion of this increase has fallen on corporate employers. In 1965 households funded 60.5 percent of the nation's health care; business, 17.0 percent; and government, 20.7 percent. By 1989 each sector paid about one-third. Employer health spending jumped from 2.2 percent of salaries and wages in 1965 to 8.3 percent by 1989 (Levit et al. 1991). In 1991 American employers spent on average $3,573 per worker on health insurance, an increase of 13 percent from 1990 (Bethlehem Steel Corporation undated). The expanding corporate share has resulted in part from cost shifting, in which governments negotiate ever lower rates for their share of health care, leaving business and commercial insurers to pay more. Someone must fund the uninsured, and this burden has increasingly fallen to business. For example, government policy transferred primary responsibility for the elderly from Medicare to employers, saving the Medicare Trust Fund $1 billion in fiscal year 1986 alone (Amkraut 1987). In 1989, the Financial Accounting Standards Board issued new accrual accounting requirements in a regulation called FAS 106. These requirements have altered the way corporations treat their future liabilities for retiree health benefits. Firms are now required to reflect these enormous liabilities on their bottom lines. This change has greatly enhanced the salience of the rising costs of the health system.

Since business purchasers of health care as a whole are getting badly stung by rising health costs, we might expect them to be major players in the reform battle. A critical mass of the business community, acting alone or in consort with other reformist forces, could provide an important counterweight to the traditional dominance of health policy by provider groups. But three constraints stand in the way of concerted corporate action: ideology, divided interests, and the option of choosing a short-term, self-interested strategy over a collective political solution.

Ideology is an initial constraint against widespread business support for government-led, national health care reform. Historically, business groups have resisted government intervention at the federal level, and have instead favored market interventions. For example, John Sloan (National Federation of Independent Business) called the Kennedy-Waxman proposal "nothing more than a first step towards socialized medicine" (Rovner 1989). Theodore Marmor, Judith Feder, and John Holahan noted in 1980 that

> national health insurance generates an ideological intensity matched by few other issues in American politics. The antagonists in the debate are well defined and well known, and they have remained relatively stable over time.

This historical antagonism has been receding, driven back by the assault of health costs on corporate profits. The number of business executives who strongly agreed that we are "facing a health care crisis" increased from 30 percent in 1985 to 54 percent in 1990 (William M. Mercer 1990). Cantor et al. (1991) found that 80 percent of the 384 Fortune 500 executives in their study believed that "fundamental changes are needed to make it [the health care system] better." Over 32 percent favored a public health insurance system either now or in the future, and 53 percent supported employer mandates. A study conducted by *Business and Health* found 30 percent of its corporate respondents in favor of and 25 percent neutral toward national health insurance (Wisnewski 1990: 36). As one corporate lobbyist put it, "Business from the far right has moved to the center in saying that the federal government needs to be involved" (interview by author, May 1991).

Although business seems more receptive to a national comprehensive solution to the health crisis, ideology may still play a role in guiding corporate America toward one reform option over another. In choosing an approach, businessmen must balance their predispositions toward market solutions with their evaluations of the relative merits and anticipated effectiveness of the plans. Single-payer systems entail the most government intervention and enjoy the least corporate support. Play-or-pay approaches have a larger share of corporate advocates, who are drawn to the aggregate limits on costs but are also reassured by the continuing hegemony of the employer-based system.

Many businessmen are instinctively drawn to the market assumptions of the Heritage Foundation and managed competition proposals; however, some worry that the cost containment measures are insufficient. The failure of market competition strategies in the eighties have made some businesspeople more open to grand solutions.[10] One participant explained his shift from a market competition approach to a national regulatory one: "Most of us recognize that the things we did in the mid-'80s didn't really work" (Polzer 1990).

A second constraint against business leadership in the struggle for health care reform is the uneven manner in which health costs affect firms. Rising health costs have a very different impact across the business community. Larger firms are more likely to fund employee health benefits and thus are more likely to feel the pain of escalating costs. Unionized firms are more motivated than nonunion companies: escalating health costs have increased labor-management conflict as employers push workers to fund a larger share of their premiums. Health benefits caused only 18 percent of strikes involving over 1,000 employees in 1986, compared with 78 percent in 1989.[11] Export companies who compete with firms from countries with national health insurance are hurt by rising costs. Health care supposedly adds $700 to the price of an American-made car, compared with only $200 to an auto made in Japan (Schneider 1990). Health costs for each Canadian steelworker on hourly pay are $3,200 a year; for his or her American counterpart, it costs $7,600 a year.[12] Firms with older employees also pay higher rates. Small firms that provide health insurance pay very high premiums, since their small pools limit their ability to negotiate favorable rates. Because firms have fairly diverse patterns of health care financing, they want different things from the reform process.

A related problem is that many more companies have now entered the business of providing health care services, especially with the expansion of for-profit facilities in the past decade (Salmon 1987). Conglomerates often experience internal dissension on the issue of cost containment, torn

---

10. Indeed, paradigm shifts are often related to the failure of the dominant paradigm to solve the problems of the day (Hall forthcoming).

11. A national health plan has been viewed by both sides of the bargaining table as a way to end battles between labor and management over who pays the bill (Victor 1990).

12. Part of the costs go to retiree benefits (Williams 1991). Critics charge that this number does not reflect the different factors that are included under the rubric of wages in the United States and Japan.

between divisions that are consumers of health care and those that are providers.

A final constraint against the political participation of business in the reform effort is the availability of short-term, self-interested alternatives. If firms are able to engage in cost shifting, passing their health care costs on to their employees, they will be less likely to pursue a collective political solution. Cost shifting may help individual firms for the short term, but it will do little to limit the aggregate costs of health over the long term.

Two Theories of Business Mobilization

The critical question, of course, is whether business can overcome these constraints and emerge as a positive force in the health reform effort. One's optimism on this point depends on one's views of human nature and political action: how corporate preferences for public policy are formed, and what it takes to mobilize the business community.

The literature on corporate involvement in public policy is dominated by the economic view of "preference." According to this approach, people in business have stable preferences, based on the material circumstances of their firms. These interests are readily apparent. In other words, businessmen know what their interests are; one can calculate their political preferences from the economic structures of their firms (Frieden 1988; Jacobs 1988; Kurth 1979).

The economic view is that mobilization of businessmen around collective issues occurs when their self-interests can also be gratified through selective side benefits of the proposal.[13] Sometimes a firm will assume the costs of political action without side benefits, but only when it expects to receive so much from the collective outcome that it is willing to bear the entire cost itself (Olson 1965; Stigler 1971). Political mobilization in any policy area typically involves those with the most narrowly focused interests. Producers have more focused interests than consumers, since the policy is key to the former's livelihood. Thus, producers are more willing than consumers to dedicate resources to influencing public policy.

The economic approach offers only limited hope that the constraints against business mobilization for national health reform can be overcome. First, the economic view of interests has difficulties accounting for the

13. Claus Offe (1985) argues that business can rely on an "individualist and purely instrumental form of collective action," whereas for workers "interests can only be met to the extent they are partially redefined."

persistence of ideology or suggesting ways to overcome it. Second, if corporate preferences are relatively fixed by the material conditions of the firm, then there is little room for compromise between divided interests. Unless interests can be partially redefined, a consensus position is unlikely. Finally, the economic view is pessimistic about getting firms to pursue a collective political solution instead of cost shifting. National health reform is a collective benefit; it purports to solve health care problems for everyone, whether or not they participate in the events leading to its enactment. This is a disincentive for firms to commit resources to the legislative process, since if they succeed in bringing about reform, all will enjoy the benefits of that reform, whether or not they worked to achieve it. Also, business consumers of health services might be reluctant to devote considerable resources to a campaign that addresses only one component of their total costs (Olson 1965).

Before we declare defeat and go home, I would suggest an alternative view of corporate preference and mobilization, one that allows us greater hope for our political project. It is the institutional view.[14] This approach takes issue with a purely material definition of interests, not because economic circumstance is unimportant, but because it can be interpreted in varied fashion. Groups have multiple objectives: the firm itself should be viewed as a "nonunitary actor" with conflicting and ambiguous interests (Thompson 1982: 233; Plotke 1992). With such indeterminacy, social context becomes critical in helping us interpret our situations and arrive at our objectives (Moe 1987: 277; Fligstein 1990: 102; Hall 1986). Ideas are vital in the interpretation of a problem; these ideas are disseminated through institutions and social networks (Eckstein 1988; Snow et al. 1986; Klandersman 1988: 173–76). Preferences are developed in collective institutional settings.

The institutional context is also essential to the mobilization of interests. The economic approach conceptualizes political mobilization as a decision made by rational individuals who calculate the costs and benefits of such action. By comparison, institutionalists perceive the cauldron of political mobilization to be the small groups in which people endlessly air their grievances and then, at a magical moment, decide to do something about them (McAdam 1988). Institutions and organizational networks are also critical to the swelling of the mobilization effort as the core group

14. My institutional approach represents a composite approach in that it draws from several traditions: state-centered theory, public choice new institutionalism, and new social movement theory. All share the assumptions that preferences are developed collectively within institutional settings and that institutions and networks provide the building blocks for political mobilization.

attracts others sympathetic to the cause. Contacts are generated through the organizational networks in which the core group is located. These networks spread the ideas of the movement, enable the recruitment of new members, and constitute a resource in political battles (Klandersman and Tarrow 1988). Just as decision makers in state institutions are influenced by policy legacies, actions of groups in society must be guided by previous political experiences and attitudes. Thus an institutional analysis looks at the group's makeup and the organizational strength of groups from which members are drawn.

Public institutions as well as private ones can be critical to rallying business. An economic view of corporate mobilization all too often neglects government leadership in the political organization of business. But the interests of political entrepreneurs may converge with interests of groups in society. Government leaders can augment their power against their own political enemies by mobilizing interest groups who will support their policy position.[15] Alliances cutting across the private-public divide can, thus, facilitate reform.

The institutional approach offers some optimism about overcoming the constraints against business participation in health care reform. First, institutionalists argue that individuals can reinterpret the ideological content of a policy collectively; organizational networks provide the avenues of change. Second, an institutional view of business preference suggests that, sometimes, groups with different material situations can redefine their interests and locate common ground. Finally, the institutional approach is sanguine about the possibility of collective action. Business-people become mobilized around health reform through the small groups or networks in which they formulate their political identities.

The institutional approach suggests that mediating institutions and organizational networks can help the business community become a positive force for national health reform. But in order to evaluate the likelihood that business will mobilize in the health area, we must identify the specific institutional characteristics that facilitate such action. Corporate involve-

---

15. In an important corrective, state-centered theorists have focused on the role of relatively autonomous politicians and bureaucrats in bringing about policy reforms. Reform efforts occur when government bureaucrats link their ambitions, interests, or good policy goals to that reform. They create the political space to achieve the reform by insulating themselves from private pressures. According to this view, the business community has little to offer the reform effort, since the impetus for reform is located within the state. I would suggest, however, that business groups may have more to offer government reformers than the state-centered folks admit. The options for government actors are not only being captured by private interests or insulating themselves from those interests (Martin 1989).

ment in public policy-making is significant at two stages of the process: issue development and legislation. First, at the issue development stage, a critical mass of businesspeople must develop preferences for national health reform; health must become an issue in the corporate community (Kingdon 1984). Businessmen must set a high priority on solving the health problem and determine that government regulation is an appropriate solution. Second, a critical mass must mobilize around a given proposal and fight for that proposal during the period of legislation.

The institutional characteristics important to the two stages are somewhat different. The issue development stage requires considerable commitment from a core organization (or organizations), which will focus business attention on the health problem and engineer a transformation of preference in the larger business community. I would suggest that organizations that spearhead policy transformations in the business community are usually new additions to the pattern of groups representing business interests. But these groups must also be at least somewhat connected to the preexisting institutional network of interest intermediation. Thus these new groups maintain a delicate balance between independence of prior policy positions and connection to established networks.

Independence is necessary because traditional trade associations tend to be fixed in the old mode of thinking about the issue. The new group leading the effort must be free from past commitments in order to move corporate thinking in a new direction. This group can help businessmen to rethink their interpretation of their material circumstances and to review the ideological content assigned to the policy problem and its solutions. But connection is equally important, since the group must be able to tap into the existing networks of intermediation within the business community. These preexisting networks allow corporate reformers to disseminate the reform concept and to link the health reform issue to other areas of corporate concern.

The legislative mobilization stage has different strategic objectives and requires different institutional characteristics. As the issue moves toward the legislative stage, organizations need to focus more narrowly on one concrete proposal and to widen membership or organizational scope. Focusing requires leadership—it takes leadership, from either the public or private sector, to focus enthusiasm for the chosen option and coordinate the campaign for legislation (Schattschneider 1960). To mobilize political resources for legislating the proposal requires a large membership or wide organizational scope. Organizational scope brings together diverse political factions and reduces infighting at the point of legislation; and organizations with many members, aggregating a broad cross section of business, are better positioned to concentrate attention on higher-order universal concerns. This can be a means to reconcile seemingly contradictory interests.

The general institutional structure of corporate interest intermediation in the United States makes it difficult to get leadership from business in policy change. The political representation of business is fragmented into single-sector trade associations (Maitland 1983).[16] Umbrella organizations lack jurisdictional monopoly and tend to cater to minority interests.

Leadership in the United States, instead, often comes from political entrepreneurs, who help businessmen to crystallize their support for a given policy alternative and to overcome the resistance to collective action by organizing the movement from above. Although umbrella business groups find it difficult to resolve intrabusiness splits, the packaging of a proposal measure by political entrepreneurs may overcome these limitations and unify diverse factions.[17] When big omnibus proposals bring diverse interests together, companies are forced to swallow bitter pills in order to get their own concerns met. The ability of the government to organize business is furthered by a "follow-the-pack" syndrome: the desire for business groups to be players may overwhelm their points of contention with various aspects of the bill. As one lobbyist put it, "Divisions may seem insurmountable, but once the legislation gets rolling anything can happen" (interview by author, September 1992). The success of pulling together a broad coalition, a process subject to many political contingencies, thus greatly affects the potential for reform.

Building Business Consensus

I will now examine the institutional terrain in which corporate preferences for health policy have been constructed and mobilized in order to evaluate the corporate contribution to the reform process. Health reform emerged as an important issue for many in the business community in the eighties. This process was fostered by several key groups, the most important being the Washington Business Group on Health (WBGH). WBGH was led by

16. Business is divided in America for reasons apart from the institutional mechanisms of interest intermediation identified here. The historical division between manufacturing and finance in this country is reinforced by our method of financing corporate growth (Zysman 1983). Also, the general weakness of labor has increased corporate infighting.

17. Examples of state-led coalition built around reform can be found in tax, trade, and environmental policy. See for example, Martin 1991.

Willis Goldbeck, a man generally acknowledged by both admirers and critics to be ahead of business on most health issues. In the seventies the group worked with local communities to set up purchaser coalitions. In the early 1980s WBGH opposed Reagan's deregulatory efforts to phase out health planning and physician peer review (Demkovich 1983). Goldbeck's endorsement of progressive principles in health offended many in conservative corporate corridors; yet his boundless enthusiasm for health reform attracted a sizable business following. As of 1990, 185 Fortune 500 companies belonged to WBGH (Burke 1990: 32). But Goldbeck's departure in 1989, combined with the increasing presence of provider groups in the organization, eroded the organization's leadership capability, though it has recently become more active again in its support for managed competition.

Another forum for enhancing employer awareness of the health issue was the Dunlop Group of Six. John Dunlop, a former secretary of the Department of Labor, organized this group as a meeting place for the heads of the primary business, labor, insurer, and provider associations. Dunlop's semicorporatist approach sought to deliver collectively beneficial outcomes by bringing all to the bargaining table. To this end, the group encouraged the development of coalitions at the community level (Bergthold 1990: 47–50).

Also important to the development of corporate awareness have been the health foundations. The Pew Foundation funded a number of programs to heighten corporate awareness, such as the corporate fellows program at Boston University. Developed by Richard Egdahl, the program brought benefits managers together to discuss a variety of problems facing corporate America. Many of the business activists currently involved in the national reform effort describe their participation in the Pew program as a critical formative experience.

The Robert Wood Johnson and Hartford Foundations also worked to heighten corporate awareness, largely through their contributions to the local health care coalition movement (Craig 1983). The coalitions have been criticized for failing to contain costs, in part because voluntaristic, community-based efforts do not have the scope to address the structural sources of cost increases (Brown and McLaughlin 1990). But the coalitions did provide forums in which local executives could come to learn about health issues.

These organizations fit the criteria of being both independent of and connected to the important political institutions of the business community. The origin of WBGH is emblematic of the balance between independence and connection. In 1973 the Business Roundtable hired Willis Goldbeck as the staff for a new task force on health reform. Goldbeck quickly determined that a separate organization dedicated to health reform was necessary in order to make big business "a credible participant in national health policy" instead of simply a force lobbying in the health field. Goldbeck wanted the entire Roundtable to be members (in addition to others) yet wanted independence from the parent organization (Bergthold 1990).

As the health issue has moved toward the second stage, that of unifying business consensus around a specific legislative proposal, institutions of interest intermediation have had less success. The experience of the National Association of Manufacturers (NAM) exemplifies the difficulty faced by umbrella organizations in providing leadership in health care reform. NAM members as a group pay very high health costs and are big losers in the cost-shifting game. A 1989 NAM study, conducted by Foster Higgins, found that health care costs in 1988 represented 37.2 percent of employers' profits; 99.3 percent of employers surveyed offered employee health care benefits.[18] In 1990 the board set up a health care task force to develop a reform position. After meeting for a year, the task force presented a play-or-pay plan, but the board voted against it. The plan was killed by a confluence of interests and ideology. NAM's tax task force fought the proposal on ideological grounds, seeing play-or-pay as a tax on firms. Other influential actors opposed, because their interests could be hurt by health care reform. NAM supporters of reform have now commissioned another survey, hoping to use member opinion to move the organization toward a more dominant reform role. But to date, despite majority interests in reform, no action has been taken.

The ERISA Industry Committee (ERIC), a benefits organization with a wide corporate membership, experienced difficulties similar to NAM's in trying to develop a health reform position. ERIC was founded in 1976 to respond to the increased regulations created under the Employment Retirement Income Security Act (ERISA). Although the group was originally primarily concerned about pensions, in recent years the focus has shifted to health benefits. In the final months of 1991, the organization set up a separate task force on health care benefits, which leaned toward play-or-pay. However, the board rejected the task force's recommendations and instead issued an "Interim Policy Statement" outlining a broad

18. The average cost hike was 19.1 percent for the largest companies (those with 5,000–20,000 employees), but 33.3 percent for the smallest companies (those with fewer than 25 employees) (DiBlase 1989).

list of goals, few of them specific. Despite this earlier deadlock, ERIC is continuing to try to formulate a more developed position, and seems to be heading toward an endorsement of managed competition.

The National Leadership Coalition tried to overcome the limits on umbrella organizations by emphasizing focus over scope. The coalition grew out of an earlier group of thirty-six individuals (mainly providers) called the National Leadership Commission, funded by the Pew Foundation in 1986 and conceptualized by Henry Simons, the current chairman. The commission produced a report in 1989 entitled *For the Health of a Nation* that argued that access, cost, and quality problems in health demanded systemic reform. Press coverage was considerable and the coalition's staff began to meet with corporate boards, labor organizations, state legislators, hospitals, and "anyone else who would listen" (interview by author with a National Leadership Commission executive, June 1992).

Although the original coalition was scheduled to end, the speaking series generated considerable enthusiasm for the group to continue. By the spring of 1990 a new coalition had come together, this time composed of business, labor, and consumer groups.[19] A number of companies and trade associations joined with their unions, especially in sectors where labor-management accords committed both sides to participating in the national policy debates. Member firms also recruited others from their industrial sector: Bethlehem Steel displayed early, avid interest in the health care cost problem and sensitized others in the steel industry.[20] In like manner, Chrysler was a leader in the auto sector; James River Company, in the paper industry; and Safeway, in the food retail sector.[21] New members were also drawn by the full-page advertisement in the *New York Times* in January 1992, which stated, "National health care reform without cost control is like moving furniture into a burning house."

19. Participants include Bethlehem Steel, Chrysler, Southern California Edison, Dayton Hudson, Georgia-Pacific, International Paper, Meredith Corporation, Northern Telecom, Pacific Gas and Electric, Safeway, Time Warner, Westinghouse, Xerox, and various unions.

20. Bethlehem persuaded its trade association, the American Iron and Steel Institute, to set up a task force to deal with the issue (interview with steel industry representatives, June 1992).

21. Joseph Califano established a task force on the board of Chrysler in the early eighties, including Lee Iacocca, Bill Milliken (former governor of Michigan), Doug Frazier (president of United Auto Workers), Jerome Holland (American Red Cross), and Wally Maher (head of employee benefits). The task force recommended to the board that there was a limit to what the company could do and what the private sector as a whole could do. The recognition of a need for greater involvement in national policy resulted in the creation of a permanent health person in Washington, D.C.—Wally Maher. This health person would "work to try to sensitize the business community, to develop coalitions, and to impress the public sector that health costs were hurting the competitiveness of private industry" (interview by author with auto industry representative, June 1992).

In the fall of 1991, the newly organized coalition formally presented a detailed plan for systemic reform of the health care system (National Leadership Coalition 1991). The coalition aimed to reduce the growth rate in health costs by 2 percent per year until the annual increases matched GNP growth (Couch 1992). The proposal endorsed play-or-pay to curb costs.[22] The states would run an expanded public program, Pro-Health, and would be responsible for making sure it met its spending target.

The National Leadership Coalition deserves points for focusing attention on a single proposal. Its success in avoiding the policy stalemates which plague umbrella groups can be attributed to an important organizational rule. In order to belong to the coalition one must agree to its charter and plan. Unlike other organizations that have been hampered in action by the desire not to give offense, the coalition is more willing to take tough positions. If a member objects to a proposal but has no alternative, the objection is ignored. The group is prepared to have members walk away (interview by author, September 1992).

There have been costs to this strategy. The rule has helped to prevent deadlock, but members have been lost in the process. Some corporations departed because they felt the coalition's position was too radical. As David Helms (senior benefits consultant at Du Pont) put it, "Maybe someday we can look at prices and mandates, but we have not exhausted all of the less radical solutions yet." [23] Others felt that Henry Simons had a preset agenda: play-or-pay was destined to be the group's choice from the beginning, and employer input was an exercise in legitimization. Labor groups were put off by the tax on workers' income, which would fund the public parts of the plan. Many unions were also unwilling to support anything other than a single-payer plan (Burke 1992).

Some companies who left the National Leadership Coalition formed a new group, the Corporate Health Care Forum, "in order to address

22. Details of the plan are as follows: Employers must either provide health care or opt out and pay a payroll tax of 7 percent; employees would pay 1.75 percent of their wages. To fund those not included in the employment-based system, the proposal would create the expanded public plan, Pro-Health. The public plan would be partially paid for by the 7 percent tax on noninsuring firms and by a fee of 0.5 percent applied to *all* companies' payroll and to workers' wages up to $125,000. Employer health plans would have to have maximum deductibles of $200 for individuals and $400 for families and would have to cover 80 percent of the costs of health care interventions. The out-of-pocket expenses would be capped at $1,500 for individuals and $3,000 for families. A National Health Review Board would be created to regulate rates and to restrict aggregate spending by setting annual targets for total expenditures tied to annual GNP growth (Geisel 1991). The coalition also called for expanding health maintenance organizations and other forms of organized care.

23. These firms included AT&T, Du Pont, Arco, Eastman Kodak, 3M, and Burger King (Garland 1991).

the interests and concerns of companies that believe that play or pay and global budgeting is not the way to go." [24] To these firms, an obvious forum for their interests was lacking. One participant explained that he did a presentation of the play-or-pay approach to the top management of his company. The top executives were troubled by the mandate on small business and shared the Urban Institute's analysis that play-or-pay constituted an avenue to the single-payer system. His company is enormously capital-intensive with high profit margins and would be hurt by that part of the payroll tax assessed on corporate earnings to cover the uncompensated care pool. In addition, it has a very low rate of unionization. Thus, its interests are markedly different from the interests of the unprofitable, heavily unionized auto and steel manufacturers (interview by author, December 1992). Although the Corporate Health Care Forum does not yet have a formal position, it is sympathetic to managed competition.

Despite the National Leadership Coalition's strength in focusing, it has been less successful in widening its organizational scope in the business community. Although the group claims to represent a fairly broad spectrum of business and labor, important gaps remain. A major gap has been the absence of support from small business. The National Small Business United (NSBU) participated at the beginning but ultimately was unable to support employer mandates. [25]

The divide between large and small business is formidable, for reasons of ideology and interest. Ideology prejudices small business groups against the active government role in play-or-pay. According to one association representative, small businessmen have "a basic mistrust in government and strong, an almost visceral belief that the market will produce a better solution" (interview by author, June 1992). Only about 25 percent of a National Federation of Independent Business sample supported government mandates or wanted government to pay premiums for those unable to pay (Hall and Kuder 1990: 11, 13, 37). But ideology seems to be slowly changing among small businessmen. The NFIB reports that "health insurance ranks twice as high as the second most important concern of small business" (National Federation of Independent Business 1992). Sixty-nine percent of NFIB's membership believes that health care is a basic right (Hall and Kuder 1990: 12).

24. The group now includes, among others, Alcoa, ARCO, Allied Signal, Amoco, Ameritech, AT&T, Bell Atlantic, Chevron, DEC, Du Pont, IBM, Kodak, MCI, Motorola, Nynex, Southwestern Bell, US West, USX (interview by author with industry representative, December 1992).

25. Also, the NSBU pointed out that most small businesses already pay 11 to 20 percent of their payroll for health insurance (Burke 1992: 53).

Interests are difficult to reconcile, since the issue has been framed in redistributive terms, and has taken on the aspect of class warfare. The uninsured come largely from the population of the working poor: those with low-wage jobs and no benefits, who work for small business and service firms. The costs of treating the uninsured are shifted, in the form of higher hospital rates, to large, privately insured companies. Thus, many big businessmen see mandates as a mechanism to force small business to accept responsibility for their workers' health costs. Small businessmen, many operating at the margin, experience these mandates as a direct attack on their profits and ability to stay in business. Small businessmen have retaliated with a proposal to cap employer tax deductions for health benefits. They argue that large firms' provision of rich benefits to their workers should not be subsidized by the government (interviews by author, September 1992).

Despite the distributive consequences of health reform, there may be some room for compromise. Making the payroll tax for the public program graduated and offering 100 percent employer deductibility for health premiums would lessen the burden on very small firms. Small business groups have not yet taken defined positions on issues like global budgeting and all-payer rates. Mandates are the central sticking point, but creative solutions to the impasse may be possible (interview by author 1992).

In the fall of 1991 an organizational development occurred that widened the gap between large and small business and made the prospects of a comprehensive reform bill in the short term more remote. Major small business trade associations entered into an alliance with insurers and providers to fight the trend toward comprehensive national reform, forming the Healthcare Equity Action League (HEAL). Over 600 firms and groups currently belong to the coalition, and 110 belong to the Steering Committee, which costs $1,000 to join (HEAL 1992).[26] HEAL has an aggressive membership drive, working especially to attract big business firms who dislike "play-or-pay."

The organization takes the middle road between fundamental reform and the status quo, calling for a variety of incremental reforms that enjoy widespread support from all parties.[27] HEAL argues that incremental reforms are more politically feasible than sweeping change:

26. Pamela Bailey (Healthcare Leadership Council) and Mark Gorman (National Restaurant Association) are the cochairs of HEAL, representing respectively the insurer/provider and small business sides on which the organization is based (PR Newswire 1992a).

27. These changes include insurance underwriting reforms, revocation of state mandates, full deductibility of health insurance premiums, medical malpractice reforms, and legal changes to encourage the proliferation of managed care (HEAL 1992).

A lot of the grand solutions produce gridlock. . . . We have settled on a first pass to do things that are doable. When something is on fire, you continue to try to design the perfect fire engine, but in the meantime you throw water on the fire." (Interview by author with HEAL representative, May 1992)

HEAL was organized by the National Association of Wholesaler-Distributors, the National Federation of Independent Business, the Food Marketing Institute, the Healthcare Leadership Council, and the National Restaurant Association. The small business founders, considering health issue in an informal group called the Powers Court Group, became aware that the Healthcare Leadership Council, a group of providers and insurers, was organizing a coalition in the health area.

The small business group determined that it was to their advantage to enter into dialogue with the medical group for two reasons. First, they favored reforms to help small businesses buy group health insurance but opposed employer mandates (Geisel 1991); they wanted to cultivate alliances but felt uncomfortable with the solutions generated by big business groups. Second, they felt that they could not afford to wait for fundamental reform. John Motley (of NFIB) explained, "Small business can't wait another year to begin to resolve this issue. They're getting hit with astronomical health insurance increases constantly. When you combine this with the effects of a national recession, everyone loses, especially employees" (PR Newswire 1992b). Also, small business had only recently begun to think about health care and had not been pushed to fundamental reforms out of frustration with incremental action. One member explained:

Some firms tend to want to create the totally perfect solution. It has become a lifelong chase for them. They are the ones who felt the pain before others because they were committed to a benefits package or engaged in international competition. The folks who got to the table first began to work on it first. It has been an incremental process for them. We only came to the process about a year ago. (Interview by author, June 1992)

Insurers joined the HEAL coalition for two reasons. First, incremental reforms offer a way of preventing more sweeping changes. Second, HEAL allowed insurer-provider groups to join forces with part of the consumer base (interview by author, September 1992).

Although tensions between the two sides have been restrained, they may yet emerge as the process progresses.[28] One source of instability is the split within the insurance industry itself. The large insurers, who have largely moved into the managed care business in recent years, are solidly behind small market reform and the managed competition approach. The "Gang of Five" has worked intensely behind the scenes to advocate managed care networks as a central part of any reform proposal. This faction also believes that the creation of large-scale networks will help to weed out small companies, who have given the industry a bad name.[29] By comparison, the small insurers oppose managed care networks and small market reform because they fear that these innovations will put them out of business.

The Health Insurance Association of America (HIAA), the main industry association, has suffered under the strain of these divisions. Several of the largest companies left the HIAA, when the industry association refused to go along with their wishes. The HIAA has been dominated by smaller companies, and until recently it concentrated its energies on resisting all types of fundamental reforms. It waged a state-level offensive with its $4 million "Campaign to Insure All Americans." This included a series of polls showing public support for retaining the private insurance system.[30]

In a surprising turnaround, however, HIAA recently proposed mandated basic benefits, community ratings, and limits on tax breaks for insurance premiums. It continued to oppose both global budgets and managed competition. How can we explain this sudden enthusiasm for a rate-regulation approach to health reform? The step marks a realization by medium-sized insurance companies, the major constituents of HIAA, that reform was imminent. Managed competition could put them out of business, since companies would bid to administer the networks and the larger companies would have a competitive advantage. Rate regulation, by comparison, could preserve a role for the smaller insurers. Also, community rating helps the smaller insurers stay in business because they tend

28. Small business groups support rating bands, or set ranges between which premiums are allowed to fluctuate, as a mechanism for keeping firm costs down. The insurers are not enthusiastic about any restrictions on premiums (interview by author with industry representative, June 1992).

29. The Gang of Five comprises CIGNA, Prudential, Metropolitan Life, Aetna, and Travelers (Garland 1992).

30. So far twenty states have passed health reform legislation, and the industry's proposal has been adopted by sixteen of them. HIAA achieved these legislative victories in part with strategically timed "fax alerts" sent to small businessmen, asking them to flood the telephone lines of their state legislators (interview by author with industry representative, September 1992).

to have smaller risk pools and to pay higher rates (Pear 1992b; interview by author with industry representatives, September and December 1992).

HEAL's future may be uncertain, yet its creation placed two obstacles in the way of national reform. First, the small business alliance with insurers created institutional constraints against a small business coalition with big business. Second, the insurers and the small business participants of HEAL have much greater lobbying capabilities than the National Leadership Coalition. For example, the strength of the small business lobby in the past decade has become legendary. A Washington observer remarks:

> The slash-and-burn approach makes political enemies, but here small business has an advantage: It is so ubiquitous that most elected officials find it counterproductive to stay angry. "These folks are intimately acquainted with members of Congress," grouses Rostenkowski, who once banned NFIB lobbyists from testifying before his committee. "If members don't play golf with them, they play tennis with them." Their grass-roots operation can flood the Congress with calls and mail almost effortlessly. (Borger 1992)[31]

By comparison the National Leadership Coalition emphasizes education over lobbying. Its staff explains that they "don't want to move the system too quickly. Any bill that passes must have bipartisan support." Although members testify before committees, the group has no organized, grass-roots lobbying operation. The limits of this legislative strategy become clear when compared with the considerable organizational power of the other side.

HEAL had considerable influence with the Bush White House in urging action and in helping to develop the Republican proposal.[32] The group convinced the Bush team that the administration could become a player in health reform without having to support a radical solution: "The issue could be controlled" (interview by author, June 1992). The president seemed reassured when he remarked, "When you see a coalition of this magnitude working for this common end, it gives me great confidence we can get something done" (Bureau of National Affairs 1992). HEAL also

---

31. HEAL has also brought in outsiders for spin control, the public relations firm of Burson Marsteller. They published an ad in *USA Today* costing $60,000, which said, "Everyone knows that we need health care reform . . . [but] we cannot afford to scrap the current system for a costly new federal bureaucracy" (Lee 1992).

32. The decision to remove from an earlier draft the proposal eliminating the tax deductibility of health insurance premiums has been credited to HEAL members (interview by author with industry representative, June 1992).

worked closely with the conservative Democrats. The group's influence with Clinton remains to be seen.

Leadership from the State

I argued earlier that mobilization of the business community at the legislative stage usually depends on leadership from political entrepreneurs. Parts of the business community can be brought into a state-led coalition to engineer radical policy change. Peterson (1992) suggests that there is more policy entrepreneurial capacity than ever before in the domain of health reform. But until the election of President Clinton, the political landscape of health reform included limited government leadership on either side of the partisan aisle.

Democratic leadership in Congress tried hard to produce a consensus proposal but remained fragmented on health reform. The fragmentation within the Democratic Congress cannot be blamed on a lack of effort to find common ground. Indeed, after Harris Wofford's election in Pennsylvania, the Democrats chose health care to be a central issue of the 1992 presidential campaign. In the Senate a special Democratic caucus was appointed to develop a consensus position.

The split was over the appropriate form of reform: both chambers contain proponents of single-payer, play-or-pay, and market reform. On the Senate side play-or-pay enjoyed front-runner status, although the party's right wing supported a market reform approach.[33] David Pryor (D-AR) and Lloyd Bentsen both feared the effect of play-or-pay on small business. Turf conflicts also existed, as over whether the leadership bill would be handled through the Labor Committee (headed by Kennedy, who favors play-or-pay) or the Finance Committee (headed by Bentsen, who favors market reform). A Senate aide remarked, "Trying to bring all the Democrats under the same umbrella on this issue is like trying to bring all the Republicans under the same umbrella on abortion" (Rovner 1991b).

On the House side, Speaker Tom Foley's (D-WA) promise to produce a leadership proposal by the end of 1991 failed. To mask the divisions plaguing the party and perhaps to solve those divisions, the Democrats

---

33. This was captured in the Senate Finance Committee bill (S. 1872) sponsored by Lloyd Bentsen (D-TX) and several Republicans. It did not constitute fundamental overhaul of the system but would nonetheless dramatically change the climate for small business employers. It would impose caps on the costs of health insurance policies for small businesses (with fifty employees or fewer). It would allow the self-insured to deduct their total costs of their health insurance premiums (instead of the current cap at 25 percent) (Rovner 1992d).

organized a series of "town hall" meetings on the "health care crisis in America" during a week in January of 1992. The meetings attempted to show how much the Democrats cared about the issue, in obvious contrast to the president. They also were designed to help the Democrats avoid another fiasco like the Catastrophic Coverage Act, in which the Congress believed that people wanted one thing but quickly encountered widespread resistance. Vic Fazio (D-CA) explained, "One of the ideas that we have here is going out and trying to find out what the American people think before we go forward" (Rovner 1992a).

In the spring of 1992, the House majority leader, Richard Gephardt (D-MO), and the Ways and Means chair, Dan Rostenkowski (D-IL), began pushing hard for a "first-step" bill that combined regulation (global budgeting) with market reform provisions to help small business. Yet some worried that this incremental approach might delay sweeping reform and give too much credit to the Republicans (interview by author with congressional staffers, June and September 1992).

Energetic fragmentation in the Democratic Congress was matched by complacent inaction by the Bush administration. Bush ignored health reform until it became clear that he needed a new domestic initiative. Despite considerable pressure to "do something," the administration initially felt that the health issue was not a winning political issue. William Roper noted in 1990 that health care was not yet a mature issue: "The candidate who made universal access to health care a central theme of his campaign did not win the 1988 election" (Rovner 1991a). Even after the president announced his market reform proposal in February, the administration did nothing to push his agenda. Robert Mosbacher (campaign chairman) explained, "Health is not a first-tier issue for us, like education" (Dowd 1992).

The president's Comprehensive Health Reform Program was finally presented to the public on 6 February, after much foot-dragging. The Bush plan met certain ideological requirements. It was designed to build on the existing system, what the president calls "the best in the entire world," rather than radically reform it. It promised to preserve choice. Finally, Bush vowed to implement the system without new taxes, although it was projected to cost $100 billion over five years (Rovner 1992b).

With the election of President Clinton, these dynamics have changed dramatically. Clinton's commitment to health reform in the campaign signaled to Washington and to the business community that a significant piece of legislation would be proposed and probably passed. The president's choice of managed competition also helped to end the deadlock over play-

or-pay, the earlier favorite. Whether or not one believes that managed competition will fulfill its manifold promises, it has brought new language into the process that may reduce some of the objections to mandates and expenditure caps (Kuttner 1993).

Clinton's choice of managed competition illustrates the complicated involvement of business in policy reform. On the one hand, the president's decision to highlight this approach in the campaign was a reflection of its acceptability by the business community and the major insurers. It demonstrates the importance of business in the development and the packaging of the issue. On the other hand, Clinton's election and the showcasing of managed competition has suddenly inspired a flurry of activity among American firms. Companies have been prompted to take a closer look at the issue and have begun to formulate a position. Where business associations before had difficulty arriving at consensus, they can now more easily take action in response to the government's agenda.

Conclusion

This paper considers the corporate role in the health care reform process. I argue that corporate employers could counteract the traditional provider opposition to the legislation of stringent cost control measures in health care financing. But the positive participation of the business community is by no means certain. Business typically does not get involved in collective issues, unless as producers they hold narrow, concentrated interests in the area. Ideological misgivings, divided interests, and self-interested alternatives also combine to hinder a show of force from corporate America.

I argue that the constraints against corporate action can be overcome with the right institutional developments in the organization of business interests. The issue stage requires committed core groups to heighten corporate awareness about health problems. These groups guide businessmen in redefining their preferences for health policy and in making the issue a high priority. Second, the legislative stage requires organizational leadership to help business agree on a particular policy option and to build a broad coalition around the chosen proposal.

Institutional developments within business at the issue stage have been fairly successful. A core band of corporate reformers has generated greater business and public awareness about the issue. Corporate energy has helped to push health reform to the top of the public agenda.

But the vast majority of companies are largely reactive, remaining silent until perceived action by government forces them to confront the issue. At the legislative stage, this corporate inertia interferes with the project of building consensus and mobilizing a coalition around a specific reform proposal. Until recently, the poor strategies and inadequate organizational development of both public and private reformers delayed legislative action. The inherent difficulty of industry to coalesce around a specific health bill was matched by a lack of focus within the state.

We are now at a critical juncture, the outcome of which is yet to be determined. A dynamic new president who is committed to the issue could make a difference. The managed competition proposal has generated considerable enthusiasm. Whether or not one believes that managed competition can really contain costs, it has introduced new language into the debate and has broken the political logjam. President Clinton seems committed to combining aspects of play-or-pay with managed competition. In a sanguine view of the future, we will get the best of each: expanded access to all Americans, vigorous caps imposed by global budgets, and long-term movement out of fee-for-service arrangements and into more cost-effective patterns of care.

For those committed to reform, the worst-case scenario would be an opportunity lost. Clinton might decide to move incrementally and lose the momentum enjoyed by presidents in their first few months. Or we could all jump on the wrong bandwagon and enact legislation that takes us no closer to solving the issue.

If corporate action depends on presidential leadership, does business really make a difference? In other policy areas, business supporters have worked to bring Republicans in line and bring about legislative victory. In the recent health battle one Democratic legislator was told, "If you deal with us, we will deal with the Republicans" (interview by author, June 1992). Business groups legitimate policy with parts of the country that are less than sympathetic to social initiatives: the Joe Managements of Main Street America.

But there is a cost to such support: business groups inevitably demand self-interested concessions. The ultimate paradox of reform is that it requires the mobilization of countervailing powers to neutralize the opposition of dominant interests. Yet these countervailing powers, losers under the old regime, demand special dispensations under the new. Reform is compromised in the process.

References

Abramowitz, Michael. 1992. Pushing Bush to a Market-led Health Solution: Enthoven Sees Competition as Best Antidote for Rising Costs. *Washington Post*, 26 January, p. H1.

Amkraut, Cathy. 1987. More Cost Shifting from Medicare Poses Management Challenge. *Business and Health* 4 (7): 50–51.

Bauer, Raymond, Ithiel De Sola Poole, and Lewis Dexter. 1972. *American Business and Public Policy*. New York: Aldine.

Bergthold, Linda. 1990. *Purchasing Power in Health*. New Brunswick, NJ: Rutgers University Press.

Bethlehem Steel Corporation. Undated. *Health Policy Briefs* 1 (6): 1–4.

Blendon, Robert. 1988. The Public's View of the Future of Health Care. *Journal of the American Medical Association* 259 (24): 3587–93.

Borger, Gloria. 1992. Small Business Pulls the Strings. *U.S. News and World Report*, 20 January, p. 26.

Brown, Barry. 1989. How Canada's Health System Works. *Business and Health* 7 (7): 28–30.

Brown, Lawrence. 1990. The Merits of Mandates. *Journal of Health Politics, Policy and Law* 15 (4): 793–96.

Brown, Lawrence, and Catherine McLaughlin. 1990. Constraining Costs at the Community Level: A Critique. *Health Affairs* 9 (4): 5–28.

Bureau of National Affairs. 1992. *Health Care Reform Group Urges Bush to Embrace Modified Package This Year*. No. 63, p. G-13.

Burke, Marybeth. 1990. Business Leaders Bring Their Clout to Washington. *Hospitals*, 20 April, p. 32.

———. 1992. Business and Labor Move Forward via Joint Health Care Reform Plan. *Hospitals*, 20 February, p. 53.

Cantor, Joel, Nancy Barrand, Randolph Desonia, Alan Cohen, and Jeffrey Merril. 1991. Business Leaders' Views on American Health Care. *Health Affairs* 10 (1): 99–101.

Catholic Health Association. 1992. Setting Relationships Right: A Working Proposal for Systemic Healthcare Reform. Unpublished paper. St. Louis, MO: Catholic Health Association.

Couch, Robin. 1992. A Health Care Plan with No Loopholes—Promises, Promises? *Financial Executive* 8 (1): 5.

Craig, John, Jr. 1983. Private Foundations' Role in Coalitions. In *Private Sector Coalitions: A Fourth Party in Health Care* (1982 National Forum on Hospital and Health Affairs), ed. B. Jon Jaeger. Durham, NC: Duke University Department of Health Administration.

Cronin, Carol. 1988. Business Wields Its Purchase Power. *Business and Health* 6 (1): 4–7.

Demkovich, Linda. 1983. On Health Issues, This Business Group Is a Leader, but Is Anyone Following? *National Journal*, 18 June, pp. 1278–80.

DiBlase, Donna. 1989. Group Health Bills Equal a Third of Profits. *Business Insurance* 23 (22): 37–38.

Dowd, Ann Reilly. 1992. Will George Bush Really Change? *Fortune*, 29 June, p. 64.

Eckstein, Harry. 1988. A Culturalist Theory of Political Change. *American Political Science Review* 82 (3): 790–91.

Faltermayer, Edmund. 1992. Let's Really Cure the Health System. *Fortune* 23 March, p. 58.

Ferguson, Thomas. 1984. From Normalcy to New Deal: Industrial Structure, Party Competition, and American Public Policy in the Great Depression. *International Organization* 38 (1): 41–94.

Fligstein, Neil. 1990. *The Transformation of Corporate Control*. Cambridge, MA: Harvard University Press.

Foster Higgins. 1992. *Health Care Benefits Survey: Managed Care Plans*. Princeton, NJ: A. Foster Higgins and Co. Inc.

Frieden, Jeff. 1988. Sectoral Conflict in U.S. Foreign Economic Policy, 1914–1940. *International Organization* 42 (1): 59–90.

Friedman, Thomas. 1993. Hillary Clinton to Head Panel on Health Care. *New York Times*, 26 January, p. A1, 20.

Fuchs, Victor. 1988. The "Competition Revolution" in Health Care. *Health Affairs* 7 (3): 5–24.

Garland, Susan. 1991. Already, Big Business' Health Plan Isn't Feeling So Hot. *Business Week*, 18 November, p. 48.

―――. 1992. Health Care Reform: It's Insurer vs. Insurer. *Business Week*, 4 May, pp. 62, 66.

Geisel, Jerry. 1991. Employers, Unions in Coalition Endorse Play-or-Pay Mandate. *Business Insurance*, 18 November, p. 73.

Gosselin, Peter. 1993. Clinton Told Health Plan Will Carry Steep Price. *Boston Globe*, 24 January, pp. 1, 10.

Haislmaier, Edmund. 1992. The Principal Culprit in Health Insurance Is the Current Tax Treatment of Benefits. *Roll Call*. New York: Levitt Communications Inc.

Hall, Charles, Jr., and John Kuder. 1990. *Small Business and Health Care*. Washington, DC: National Federation of Independent Business Foundation.

Hall, Peter. 1986. *Governing the Economy*. New York: Oxford University Press.

―――. Forthcoming. Keynes in Political Science. *History of Political Economy* 26 (1).

HEAL (Healthcare Equity Action League). 1992. *Solving the Health Care Crisis: Statement of Basic Principles*. Washington, DC: National Association of Wholesaler-Distributors.

Jacobs, David. 1988. Corporate Economic Power and the State: A Longitudinal Assessment of Two Explanations. *American Journal of Sociology* 93 (4): 852–81.

Jaeger, B. Jon, ed. 1983. *Private Sector Coalitions: A Fourth Party in Health Care*. 1982 National Forum on Hospital and Health Affairs. Durham, NC: Duke University Department of Health Administration.

Kennedy, Edward. 1991. An Affordable Health-Care Plan for All. *Boston Globe*, 6 June, p. 21.

Kingdon, John. 1984. *Agendas, Alternatives, and Public Policies*. Boston, MA: Little, Brown.

Kinsley, Michael. 1992. Quack. *New Republic* 206 (9): 4.

Klandersman, Bert. 1988. The Formation and Mobilization of Consensus. In *International Social Movement Research*, ed. Bert Klandersman, Hanspeter Kriesi, and Sidney Tarrow. Greenwich, CT: JAI.

Klandersman, Bert, and Sidney Tarrow. 1988. Mobilization into Social Movements. In *International Social Movement Research*, ed. Bert Klandersman, Hanspeter Kriesi, and Sidney Tarrow. Greenwich, CT: JAI.

Knox, Richard. 1991. Senate Democrats Unveil Universal Health Care Plan. *Boston Globe*, 6 June, pp. 1, 28.

Kosterlitz, Julie. 1992. Survival Tactics. *National Journal*, 24 October, pp. 2, 428–32.

Kurth, James. 1979. The Political Consequences of the Product Cycle: Industrial History and Political Outcomes. *International Organization* 33 (1): 1–34.

Kuttner, Bob. 1993. A Plan to Cure the Nation's Health Care Ills. *Boston Globe*, 4 January, p. 11.

Lee, Gary. 1992. Health Industry Lobbyists Boost President's Plan. *Washington Post*, 7 February, p. A23.

Levit, Katherine, Helen Lazenby, Suzanne Letsch, and Cathy Cowan. 1991. National Health Care Spending, 1989. *Health Affairs* 10 (1): 117–30.

McAdam, Doug. 1988. Micromobilization Contexts and Recruitment to Activism. In *International Social Movement Research* ed. Bert Klandersman, Hanspeter Kriesi, and Sidney Tarrow. Greenwich, CT: JAI.

Maitland, Ian. 1983. House Divided: Business Lobbying and the 1981 Budget. In *Corporate Social Performance and Policy*, vol. 5. Greenwich, CT: JAI Press.

Marmor, Theodore. 1993. Coalition or Collision? Medicare and Health Reform. *American Prospect* 12:53–59.

Marmor, Theodore R., Judith Feder, and John Holahan. 1980. *National Health Insurance: Conflicting Goals and Policy Choices*. Washington, DC: Urban Institute.

Martin, Cathie Jo. 1989. Business Influence and State Power: The Case of U.S. Corporate Tax Policy. *Politics and Society* 17 (2): 189–223.

———. 1991. *Shifting the Burden: The Struggle over Growth and Corporate Taxation*. Chicago: University of Chicago Press.

Moe, Terry. 1987. Interests, Institutions, and Positive Theory: The Politics of the NLRB. In *Studies in American Political Development*, vol. 2. New Haven, CT: Yale University Press.

Morone, James A., and A. Dunham. 1985. Slouching towards National Health Insurance: The New Health Care Politics. *Yale Journal on Regulation* 2 (2): 263–91.

National Federation of Independent Business. 1992. *NFIB View on Small Market Reform*. Washington, DC: National Federation of Independent Business.

National Leadership Coalition for Health Care Reform. 1989. *For the Health of a Nation*. Washington, DC: National Leadership Coalition for Health Care Reform.

———. 1991. *Report from the National Leadership Coalition for Health Care Reform*. Washington, DC: National Leadership Coalition for Health Care Reform.

Offe, Claus. 1985. Two Logics of Collective Action. In *Disorganized Capitalism: Contemporary Transformations of Work and Politics*, ed. John Keane. Cambridge, MA: MIT Press.

Olson, Mancur. 1965. *The Logic of Collective Action*. Cambridge, MA: Harvard University Press.

Pear, Robert. 1992a. Doctors' Group Offers Plan to Curb Health-Care Costs. *New York Times*, 15 September, p. A1.

———. 1992b. In Shift, Insurers Ask U.S. to Require Coverage for All. *New York Times*, 3 December, pp. A1, 22.

———. 1992c. Budget Official Sees No Savings in Clinton's Health Care Plans. *New York Times*, 3 December, p. A16.

Peterson, Mark. 1992. Leading Our Way to Health: Entrepreneurship and Leadership in the Health Care Reform Debate. Occasional Paper 92:6 (August). Cambridge, MA: Harvard University.

Plotke, David. 1992. The Political Mobilization of Business, 1974–1980. In *The Politics of Interest*, ed. Mark Petracca. Boulder, CO: Westview.

Polzer, Karl. 1990. Strategies to Contain Health Care Costs. *Business and Health* 8 (9): 30.

PR Newswire. 1992a. HEAL Supports President's Health Care Reform Proposal. New York: PR Newswire Association, Inc., 3 March.

———. 1992b. Bush Health Plan Will Gain Support from Small Business, NFIB Predicts. New York: PR Newswire Association, Inc., 6 May.

Rosner, Jeremy. 1993. A Progressive Plan for Affordable, Universal Health Care. In *Mandate for Change*, ed. Will Marshall and Martin Schram. New York: Berkley Books.

Rovner, Julie. 1989. Kennedy-Waxman Introduce Insurance-for-All Proposal. *Congressional Quarterly* 47 (15): 286.

———. 1991a. Congress Feels the Pressure of Health-Care Squeeze. *Congressional Quarterly* 49 (7): 414–21.

———. 1991b. Complex Issues, Turf Battles Delay Democratic Overhaul. *Congressional Quarterly* 49 (22): 1450.

———. 1992a. Health-Care Grievances, Fears Aired at Nationwide Meetings. *Congressional Quarterly* 50 (3): 114–16.

———. 1992b. Play-or-Pay Gains Momentum as Labor Panel Marks up Bill. *Congressional Quarterly* 50 (4): 172–74.

———. 1992c. Bush's Plan Short on Details, Long on Ambition, Critics. *Congressional Quarterly* 50 (6): 305.

———. 1992d. Insurance Reforms Slide by Senate Finance in Tax Bill. *Congressional Quarterly* 50 (10): 536–37.

Salmon, Warren J. 1987. Introduction—Special Section on the Corporatization of Medicine. *International Journal of Health Services* 17 (1): 1–6.

Sapolsky, Harvey, Drew Altman, Richard Greene, and Judith Moore. 1981. Corporate Attitudes toward Health Care Costs. *Health and Society* 59 (4): 561–85.

Schattschneider, E. E. 1960. *The Semisovereign People*. New York: Holt, Rinehart and Winston.

Schneider, William. 1990. Is There a Cure for America's Medical Inflation? *National Journal*, 21 April, p. 983.

Skocpol, Theda. 1985. Bringing the State Back In: Strategies of Analysis in Current Research. In *Bringing the State Back In*, ed. Peter Evans, Dietrich Rueschemeyer, and Theda Skocpol. New York: Cambridge University Press.

Snow, David, E. Burke Rochford, Jr., Steven Worden, and Robert Benford. 1986. Frame Alignment Processes, Micromobilization, and Movement Participation. *American Sociological Review* 51 (4): 464–81.

Starr, Paul. 1992. *The Logic of Health Care Reform*. Knoxville, TN: Whittle Direct Books.

——. 1993. Healthy Compromise: Universal Coverage and Managed Competition under a Cap. *American Prospect* 12:44–52.

Stigler, George. 1971. The Theory of Economic Regulation. *Bell Journal of Economics and Management Science* 2 (1): 3–21.

Swartz, Katherine. 1990. Why Requiring Employers to Provide Health Insurance Is a Bad Idea. *Journal of Health Politics, Policy and Law* 15 (4): 779–92.

Thompson, Graham. 1982. The Firm as a "Dispersed" Social Agency. *Economy and Society* 11 (3): 233.

Tower Perrin. 1992. Managed Care: Employer Perspective. *1992 Profile* 1 (2): 2. New York: Tower Perrin, Inc.

Victor, Kirk. 1990. Gut Issue. *National Journal*, 24 March, pp. 704, 706.

Wilensky, Gail. 1989. The Real Price of Mandating Health Benefits. *Business and Health* 7 (3): 32–36.

William M. Mercer. 1990. *Employer Attitudes toward the Cost of Health Care*. New York: William M. Mercer, Inc.

Williams, Walter. 1991. United States Senate Committee on Finance Hearing on Health Care Costs, April 16, 1991. *Healthwise* 2 (2): 2.

Wisnewski, Robert. 1990. The 1990 National Executive Poll on Health Care Costs and Benefits. *Business and Health* 8 (4): 25–38.

Woolhandler, Steffie, and David Himmelstein. Undated. To Save a Penny Two Are Spent. Unpublished paper. Cambridge, MA: Harvard University, Division of Social and Community Medicine.

Zedlewski, Sheila, Greggory Acs, Laura Wheaton, and Colin Winterbottom. 1992. *Exploring the Effects of Play-or-Pay Employer Mandates: Effects on Insurance Coverage and Costs*. Washington, DC: Urban Institute.

Zysman, John. 1983. *Governments, Markets and Growth*. Ithaca, NY: Cornell University Press.

Can an Employer-Based Health Insurance System Be Just?

Nancy S. Jecker

Abstract It is America's distinctive practice to tie private health insurance to employment, and recent proposals have tried to retain this link through mandating that all employers provide health insurance to their employees. My primary approach to these issues is neither economic, nor historical, nor political but *ethical*. After a brief historical overview, I outline a general approach to evaluating the ethical significance of linking the distributions of distinct goods. I examine whether an *unjust* distribution of jobs spoils justice in the distribution of health insurance, taking as a central example gender inequities in employment and exploring their impact on job-based health insurance. Second, I explore the possibility that *justly* awarding jobs guarantees justice in employment-sponsored insurance. However, linking the distributions of different goods remains problematic, because such links inevitably undermine equality by enabling the same individuals to enjoy advantages in many different distributive areas. Finally, I examine recent proposals to reform America's health care system by requiring all employers to provide health insurance to their employees. I argue that such proposals lend themselves to the same ethical problems that the current system does and urge greater attention to alternative reform options.

America's distinctive practice of linking private health insurance to employment is coming under increasing fire. Critics charge that the system produces inequities because it misses so many people. They also fault job-based insurance as inefficient, claiming that it feeds the problem of rising health care costs by distancing consumers from health care costs and thereby encouraging overuse; they argue that employer-based insurance restricts opportunity and lowers productivity because workers feel locked into current jobs for fear of losing benefits. Others worry that employment-sponsored insurance reduces American competitiveness in world markets by raising the cost of American products: in 1990, fully

26 percent of the average company's net earnings went for medical costs (Freudenheim 1991).

Since reform of America's health care system is very much on the political agenda today, if employment-based proposals are flawed it is important to state clearly and forcefully why they are. After exploring how the current system of linking health insurance to jobs arose, I argue that employment-related insurance contains built-in inequities. Whereas many other objections to employer-sponsored health insurance can be met without abandoning an employer-based framework, the objections I raise are *endemic* to any employment-sponsored system. The objections I put forward constitute an ethical critique of any job-based insurance framework.

Tying health insurance to employment raises two distinct justice questions. First, is the distribution of jobs itself just? Second, is it just to allow the distribution of jobs to determine the distribution of health insurance? My argument proceeds in two stages. The first stage shows that if jobs themselves are unfairly awarded, this spoils justice in the distribution of health insurance tied to jobs. Second, even if jobs are awarded in a fair and unbiased fashion, tying health insurance to employment undermines equality. In the final sections of the paper, I argue that recent proposals to expand employer-sponsored health insurance fall short of justice standards: although expanding employment-based insurance may prove politically attractive because the current system is so deeply entrenched, from a moral point of view it has significant drawbacks.

Historical Overview

The present system of employer-sponsored health insurance came into existence after the defeat of national health insurance proposals during the 1930s and 1940s. Before this time, private health insurance plans largely offered contracts for the provision of services by a single physician to a group of subscribing individuals. These early plans were paid for by the individual but were sponsored by employers for their employees, or by labor unions, lodges, fraternal orders, and consumer groups. Coverage was generally limited to physician services and excluded hospital care. Under the plans, physicians were prepaid a fixed amount per enrollee per year. Such programs were not available on a large scale and depended on a special circumstance: a strong union, a forward-looking employer, or a cohesive immigrant group (Fein 1989). Few companies entered the health insurance market because they were concerned that providing health insurance on a large scale would not prove profitable. Many assumed that only the sick would subscribe to private insurance, that it would be difficult to monitor abuse, and that high acquisition and collection costs would cut into profits (Starr 1982).

Shortly after World War II began, employers developed an interest in offering group health plans. Civilian labor was in short supply when, in 1942, the War Labor Board imposed a ceiling on wages to prevent inflation. The board also decided that fringe benefits up to 5 percent of wages would not be considered inflationary. In response, employers expanded employee benefits to include health insurance. This was a way of luring new workers and retaining present employees in a competitive market. Soon after this development, the federal tax code made health insurance packages even more attractive.[1] The code permitted employers to treat health insurance contributions like wages and to deduct them from profits, and it allowed employees who obtained health insurance paid for by an employer to receive a nontaxable benefit. Thus, part of the cost of health insurance was underwritten by government: a dollar contributed to health insurance lowered the employer's federal income tax, but did not raise the employee's federal income tax. The impetus behind the federal tax subsidy came from many sources: those concerned to assure the financial solvency of hospitals, sustain physicians' incomes, or provide financial security to individuals and families banded together with others whose main purpose was undercutting efforts to introduce a government-sponsored health insurance program (Fein 1989).

In this manner, our present system of linking health insurance to jobs was born. Although the tax code stimulated and subsidized the development of health insurance linked to jobs, it did nothing to encourage or assist insurance coverage plans for individuals or for groups such as neighborhoods and religious or fraternal organizations. By subsidizing the purchase of health insurance only when the employer paid the premium, the tax code extended benefits to some while denying them to others. As others have noted, the code might have been more inclusive, permitting a tax deduction or tax credit for premium payments made by individuals on their own behalf or made by community-based groups not linked to employment.

Those who were left out—the poor and unemployed—did not rep-

---

1. The decision to allow employers' contributions to employee health plans to count as wages and be deducted from profits was made by the U.S. Treasury Department (1961).

resent an organized or powerful opposition. Thus, employment-related health insurance spread. During World War II, total enrollment in group hospital plans grew from fewer than 7 million to about 26 million subscribers, representing approximately one-fifth of the population (Starr 1982). The postwar expansion was even more impressive, largely because labor unions gained the right to bargain collectively for health care benefits. Once employers' refusal to bargain over health care coverage was defined as an unfair labor practice, health insurance was no longer viewed as a gift that employers gave at their discretion. In the postwar period, health insurance coverage expanded from 32 million in 1943, to 53 million two years later, and to 77 million by 1951. By 1954, over 60 percent of the population had some type of hospital insurance, 50 percent some type of surgical insurance, and 25 percent medical insurance (though often only for in-hospital services) (Anderson and Feldman 1956).

Today, workplace health insurance represents the dominant form of private health insurance. Obviously, employment-sponsored health insurance leaves out the unemployed and their dependents. Yet employment itself is by no means a guarantor of health care access. In 1987, 76.8 percent of the uninsured were employed or were nuclear family dependents of the employed; in 1988, 85 percent of the uninsured population consisted of workers or their family members (Friedman 1991). Thus, employment-related insurance leaves out many employed persons. In general, workers in smaller and nonunionized firms are less likely to receive health insurance benefits through the workplace. Even among those who are both employed and insured, health care benefits and access are not uniform. For example, low-wage firms tend to pay a smaller percentage of premium costs and to offer policies with fewer benefits, placing employees at triple jeopardy: they receive less pay, poorer protection, and less tax-exempt employer assistance to defray premium costs (Fein 1989). In addition, the federal tax exclusion subsidy is regressive because it offers the most generous after-tax benefits to those with the highest incomes, who would have paid the highest marginal tax rates for their health benefits. Persons with the lowest incomes, who are in the lower marginal tax brackets, receive the smallest after-tax benefits (Cantor 1990).

Increasingly, employers themselves express concern about the rising costs of health insurance and shift costs to employees or hire part-time and temporary workers for whom insurance benefits need not be provided. The recessionary periods of the 1980s and early 1990s have increased the pressure on employers to reduce health care expenditures. The diminished power of labor in collective bargaining has made it easier to achieve such reductions. Increasingly, workers pay for rising health care bills through the slower wage growth that results when companies subtract health care cost increases from the money available for wages. Despite cost shifting, employers continue to feel pressure and dissatisfaction. In a recent survey of chief executives of Fortune 500 companies, 91 percent expressed the belief that basic change or complete rebuilding of the present system is needed (Cantor et al. 1991). The leading critics of job-based insurance tend to be large, long-established companies whose work forces are made up of people in their forties and fifties, who require relatively more health care than younger workers; companies whose health plans insure a large portion of retired workers; and companies whose products compete on world markets (Uchitelle 1991).

The Domino Effect

To an increasing degree, doubts about the present system raise a more fundamental question: Is America's virtually unique system of linking health insurance to paid labor inherently unjust? Or is it possible to remedy justice problems within the framework of a job-based system? To address such questions, I begin by invoking the familiar idea of a domino effect. One way a domino effect can operate is when injustices in one distributive arena are compounded by linking that arena to another. For example, suppose that access to higher education was determined by invidious racial discrimination. If access to some other good, such as the right to vote, was tied to having an undergraduate degree, then injustice in education would infect the voting area as well. Assuring justice in the political sphere may then require *separating* the distribution of voting rights from the awarding of undergraduate degrees. Of course, distributive domains are never wholly distinct, and what happens in one distributive arena influences outcomes in other areas. But the effects of one distribution on another can be relatively strong or weak. To prevent injustice in one area from spilling over into another domain, the discovery of injustice in one area calls for a policy of containment, in which the goal is to isolate the unjust distribution as much as possible and prevent it from infecting other distributions (Walzer 1983).

The relevance of the domino effect to health care is straightforward. The distribution of private health insurance is based almost entirely on participation in the paid labor force. If it can be shown that those jobs that provide health insurance are distributed in an unjust way, then tying health insurance to jobs compromises justice in health care. Since the jobs that tend to provide health insurance fall into identifiable categories, we need to examine whether the distribution of these kinds of jobs is just or whether it instead imposes disproportionate burdens on certain groups.

Clearly, there are numerous perspectives from which to evaluate justice in jobs providing health insurance. In making this evaluation, I will focus primarily on inequalities between men and women. The impact of health care financing on men compared with women is a neglected topic but an increasingly important one in light of differences in their socioeconomic status, labor force participation, and health care needs and utilization patterns. Although I use the example of sex-based discrimination, my broader aim is to show that workplace discrimination of *any* sort, whether based on race, ethnicity, religious affiliation, age, or sexual orientation, creates corresponding injustices in employment-based insurance.[2]

It should come as no surprise that the workplace insurance system, developed in the 1940s, was based on the assumption that working women are economically dependent on a wage-earning male head of household who shares his higher earnings and retirement and health insurance benefits with her. Although more women today receive health insurance directly from an employer than ever before, employed women are less likely than employed men to receive private health insurance through their job. In 1980, of the 58.4 million men aged fifteen and over who had wage and salary income, 65.4 percent (38.2 million) had an employer or a union that paid all or some of the cost of health insurance; but of the 50.1 million female workers, only 49.7 percent (24.9 million) had an outside contribution (Muller 1990). The entire cost of health insurance was paid for 29.6 percent of men but for only 22.9 percent of women (Muller 1990).

Working women less often receive private insurance through their employer, first, because eligibility rules continue to reflect a male model of work and male patterns of labor force participation. Full-time, full-year workers more often receive health insurance coverage through the workplace. But, partly as a result of assuming caregiving responsibilities for children and aging relatives, women are more likely to work on a part-

2. For example, critics of job-based insurance note that blacks enjoy less access than non-blacks to job-based insurance because they often live in nontraditional family structures and do not qualify for coverage as married spouses or dependent offspring (Long 1987). Other groups that fare particularly poorly include gay couples, because the uninsured partner does not qualify for family medical benefits through the employed partner, and illegal immigrants, who are not eligible for Medicaid even if they lose their jobs and become destitute.

time or part-year basis (Kasper and Soldinger 1983). Full-time, full-year employees represent two-thirds of all male workers aged fifteen and over, but only half of all female workers (Muller 1990). Whereas men average 1.3 years outside the paid labor force, women average 11.5 years (Older Women's League 1989). And, in both 1981 and 1987, nearly one in four employed women aged forty-five to sixty-four held part-time jobs (Older Women's League 1988). Women who combine child care with paid work by making themselves available as independent contractors, rather than as salaried employees, are also excluded from employer benefit plans. Although these "peripheral workers" help to meet firms' peak demands for administrative and clerical work, they make the worker the risk taker for health needs (Muller 1990).

Second, working women predominate in nonunion jobs, and this job category is less likely to provide health insurance coverage. In the twenty-five-to-thirty-four age group, 13 percent of women workers belong to unions, compared to 19 percent of men workers; at ages thirty-five to fifty-four, the gap between women and men widens, with 19.2 percent of women and 29.8 percent of men union-affiliated; by age fifty-six, union membership declines for both men and women, but more rapidly for women. Not surprisingly, unionized workers generally fare much better with respect to wages and benefits than their nonunionized counterparts, because they have an organized labor force that bargains on their behalf.

A third factor that reduces women's employment-related coverage is that the rate at which women change jobs has greatly increased over the past two decades, while the rate for men has held constant (Schorr 1991). Partly as a result of child rearing and other caregiving roles, women workers are more likely to enter and leave the work force. They are therefore increasingly vulnerable to clauses in employer insurance plans that exclude or limit coverage for preexisting conditions. A 1987 survey found that 57 percent of employers who offer health insurance have pre-existing condition clauses in the policies they offer (Cotton 1991). The insurance industry uses these clauses to apply higher premiums, waiting periods, condition-specific payment denials, or complete denial of coverage to people with previously existing medical problems. In principle, these clauses are meant to control insurance industry costs by preventing adverse selection—the purchasing of insurance by people who want to pay for insurance only when they need to use it. Yet preexisting condition clauses also block access to care for women and others who participate in the paid labor force intermittently.

Fourth, low-paying jobs are less likely to offer health insurance benefits, and women predominate in such jobs. When health insurance premiums rise, many companies with a large proportion of low-wage workers find it increasingly difficult to divert money from wages to health care without reducing wages to unacceptably low levels. As a result, companies such as fast-food restaurants, gasoline stations, and other service jobs keep wages competitive by dropping benefits, including health care (Uchitelle 1991). Low pay is a marker for women's wages, partly because of the child and elder care responsibilities women assume. When women who are caregivers remain in the paid labor force, they often choose jobs with fewer demands and less pay because of caregiving duties. Thus, the average earnings of a woman who gives birth drop $3,000 the first year and stay about $5,000 below what they would otherwise be for the next two years (Muller 1990). The wage gap between women and men is greatest between the ages of forty-five and sixty-four, when full-time male workers are at the height of their earning power and women are earning basically what they did in younger years. During this period (ages forty-five to sixty-four), women working full-time earn less than two-thirds of wages of men working similar hours (Muller 1990).

In addition to gender disparities within employment-sponsored insurance, women who work at home without pay, whether because they have very young children or because they are caring for a frail elderly relative, are often denied access to private health insurance unless they are married to someone who provides it for them. The U.S. Long-Term Care Survey of 1982 found that 44 percent of daughter caregivers were not married, either because they had never married, were widowed, or were divorced or separated (Stone and Cafferata 1987). Even among married caregivers, a 50 percent divorce rate makes reliance on a spouse's health care benefits risky, and economic dependence makes women vulnerable to inequalities within the family (Weed 1980).

The significance of the sex differential in employer-based insurance lies in the fact that the *public* insurance for which working-age women are eligible is likely to be far less generous than private insurance offered through an employer. Working-age women typically are too young to qualify for Medicare, but often they are not too rich to qualify for Medicaid, the state- and federal-financed health entitlement program for the poor. For every male eighteen years of age and older covered under Medicaid, there are two females aged eighteen and over (Muller 1990). But Medicaid is a mixed blessing for women. The health benefits women receive through Medicaid are notoriously meager and inconsistent from one state to the next. Moreover, Medicaid eligibles frequently lack access to mainstream providers, because reimbursement rates are set below costs (Pare 1991). Over 25 percent of the nation's privately practicing physicians refuse to treat Medicaid patients; and participation by obstetrician-gynecologists and other key specialists is even lower (National Pharmaceutical Council 1986). Hospital admissions under the care of a personal physician, the norm for insured and self-pay patients, are precluded when Medicaid clients are not accepted by practitioners (Muller 1990). Hence, even though women are slightly more likely than men to be insured (they make up only 40.6 percent of the uninsured [Muller 1990]), the insurance benefits they receive provide only limited access to the health care system. Gender inequities will persist so long as public insurance for working-age adults remains inferior to private insurance, and the main route to private insurance continues to be through job categories in which men predominate.

The above discussion reveals quite clearly that women and men do not participate at equal levels in jobs providing health insurance benefits. Although employer-based insurance is not explicitly gender-biased, the society to which such a policy is applied is pervasively gender-structured. Women's health care access is reduced because women tend to work in lower-paying and lower-status jobs that offer fewer benefits, and they are more likely than men to work on a part-time, part-year basis. Women who stay at home to serve as caregivers for family members become dependent on a male head of household for health insurance, with women representing 70 percent of those who receive employment-based insurance through a relative (Swartz 1990). Unmarried caregivers go without health insurance or rely on inadequate public programs. To the extent that employment disparities between men and women reflect injustice, the link between employment and health insurance merely amplifies this injustice.

The Problem of Dominance

Of course, showing that men are more likely than women to fill jobs that offer health care benefits does not yet establish that such jobs are awarded *unjustly*. Some have argued, to the contrary, that gender differences in employment reflect differences in women's and men's preferences in a free market, rather than invidious discrimination. According to this line of thinking, women voluntarily forgo jobs offering higher salaries and benefits in order to pursue goals outside the paid labor force (Fuchs 1988). Yet whether or not women make such choices armed with full information and freedom is hotly debated. A growing body of feminist scholarship challenges this account, by arguing that unequal treatment begins early in life and has the effect of limiting women's aspirations to pursue careers and reducing their odds of competing successfully (Faludi 1991; Hollard and Eisenhart 1990; Gilligan 1982; Willard 1988; Abir-Am and Outram 1987). Moreover, when high-paying and prestigious occupations are heavily sex-segregated, women seeking employment in them must bear whatever stigma the society associates with being different from other, more traditional women (Goldin 1990).

To sidestep this debate, let us suppose for the purposes of argument that jobs providing health insurance coverage are justly distributed among men and women and among all groups in the society. Suppose that such jobs are allocated in conformity with ideal justice standards to which all agree. Would it then be appropriate or desirable to link the distribution of other social goods, such as health care, to the distribution of jobs?

The strongest argument against linking the distribution of one social good to another involves the problem of dominance. Michael Walzer (1983), who has written extensively in this area, describes dominance as a pattern of distributing diverse goods so that one good, or one set of goods, is determinative of value in all the different spheres of distribution. A good is dominant if the individuals who have it, because they have it, can command a wide range of other goods. For example, wealth and income are the principal dominant goods in our society because they are readily convertible into power, privilege, and position in many areas.

According to Walzer, the need to avoid dominance stems first from the observation that different social goods constitute different distributive spheres in which distinct distributive principles govern. For example, the criteria of intelligence and talent are a fair basis for awarding jobs, but it would be inappropriate to make these the standard for distributing friendship, honor, physical security, food, or shelter. Likewise, something is wrong with the wielding of political power to gain other kinds of benefits, such as superior health care or educational advantages.

If different social goods make up different distributive arenas, and specialized principles apply to each, then justice requires an "art of separation" (Walzer 1984). Separating the distribution of different goods makes it possible to tailor standards of justice to suit each kind of good. By contrast, linking the distribution of diverse goods, or allowing goods of one type to be converted into other goods, hinders ideal justice by weakening equality between persons. Although equality does not require that persons enjoy equal standing with respect to each and every good, the prospect of forming and sustaining equal relationships is diminished when the same individuals have superior standing across many different spheres of distribution. Walzer (1983: 19–20) expresses this point by noting that

> citizen X may be chosen over citizen Y for political office, and then the two of them will be unequal in the sphere of politics. But they will not be unequal *generally* so long as X's office gives him no advantages over Y in any other sphere—superior medical care, access to better schools for his children, entrepreneurial opportunities and so on. So long as office is not a dominant good, is not generally convertible, office holders will stand, or at least can stand, in a relation of equality to the men and women they govern.

The conclusion of this argument forbids any good from serving as the basis for access to other goods with which it has no inherent connection.

Applied to health care, this reasoning suggests that even if jobs are awarded justly, the standards for giving out jobs are not the appropriate standards for apportioning health care. Whereas criteria such as education, work experience, job skills, and freedom from caregiving responsibilities are relevant to evaluating job candidates, these factors should not determine entitlement to health care. Of course, jobs were not made convertible into health care on these grounds. But in hindsight, the de facto effect of an employer-based insurance system has been to make health care available in accordance with the standards used for distributing certain jobs.

One reply to the dominance argument might be that to reject employer-provided insurance leaves open the possibility of using a person's place of employment as a *mechanism*, rather than a *standard*, for dispensing health insurance. A mechanism for distributing goods is chosen according to standards of convenience and efficiency, rather than justice, and it can be morally neutral in a way that distributive standards cannot. For instance, provided that all people are equally able to exercise their right to vote, the difference between registering voters through driver license bureaus or through mail-in forms is morally neutral.

Yet the reply to this suggestion is that voter registration and enrollment in health insurance are different in an important sense. Whereas the right to vote is an all-or-nothing phenomenon, health insurance can be more or less generous. Even assuming that everyone has access to health insurance through workplace insurance, or through a public insurance system, *adequate* health insurance may not be universally available. So long as public insurance is inferior and adequate health benefits remain tied to jobs, labor force affiliation still functions as a standard, rather than merely a mechanism, for distributing health insurance.

A second objection to the argument based on dominance notes that we already tie many other benefits to employment, such as vacations, retirement pensions, unemployment compensation, life insurance, and child care. Are all of these ties equally unjust because they raise the problem of dominance?[3] To answer this question, it is important to note that many of these connections are troubling for the very same reason that connecting health insurance to jobs is: such connections compound inequalities that are already endemic in American society. For instance, when a good job is readily convertible into good child care services or a generous old age pension, this spreads inequalities from jobs to other areas. Rather than establishing that the link between jobs and health insurance is benign, the presence of other job-related advantages makes the connection between health insurance and jobs more worrisome. It shows that the jobs to which health benefits are linked *already* approximate a dominant good and *already* are associated with advantages in many other areas.

Yet, notwithstanding these similarities, it is crucial to see why the coupling of jobs and superior health insurance is especially pernicious and raises unique justice concerns. Unlike the loss of other job-related perks, the loss of adequate health care coverage has potentially devastating effects in all other areas of life. For example, when persons lack access to preventive screening for various diseases, they may develop more serious forms of illness that could have been easily treated or controlled at an earlier stage. A delay in receiving treatment may result in lifelong disabilities or premature death. The loss of other job-related benefits, by contrast, does not ordinarily cause such profound losses. For example, although persons forced to go without vacations or child care benefits may find their opportunities limited, these deprivations do not have widespread effects that impinge so fundamentally upon individuals' opportunities (Daniels 1988).

---

3. Professor Leslie Francis called this objection to my attention.

Recent Proposals for Health Care Reform

In light of the preceding discussion, one might wonder whether recent proposals to reform America's health care system while retaining a link between jobs and health care can avoid the problems presented here. However, I will argue that both the domino effect and dominance would persist under mandatory employer health insurance. This conclusion is particularly significant in view of the fact that many people who are convinced of the irrationality and injustice of our *present* job-based system nonetheless feel that its problems can be averted without giving up on an employment-based framework. For example, despite the dissatisfaction that employers express with job-based insurance, a solid majority (75 percent) of executives at the nation's largest companies prefer to retain employers as the main source of health insurance. Many distrust proposals for government-sponsored national health insurance, and view with suspicion health care reforms that allow government to encroach upon the private sector. Thus, many proposals for reforming the nation's health care system continue to make the workplace a pathway to private insurance but seek to expand access by requiring that all employers provide health insurance for their workers.

The Nixon administration was the first to propose mandatory employer-provided insurance. More recently, the Kennedy-Waxman Mandated Coverage Bill called for employers to enroll all employees and their families in a health insurance plan offering a minimum set of benefits. Senator George Mitchell introduced a bill on behalf of Senate Democrats in June of 1991. It combined annual targets for health care spending with a requirement that all employers provide health insurance for their employees or pay a payroll tax to help pay for a new public health care plan for people without health insurance. As a presidential candidate, Governor Bill Clinton proposed a similar plan, with the addition of a National Health Board to establish annual budgets and define a core benefits package (Clinton 1992). Physicians also have entered the debate about health care reform. The American Medical Association (AMA) endorses a proposal called Health Access America, in which employer health insurance is mandatory for full-time employees and their families (Todd et al. 1991).

Those who favor mandating employer insurance often call attention to its political and strategic advantages. As the vast majority of the uninsured are employed, mandating employer coverage has the distinct advantage of covering the largest subset of the uninsured. In addition, the cost of extended coverage would be born outside the federal budget and would not appear as a direct tax item. Yet how does mandatory insurance fare in light of the two problems (the domino effect and dominance) discussed above?

By itself, mandatory employer insurance would mean that vastly greater numbers of employees would receive health insurance. Yet eligibility criteria would probably continue to exclude certain categories of workers. For example, the Pepper Commission's Blueprint for Health Care Reform acknowledges that small businesses face significant barriers to voluntary purchasing of health insurance and, for the near future, would seek to reduce barriers while not requiring small businesses to cover their workers (Rockefeller 1991). A group calling itself the National Organization of Physicians Who Care proposes achieving mandatory insurance at a reasonable cost through a high deductible, perhaps $1,000 (Brown et al. 1991). This would continue to place a heavier burden on persons who occupy low-paying jobs. Health Access America, the plan endorsed by the AMA, mandates health insurance only for full-time employees and their families and initially only for large businesses. To the extent that exceptions to categorical coverage are made in job categories that women are more likely than men to fill, inequities between men and women would persist. In other words, to the extent that injustice is lifted, it would be lifted more for men than for women. In addition, even if all employed persons were eventually covered by their employers, this would not affect the 15 percent of the uninsured population that is unemployed. If the distribution of jobs per se reflects discriminatory practices, linking health insurance to jobs converts employment discrimination into discrimination in health care access. Even if mandatory employer insurance was supplemented with public insurance for the unemployed, those who rely on a public system would probably continue to receive vastly inferior care. So long as the recipients of public insurance are limited to marginal groups in society, it will remain difficult to maintain an adequate public program. Finally, even assuming that all jobs are *justly* awarded, the unemployed population should not be disqualified from health insurance on the same basis from which it is disqualified from work. Standards that are fair for excluding people from jobs are not necessarily fair for excluding people from health care coverage.

Conclusions

In conclusion, the current system of employer-based health insurance arose through historical events and accidents, rather than through a deliberate and morally thoughtful process. In its wake, patterns of injustice in the distribution of jobs linked to health insurance have compromised justice in health care. Ethical principles appropriate for distributing jobs are not the same as the ethical criteria that should govern access to health care. This more pervasive and fundamental problem provides a reason for separating the distribution of jobs and health insurance even if jobs are fairly awarded. Finally, proposals that call for mandatory employer insurance and an expanded public system for the poor and unemployed do not eliminate justice concerns. Such proposals fall short because they do not ensure that the most vulnerable members of society receive adequate protection.

Taken together, these points provide an initially compelling argument for uncoupling health insurance and jobs. If my reasoning is correct, we would be wise to explore seriously alternatives to job-based insurance. All things considered, we may then decide that future health care reforms should be fashioned without retaining a link between jobs and health care. Separating health insurance from paid labor force participation may prove a prerequisite to achieving the goal of adequate health care coverage for all.

References

Abir-Am, P. G., and D. Outram, eds. 1987. *Uneasy Careers and Intimate Lives*. New Brunswick, NJ: Rutgers University Press.

Anderson, O. W., and J. J. Feldman. 1956. *Family Medical Costs and Voluntary Health Insurance: A Nationwide Survey*. New York: McGraw-Hill.

Brown, R. S., R. A. Beltran, S. C. Cohen, P. T. Elliot, G. M. Goldman, and S. G. Spotnitz. 1991. The Physicians Who Care Plan: Preserving Quality and Equitability in American Medicine. *Journal of the American Medical Association* 265:2511–15.

Cantor, J. C. 1990. Expanding Health Insurance Coverage: Who Will Pay? *Journal of Health Politics, Policy and Law* 15:755–78.

Cantor, J. C., N. L. Barrand, R. A. Dsonia, A. B. Cohen, and J. C. Merrill. 1991. Datawatch. *Health Affairs* 10:98–105.

Clinton, B. 1992. The Clinton Health Care Plan. *New England Journal of Medicine* 327:804–7.

Cotton, P. 1991. Preexisting Conditions Hold Americans Hostage to Employers and Insurance. *Journal of the American Medical Association* 265:2451–53.

Daniels, N. 1988. *Am I My Parents' Keeper?* New York: Oxford University Press.

Faludi, S. 1991. *Backlash: The Undeclared War against American Women*. New York: Crown.

Fein, R. 1989. *Medical Care, Medical Costs: The Search for a Health Insurance Policy*. Cambridge, MA: Harvard University Press.

Freudenheim, M. 1991. Health Care a Growing Burden. *New York Times*, 29 January, pp. A1, C17.

Friedman, E. 1991. The Uninsured: From Dilemma to Crisis. *Journal of the American Medical Association* 265:2491–95.

Fuchs, V. 1988. *Women's Quest for Economic Equality*. Cambridge, MA: Harvard University Press.

Gilligan, C. 1982. Women's Place in Man's Life Cycle. In *In a Different Voice*, by C. Gilligan. Cambridge, MA: Harvard University Press.

Goldin, C. 1990. *Understanding the Gender Gap: An Economic History of American Women*. New York: Oxford University Press.

Hollard, D. C., and M. A. Eisenhart. 1990. *Educated in Romance: Women, Achievement and College Culture*. Chicago: University of Chicago Press.

Kasper, A. S., and E. Soldinger. 1983. Falling between the Cracks: How Health Insurance Discriminates against Women. *Women and Health* 8:77–93.

Long, S. H. 1987. Public versus Employment-related Health Insurance: Experience and Implications for Black and Nonblack Americans. *Milbank Quarterly* 65 (Suppl. 1): 200–212.

Muller, C. 1990. *Health Care and Gender*. New York: Russell Sage Foundation.

National Pharmaceutical Council. 1986. *Pharmaceutical Benefits under State Medical Assistance Programs*. Reston, VA: National Pharmaceutical Council.

Older Women's League. 1988. *The Road to Poverty: A Report on the Economic Status of Midlife and Older Women in America*. Washington, DC: Older Women's League.

———. 1989. *Failing America's Caregivers*. Washington, DC: Older Women's League.

Pare, R. 1991. Suits Force U.S. and States to Pay More for Medicaid. *New York Times*, 29 October, pp. A1, A10.

Rockefeller, J. D. 1991. A Call for Action: The Pepper Commission's Blueprint for Health Care Reform. *Journal of the American Medical Association* 265:2507–10.

Schorr, A. L. 1991. Job Turnover—A Problem with Employer-based Health Care. *New England Journal of Medicine* 323:543–45.

Starr, P. 1982. *The Social Transformation of American Medicine*. New York: Basic.

Stone, R., and G. L. Cafferata. 1987. Caregivers of the Frail Elderly: A National Profile. *Gerontologist* 27:616–26.

Swartz, K. 1990. Why Requiring Employers to Provide Health Insurance Is a Bad Idea. *Journal of Health Politics, Policy and Law* 15:779–92.

Todd, J. S., S. V. Seekings, J. A. Krichbaum, and L. K. Harvey. 1991. Health Access America. *Journal of the American Medical Association* 265:2503–6.

Uchitelle, L. 1991. Insurance Linked to Jobs: System Showing Its Age. *New York Times*, 1 May, pp. A1, A14.

U.S. Treasury Department. 1961. *Internal Revenue Bulletin, Cumulative Bulletin, 1956–1961*. Washington, DC: U.S. Government Printing Office.

Walzer, M. 1983. *Spheres of Justice*. New York: Basic.

———. 1984. Liberalism and the Art of Separation. *Political Theory* 12:315–30.

Weed, J. A. 1980. *National Estimates of Marital Dissolution and Survivorship, Vital and Health Statistics.* Series 3, Analytic Studies, no. 19, DHHS Publ. #PHS 80-1403. Washington, DC: U.S. Department of Health and Human Services.

Willard, A. 1988. Cultural Scripts for Mothering. In *Mapping the Moral Domain,* ed. C. Gilligan, J. V. Ward, and J. M. Taylor. Cambridge, MA: Harvard University Press.

This paper was presented at the Stanford University Institute for Research on Women and Gender (Palo Alto, CA, 1991), the American Philosophical Association Pacific Division Conference (Portland, OR, 1992), and the American Society of Law and Medicine (Toronto, Ontario, 1992). The author gratefully acknowledges the scholarly assistance of Professor Leslie Francis and the financial support of the University of Washington Royalty Research Fund.

Commentary

Revisiting the Employment-Insurance Link

Joan E. Ruttenberg

The employment-insurance link is the organizational backbone of our health insurance system. Indeed, the link has become so embedded in our worlds of work and health care and in our national assumptions that it has become difficult at times even to imagine that it might have been different, or that it might be different in the future. Yet the link is not the product of considered policy-making but of historical accident. Now that federal reform of the health care system has been given a high priority in the Clinton administration, there is both the need and the opportunity to revisit this American idiosyncrasy.

There are certainly many avenues for criticism of the organizational structure that renders access to health care for most Americans dependent upon access to private insurance obtained via employment. The system has been accused of inefficiency, of harboring gaps and inadequacies, of promoting rampant inflation in health care expenditures. Such criticisms are at the margin, however; if these are the most serious flaws in the system, we can create incentives for efficiency and patch the worst gaps, and the link itself need not be scuttled. In contrast, as Nancy Jecker argues more fundamentally elsewhere in this book, in her essay "Can an Employer-Based Health Insurance System Be Just?" the employment-insurance link by its very nature may be unavoidably unjust. If she is right, then no amount of tinkering at the margins will ever produce a fair health care system. Dr. Jecker's analysis is lucid and to the point. But in demonstrating so clearly the risk of injustice inherent in the linked system, her work suggests two further areas of inquiry.

First, Dr. Jecker's analysis succeeds in laying bare a crucial question of values and priorities that some policymakers seem to pretend does not exist. According to Dr. Jecker, if the distribution of jobs is subject to unfairness, then linking health insurance to jobs replicates and expands the unfairness. But even if jobs are fairly distributed, Dr. Jecker argues, the criteria for job distribution will prove unfair when they are used to distribute other social goods. Dr. Jecker clearly has a point here: it would be inappropriate to *assume* that the reasons we believe people ought to get jobs, particularly high-paying jobs with rich benefits, are the same as the reasons we believe people ought to have health insurance.

But while we should not assume that linking insurance to jobs assures fairness, neither can we assume that it assures unfairness. In order to reach such a conclusion, we would need some preexisting idea of what a fair distribution of insurance would look like. The logic inherent in Dr. Jecker's argument is that each independent social good ought to be allocated according to its own individual characteristics in order to maximize justice in the distribution of that good. What values then *should* govern the distribution of health insurance? Who "ought" to be insured and who "ought" not to be? And how would a distribution based on the answers to these questions compare to that achieved when health insurance is distributed via jobs?

This is not just an exercise in logic and hypothesis. As Dr. Jecker acknowledges, there are those who would argue, not simply assume for the sake of argument, that the distribution of jobs *is* fair: that (perhaps with some exceptions for egregious discrimination) jobs are distributed by a market that rewards hard work, discipline, and good ideas with high pay and rich benefits. While it is perhaps not often expressed explicitly, the evidence is all around us that many Americans are quite comfortable with the idea that health insurance ought to be distributed by this same market.

For example, the present employment link, which many favor retaining, can be seen as simply a slightly less direct way of distributing insurance according to the market. Those employees who can command higher incomes (full-time, highly skilled, and unionized workers) are the same employees who are most likely to be insured. In fact, severing the employment-insurance link without more would arguably produce little change in the actual distribution of health insurance. Presumably, that portion of employees' earnings no longer received in kind as health insurance coverage would be available as wages to be spent on employee-purchased insurance. In effect, distributing health insurance through employment is simply a proxy (albeit perhaps an imperfect one) for distributing health insurance according to the most "dominant" social goods: income and wealth. This is simply another way of describing the market.

In addition, while it may sound unduly harsh to some ears to suggest that we as a society condone limiting health care to only those who can pay the market's price, it is revealing to examine how other social goods are distributed. It is beyond dispute that adequate food, shelter, heat, and clothing are all fundamental to human survival and well-being, even more so than health insurance. And there are certainly many efforts, both nationally and locally, to assure such goods to those who would not otherwise be able to afford them. Yet at base, access to each of these goods is market-driven, the purchasers are individuals, and in most circumstances many more are unable to purchase what they need in the market than are helped by extramarket mechanisms. A market-based distribution of health insurance would not be inconsistent with the way our society has handled the distribution of most basic social goods.

The point to be made here is that merely linking health care to employment does not inexorably lead one to conclude that injustice is produced if one believes that both employment and insurance are appropriately distributed via the market. In this view, a market distribution of health insurance would be unjust only if it violated some other, independent standard of fairness: for example, that those who need medical care should get it. Despite our comfort, at some level, with allowing the market to distribute health insurance, this need-based value is also widely shared, if not always explicitly expressed. The result is a set of remarkably inconsistent attitudes toward health care. On the one hand, until very recently, we appear to have been quite tolerant of the current system in which ability to pay (or to strike a bargain with someone else to pay) has been the major determinant in access to health insurance, and hence to health care. Such persistent tolerance more than suggests endorsement. On the other hand, we are regularly outraged by anecdotes of laboring women turned away from hospital emergency rooms, senior citizens prematurely ejected from acute care settings, and whole families struggling without health insurance coverage because of their inability to pay. The obvious and inevitable outcome of a system in which health care coverage is for sale in the market is that some who need care will not get it.[1] If distribution by market (or by its

1. An alternative "safety net" for health care coverage does of course exist, but, as Dr. Jecker points out, it is on the whole far inferior in adequacy of coverage to the private insurance system. Inferior systems can always be improved. But the very fact that a system for distributing social goods is split into two or more tiers, with an obvious preference for one over the others, arguably calcifies the qualitative difference among the tiers. In such a situation, even the "safety net" will not assure that all who need care will get it.

proxy, employment) is to be desired, its advocates will have to make their peace with this reality. If, instead, a market distribution is seen as unfair, it is so by reference to a different standard of fairness: one based on need rather than on ability to pay. Whichever standard of fairness is adopted, the choice ought to be explicitly confronted. The employment-insurance link merely obfuscates this choice.

Dr. Jecker's article also invites an important historical examination. Many analysts have demonstrated that commercial health insurance, its growth fueled in large part by the employment link and concomitant federal tax policy, plays a central role in, and hence has had a dramatic influence on, the health care system itself. But has our increasing reliance on commercial health insurance as the primary social policy tool for attaining health also created biases in our most basic choices about health resource allocation?

The primacy of commercial insurance in our health care system is readily apparent. While multitudes of government programs attempt to fill in the gaps left by commercial insurance,[2] such programs are clearly considered a "safety net"; private insurance has always been regarded as the first choice for the funding of individuals' health care needs. Most proposals for health care reform in this country of necessity include extensive discussions of access to and affordability of insurance. In fact, it is an accepted truism that access to insurance is tantamount to access to health care; in many discussions of health policy, the two terms are used almost interchangeably.

It should not be surprising, then, that commercial insurance has had significant influences upon the very system in which it plays such a principal role. In many ways, the American health care system of the late twentieth century is the product of the incentives and disincentives created by the growth of private insurance (itself occasioned by the promotion, through the tax code and otherwise, of employer-based group insurance). These influences have been well documented. They range from the inflationary impact of the third-party-payer and fee-for-service reimbursement systems, to the increasing use of medical underwriting to classify risks more precisely (leading in part to larger numbers of uninsured individuals

---

2. Examples of such programs include Medicaid (for a portion of those unable to afford private insurance), Medicare (for those unlikely to be able to afford adequate coverage due to the increased risk of illness brought about by advancing age or disability), state-mandated benefits and federal COBRA (to require commercial insurers to extend benefits beyond the limits they might otherwise choose), and state high-risk "pools" (to facilitate coverage for those deemed "uninsurable" in the commercial market).

and families as risk spreading is eliminated and insurance becomes unaffordable), to a shifting in the structure of employment itself (as employers seek to avoid the burdens of insurance through increasing their part-time work force). Not the least of these influences has been a series of shifts in patterns of health care utilization: which services insurers choose to reimburse, and at what rates, tend to determine the kind of health care services people experience.

But a more subtle, and perhaps more profound, mechanism may also be at work. The dominance of commercial insurance has arguably been one of the major contributors to the concentration of social resources (financial and other) in the delivery of medical treatment for illness and injury and the shortchanging of efforts to prevent the social conditions that cause illness and injury.

It is no secret that many of the causes of ill health are both socially rooted and preventable: environmental toxins, substance abuse and addictions, poor nutrition, inadequate housing and homelessness, adolescent pregnancy, unprotected sexual relations, and violence all fall into this category. Steps taken to remedy such causes must of necessity cut across many substantive boundaries and must consist of broad-based efforts to create the social conditions conducive to good health.

Yet insurance, by definition, is the business of assuming the financial risk of adverse occurrences. Its overriding focus in the health care context is on determining who is most likely to experience illness or injury and which treatments by which practitioners ought to be reimbursed. To enhance predictability and hence profitability, insurers naturally seek to keep the range of reimbursable expenses both clearly defined and as narrow as possible, consistent with the scope of contractual benefits.[3] One way of doing this is the virtually universal contract clause requiring that, to be reimbursed, an expenditure must be for services that are "medically necessary." Medical necessity, in turn, assumes the presence of an illness, injury, or medical condition for which a medical practitioner (typically a physician) believes treatment is indicated. Commercial insurance also has its historical roots in the assurance of income flow to hospitals and physicians—in fact, at its inception such reimbursement was its raison d'être. By and large, hospitals and physicians are neither trained nor well posi-

---

3. Of course, *any* payer, public or private, will have the same economic incentives to delimit its own financial liability. The important point here is that the consequences of such an incentive may be radically different when the payer is also the entity with the power and obligation to act to protect the public health.

tioned to grapple with the social ailments at the root of much individual disease.

Thus, by definition, health care dollars routed through health insurance will inevitably be biased toward treatment after illness or injury has occurred, whether or not it would be more sensible for society as a whole to avoid adverse consequences by investing in prevention. While the growth of entities like HMOs, which combine the payer and provider functions, may increase insurer sensitivity to and expenditures for prevention, we cannot (and perhaps should not) expect insurers to underwrite the society-wide multidisciplinary programs needed to reduce the ill health effects of the social problems described above. The responsibility for more systemic investment in public health and prevention, most would say, lies with public authorities. But by so dividing responsibility for the creation and maintenance of good health between private insurers and public authorities and then elevating private insurance to the central role in our health care system, we facilitate an increasing disregard for the crucial links between prevention and treatment. By allowing ourselves to believe that health insurance alone assures health, we risk losing sight of the leverage that can be produced by earlier interventions in the development of illness.

In addition, this bifurcation spurs a cost inflation paralleling that for which the third-party-payer fee-for-service reimbursement system is famous. As the entity responsible for systemic prevention, government is several steps removed and so insulated from the actual costs of illness:[4] a clear perception of such costs is muffled by both the private insurance system, through which the cost of care is filtered, and the employer-insurance link, through which the cost of insurance is filtered.[5] An accurate cost-benefit analysis of spending to prevent illness and injury becomes impossible. The result is excessive expenditures for post hoc treatment due to inadequate expenditures for systemic prevention. We therefore find our-

4. As commercial insurance has become more expensive and difficult to get, and as public health care programs have grown in response, both federal and state governments have come to feel more directly the increasing cost of medical treatment. Yet it may be too easy for government to respond to these signals by attempting to shift participants in these programs back into the privately insured sphere, rather than by seeking to prevent poor health in the first instance.

5. It is true that, even through these screens, messages about the cost of care can filter through, as evidenced most dramatically by recent changes in political rhetoric to include statements about skyrocketing health care costs to business and the need for reform. These messages, however, are political, not economic, stemming as they do from complaints by larger and more powerful segments of the business community about the anticompetitive effects of rising health care costs. We can expect government to respond differently to such political messages than it would to a direct economic perception of the costs.

selves on the brink of the twenty-first century presiding over a massively expensive and inflationary medical treatment system that rarely underwrites the prevention of illness and an underdeveloped and underfunded public health structure with considerable untapped potential for avoiding the need for medical treatment.

The historical quirk that produced the employer link to and public subsidy of the purchase of health insurance may, as Dr. Jecker suggests, produce inevitable injustices in the distribution of health insurance. This quirk, on a larger scale, may also be a major contributor to the creation of an unbalanced and ultimately counterproductive distribution of health care resources. As policymakers in the coming years consider how to increase good health, whether within or outside the confines of the employment-insurance link, they must also consider how to reverse the most damaging aspects of this historic misallocation of resources.

The Pragmatic Appeal of Employment-Based Health Care Reform

David A. Rochefort

That employment-related health benefits have unjustly omitted many Americans from insurance coverage is easy to see. And current state-level public health insurance programs serving welfare recipients and the poor generally do not compare favorably with private insurance plans (except in the area of long-term care). But these points, properly underscored by Nancy Jecker in her essay in this volume, constitute more an indictment of *past* practices than a criticism of possible reforms. In fact, it is entirely feasible to design an employment-based health insurance program that would address such concerns, effectively marrying social justice with political pragmatism. To appreciate that such a program could be devised, however, it is necessary to set aside some major misconceptions about employer mandates that have entered into the national health policy debate.

A Crossfire of Criticism

Under a national employer mandate, the primary method for extending health insurance coverage would be to require all businesses to provide employees and their dependents with a standard basic package of benefits. Depending on the nature of this requirement, companies could do this directly or by paying a tax for employees to be covered by another source established by government. Also encompassed by the government program would be the unemployed uninsured. When the latter, indirect method of coverage is given to businesses as an option, the plans are known as "play or pay."

Such employer-mandate plans represent a middle-of-the road reform strategy between providing tax subsidies to uninsured individuals, to help them purchase their own private coverage, and a total government take-over of the health care financing system—two other prominent policy positions, associated with Republicans and Democrats, respectively. As such, mandates have been attacked both for proposing too much public intervention and for proposing too little.

From those inclined toward a tax-based solution has come a series of ominous predictions about the economic impact of mandates (White House 1992; see also Fuchs 1992; *Businews* 1988). By increasing the cost of labor to employers, it is argued, mandates will reduce wages and jobs. Particularly hard hit will be small companies, a sector that accounts for more than half of all working uninsured. Prices of goods and services, too, are expected to rise.

On a more philosophical plane, opponents of mandates question whether guaranteeing universal health care coverage is truly a social responsibility. Or, if granting the point, they maintain that it is unfair to impose this responsibility on private employers. Not entirely consistently, others on the right, including the former Bush administration, have criticized mandates as likely to "cascade into a form of national health insurance" (White House 1992: 78)—one scenario is that more and more employers would elect to pay into the publicly operated insurance fund under the play-or-pay option. Another prediction is that a steady aggregation of older and sicker workers drawing on the public fund will lead to unacceptably rising costs for government.

Just as many complaints, albeit of a different orientation, come from those who advocate the establishment of a national public health care program in the United States (see, e.g., Russo 1991; Kerrey 1991; Glaser 1991; Swartz 1990). Some, extrapolating from defects of the current employment-based insurance system, foresee an increasing fragmentation of the insurance market, with private insurance companies calibrating products and prices according to the risk profiles of a greater number of employment groups. Also, the danger of "job lock," wherein people are hesitant to leave a position for one with less generous health benefits, would be worsened if insurers excluded the coverage of preexisting conditions for new group members. In her ethical assessment, Jecker expresses concern over the special problems this practice would create for women, who are more likely to participate intermittently in the work force. And present experience casts doubt on the ability of multiple separate employers to bargain effectively with insurance companies and health care providers to control rising costs.

In general, critics on the left characterize the employer mandate approach to health care reform as "partial" and "incremental." Their worst fear is not that the adoption of such a strategy will soon lead to national health insurance, but that it will divert needed "comprehensive" and "fundamental" policy change. At last at the point of following the road taken by other Western nations that have confronted similar health system problems, America seems ready to veer off into another historical cul-de-sac. Were a large number of employers to choose to pay into the publicly sponsored insurance plan, proponents of a single national program fear the Medicaid experience writ large—a two-class system of care, which satisfies neither recipients nor providers. Jecker, for example, describes current Medicaid benefits as "notoriously meager and inconsistent from one state to the next." Finally, the financing method of an employer mandate is judged regressive in its effects, that is, it inflicts greater burdens on lower-income workers (see, e.g., Cantor 1990).

These appraisals cast employer mandates as at best ill-considered and at worst a disastrous course of health care reform. To the extent that the brief against mandates has been constructed for political debate, however, it includes the kinds of abstractions, distortions, worst-case scenarios, and straw-man arguments typical in this context. While no analysis can dispel purely ideological preferences for more or less government, careful scrutiny of these various pitfalls can put into perspective the true potential of the mandate strategy. As Brown (1990: 794) has written, "A key policy question about mandates . . . is not whether they are a good idea, or even whether they are preferable (on whatever grounds) to other approaches, but rather whether they might play a positive role in catalyzing and sustaining an effective strategic *mix*" (emphasis in original).

Disinsurance and Disemployment Dilemmas

Economic warnings about employer-mandated health insurance have a familiar historical ring. Conservative business elements have used a rhetoric of impending calamity whenever government has contemplated new regulation of the private sector. Had these claims been taken at face value in the past, however, the U.S. would not have child labor laws today. Nor would we ever risk increasing the minimum wage, even though experience shows that such mandated wage increases do not seem to lead to substantial job loss to the extent that this is directly measurable (Zedlewski et al. 1992: 64; Levitan 1990: 152). Recent business resistance to a family leave bill also centered on this issue of creating unfair and burdensome new private obligations. Here again, however, the evidence from businesses already providing leaves to their employees—for example, the businesses in Dade County, Florida, the first county in the nation to pass a family leave ordinance—is that costs are lower than anticipated, while worker satisfaction and productivity have grown (Rohter 1993).

The truth is that no one can predict with precision the economic impacts on private employers of government-mandated health insurance, as numerous health care economists agree (Zedlewski et al. 1992; Kronick 1991; Swartz 1990). Without firm estimates of such components in the calculation as the "elasticity" of the demand for labor, it is possible only to delineate a likely range of outcomes based on certain assumptions. A recent pair of sophisticated "microsimulation" studies provide this analysis.

Kronick (1991) estimated the effect of implementing the universal health care law passed by the Dukakis administration in Massachusetts in 1988, which is now in abeyance. The bill contains a play-or-pay requirement for employers, which asks them to provide health insurance or pay a 12 percent payroll tax on the first $14,000 of workers' earnings. (Certain categories of employers, like the self-employed and businesses with fewer than six workers, are exempt.) Kronick points out that while some businesses not currently providing coverage might suffer under the program, others, such as those offering health insurance and absorbing the costs of uncompensated care, would be helped. The opportunity to purchase the government-sponsored plan on a sliding income scale would also benefit the self-employed. Thus, jobs would be lost in some businesses but would increase in others, and the net economic effect is not clear.

Kronick also considered various "disinsurance" effects that could swell the government-sponsored plan, taking into account, for example, the anticipated behavior of the self-insured, of firms with low-wage workers, firms whose insurance premiums are higher than average, and firms simply eager to rid themselves of the "administrative hassle" of providing health insurance coverage, who would opt for the government plan. His conclusion was that Massachusetts could implement the universal health law, even with these increases, relying completely on revenues from the payroll tax, money saved from eliminating the uncompensated care pool, collecting sliding-scale premiums from people not covered through their employers, and anticipated Medicaid savings.

Zedlewski et al. (1992) examined the impacts of a national play-or-pay employer mandate. Some factors distinguishing this simulation from Kronick's are that the nation as a whole has different labor and wage patterns from Massachusetts and a higher uninsurance rate. In addition, this model assumed two employer premium costs, one lower than the other, based on the possible advantageous impacts of small-group insurance reform, and two alternative payroll taxes, 7 percent and 9 percent. They found that the size of the public plan could range from 35 to 52 percent of the nonelderly population. In 1989 dollars, new government costs would fall somewhere between $25 billion and $37 billion, and new employer costs between $29 billion and $44 billion. Legislative choices concerning the design of the program would directly influence where along the spectrum of possibilities these values actually land.

Who Pays What, When, and How?

One thing is certain. Under all proposed plans the buck stops the same place. Whether it's lost wages, higher prices, higher premiums, or increased taxes, the public will have to foot the bill for expanding health insurance coverage. Within the intricacies of that money trail, however, lie varying equity issues.

Businesses that insure have to pay high premiums because hospital rates are calculated to include uncompensated care of employees of noninsuring businesses. Hence, the charge rings false that to compel noninsuring businesses to offer health benefits is unfair; in this light, it is noninsuring companies that perpetrate inequity, by "free riding" on the cross-subsidies woven into the health care financing system. More and more, business and other group health insurers attempt to resist paying these added costs for hospitals' bad debt and free care—which exceeded $300 million in Massachusetts in fiscal year 1991 (Kronick 1991)—by such means as negotiated provider discounts and self-insurance. Last year in New Jersey, the courts upheld a related challenge to the state's hospital financing law, which tacks onto the hospital bills of all insured patients (excepting those on Medicare) a 19 percent surcharge to pay for the uninsured (Sullivan 1992). These trends foretell a progressive destabilization of the health care economy (Coddington et al. 1991) and the necessity of bringing all actors into a new systemwide arrangement.

A second frequent equity criticism is that employer mandates penalize struggling small businesses, which are overrepresented among the companies to be affected by new requirements. Current patterns of uninsurance make this problem a real one, although there are several mitigating factors. Any price increases and wage cuts arising from mandates should be felt by all noninsuring small businesses more or less equivalently, maintaining the competitive balance internal to that sector. Also, the leading employer mandate proposals, like HealthAmerica and the proposal of the National Leadership Coalition for Health Care Reform, contain numerous provisions specifically to soften the impact on small businesses. Included are slower phase-in schedules, small-group insurance reform, special treatment of new businesses, improved tax deductions, and new tax credits for firms with low profit margins. Zedlewski et al. (1992) indicate that government could further reduce small business expense without proportionately increasing its own outlays or the size of the play-or-pay public insurance program. Government could allow small businesses to pay less than the standard 80 percent share of the insurance premium for workers' dependents and subsidize the added expenses for all families beneath a certain income level.

The Bush administration complained about the high costs to government—and, implicitly, the unfairness to taxpayers—of an employer mandate strategy. Yet analysts have placed the public sector costs of the former president's tax credit proposal at just about the same level as an employer mandate—and this is *without* a guarantee of universal coverage under the tax credits (Kranish and Knox 1992).

Finally, there is the question of "regressivity" under employer mandates. The problem is straightforward: assuming some trade-off between new health benefits, payroll taxes, and wages, low-wage earners will be losing a greater proportion of their income. To be sure, a wholly publicly funded program supported by outlays from a progressive income tax would be more egalitarian. However, several points complicate the choice of most suitable funding for health reform.

First, there is the force of tradition to reckon with. The major social insurance entitlements of the American welfare state for unemployment, disability, Medicare, and old-age pensions are all financed primarily by payroll taxes, not general revenues. With government using a sliding-scale fee for enrollees in the publicly sponsored plan and for the premiums of low-income workers in employer plans—a provision of HealthAmerica, for example—an employer mandate would be that much more progressive than these established programs. The opportunity to reduce tax liability by making pretax health plan contributions would be another monetary bonus that mandates would give to those presently working without insurance. Second, although it may be regressive at "take-in," universal health insurance would be progressive at payout to the extent that lower socioeconomic and minority groups have greater need for health services. Third, this awkward combination of regressive and progressive principles, with the regressive dimension outermost, could be critical to avoiding the public perception of universal health care as "welfare." This, in turn, would enhance the initiative's long-term political viability.

A Trojan Horse

The idea that job lock, more extensive "redlining" of groups and individuals, and other private insurance abuses would worsen under an employer mandate system assumes a half-measure type of reform that is not under serious consideration. Current leading mandate proposals do much more than merely require universal workplace coverage, leaving present market dynamics to shape the outcome. They also embody an array of interventions to remedy the inefficiencies and ineffectiveness of that health care market. Such changes include requirements for communitywide insurance rating and no coverage exclusions on the basis of health status or preexisting conditions. Other pieces of this omnibus overhaul strategy are malpractice reform and administrative and billing simplification. Whether all of these actions will be pursued far enough and buttressed with adequate monitoring is a fair concern. Much of the legislative and administrative process will consist of bargaining with powerful interests over just these issues. Admittedly, this is not a struggle to be taken lightly. But it is simply incorrect at this stage of the national debate to portray mandate reformers as unmindful of such problems.

Another fundamental component of leading mandate plans is payment reform. Many include rate setting to establish standard reimbursements for providers from all third-party payers and an independent Federal Reserve type of health expenditure board to specify national and state spending ceilings. These cost-containment measures draw simultaneously on the lessons of national health care programs in other countries like Canada and Germany, as well as innovative state programs inside the U.S., whose impressive successes are discussed elsewhere in this issue.

The specter of a monster Medicaid program likewise misconstrues the nature of the employer-mandate strategy. If the public plan under play or pay, as is generally proposed, featured a standard package of benefits across states equivalent to basic private coverage, higher provider reimbursement levels, and substantial working- and middle-class enrollments (not to mention a different program name—AmeriCare under Health-America, Pro-Health under the National Coalition), would the resulting program still equal Medicaid?

Alternatively, instead of playing the role of direct insurer, public authorities could function like "the health benefits manager of a large employer . . . contract[ing] for health benefits with a selection of high-quality health plans," and giving a choice of these plans to those not insured by their employer (Kronick 1991: 28). Hawaii's state health insurance plan supplies a working example, albeit with limited benefits (Dukakis 1992). This approach is also consistent with current "managed competition" reforms. In short, there is no reason why a mixed private-public system of universal health insurance must perpetuate the current problem of two standards of care reflecting different sources of coverage.

Morone and Dunham (1986) have suggested that fundamental policy shifts in the American political system sometimes assume the guise of incremental changes. Reviewing the development, refinement, and spread of diagnosis-related group reimbursement from the state to national levels in the 1980s, they mused whether the country might not be "slouching toward national health insurance." Heavily regulated employer mandate plans exhibit something of this same deceptive innocuousness, appearing merely to extend current private insurance arrangements, while introducing sweeping new public controls over the health care system. They are also, in this sense, a kind of Trojan horse of reform. Terminology aside, the similarities with both the aims and means of national health insurance outweigh the differences.

Political Calculus

If mandates and national health insurance hold much in common from a policy perspective, they lie at opposite ends of a political pragmatism scale (Pollack and Torda 1991). American history teaches us that major domestic innovations require presidential leadership; but candidate Clinton frequently expressed his objections to a single-payer, all-government health reform, and he is unlikely now to throw the weight of the Oval Office behind this model. National health insurance also has the opposition of the insurance industry and a majority of top business leaders. A tax increase of hundreds of billions of dollars would be needed to finance a program of this type. No matter that this mostly represents reallocation of monies now being paid as premiums and out-of-pocket spending, the prospect is certain to be unpalatable to a society looking for tax relief.

By contrast, employer mandates hold the support of many of the very most powerful actors in the national health policy debate. For example, sponsorship of the HealthAmerica bill, introduced in Congress in July of 1991, came from the Senate Democratic leadership, including Senators Mitchell, Kennedy, Riegle, and Rockefeller. House Ways and Means Chair Dan Rostenkowski's Health Insurance and Cost-Containment Act of 1991 also features a play-or-pay device as its centerpiece. Elsewhere on the political scene, the American Medical Association, for most of the twentieth century this country's most implacable foe of national health plans, has finally cast its vote for reform with an employer mandate strategy. Former presidents Gerald Ford and Jimmy Carter support an employment route to expanded coverage, along with the numerous major business, union, and consumer organizations that came together in the National Leadership Coalition, of which they were honorary cochairs. Some other backers of this general approach—each, of course, with its own preferred variations—include the American Association of Retired Persons, the American Hospital Association, the Pepper Commission, the American Nurses Association, and the AFL-CIO.

In light of this political analysis, the heated dispute between advocates of a single-payer model and an employer mandate is one of the most unfortunate aspects of the contemporary health care debate. During recent years, no point of view has been more cogently articulated in health policy circles than the virtues of a Canadian-type national health program (see, e.g., Evans 1986; Marmor and Mashaw 1990; Woolhandler and Himmelstein 1991; GAO 1991). The influence of this argument, in turn, has been far-reaching, as witnessed in the strong regulatory mechanisms being incorporated in employer mandate proposals. Other aspects of employer mandate legislation could do even more to pave the way for national health insurance in the U.S., should that step prove necessary; they include waiver options for state single-payer programs and public "stop-loss" limits on liability per privately insured person (Aaron 1991). At the same time, an employer mandate is pivotal to leading managed competition proposals (e.g., Enthoven and Kronick 1991), now in good grace with the Clinton administration.[1]

A predominantly employment-based system is America's indigenous contribution to the international panoply of health insurance approaches. Moreover, of the roughly 35 million Americans who now lack health

1. One question, however, in blending a system of managed competition with employer mandate plans having strong public cost control mechanisms is the emphasis to be placed on market versus government price restraints.

insurance, 85 percent are workers and their dependents (Fuchs 1992), making the workplace a logical and effective vehicle for addressing the problem of no insurance for the bulk of the population affected. Labor market analysts report a rising trend in businesses' use of part-time and temporary help, "disposable workers," who can be paid lower wages with few fringe benefits (Kilborn 1993). This development makes more comprehensive regulation of privately provided benefit packages not just desirable but an absolute necessity, in order to stem rampant shifting of costs onto private households and government.

Although it is now imperfect, employment-based health insurance nonetheless offers to policymakers a ready-made structure for achieving their objectives of universality and cost constraint. We understand its operational requirements, needed adaptations, and future potential far better than any other model.

References

Aaron, H. J. 1991. *Serious and Unstable Condition: Financing America's Health Care*. Washington, DC: Brookings Institution.

Brown, L. D. 1990. The Merits of Mandates. *Journal of Health Politics, Policy and Law* 15 (4): 793–96.

Businews. 1988. Government Mandates: Will Small Business Survive? September/ October, p. 1.

Cantor, J. C. 1990. Expanding Health Insurance Coverage: Who Will Pay? *Journal of Health Politics, Policy and Law* 15 (4): 755–78.

Coddington, D. C., D. J. Keen, K. D. Moore, and R. L. Clarke. 1991. *The Crisis in Health Care: Costs, Choices, and Strategies*. San Francisco, CA: Jossey-Bass.

Dukakis, M. S. 1992. Hawaii and Massachusetts: Lessons from the States. *Yale Law and Policy Review* 10 (2): 397–408.

Enthoven, A. C., and R. Kronick. 1991. Universal Health Insurance through Incentives Reform. *Journal of the American Medical Association* 265 (19): 2532–36.

Evans, R. G. 1986. Finding the Levers, Finding the Courage: Lessons from Cost Containment in North America. *Journal of Health Politics, Policy and Law* 11 (4): 585–615.

Fuchs, B. C. 1992. *Mandated Employer-provided Health Insurance*. Washington, DC: Congressional Research Service, 24 February update.

GAO (General Accounting Office). 1991. *Canadian Health Insurance: Lessons for the United States*. Washington, DC: General Accounting Office.

Glaser, W. A. 1991. *Health Insurance in Practice*. San Francisco, CA: Jossey-Bass.

Kerrey, R. 1991. Why America Will Adopt Comprehensive Health Care Reform. *American Prospect* 2 (Summer): 81–91.

Kilborn, P. T. 1993. New Jobs Lack the Old Security in a Time of "Disposable Workers." *New York Times*, 15 March, p. A1.

Kranish, M., and R. A. Knox. 1992. Bush Offers Cost-Control Health Plan. *Boston Globe*, 7 February, p. 1.

Kronick, R. 1991. Can Massachusetts Pay for Health Care for All? *Health Affairs* 10 (1): 26–44.

Levitan, S. A. 1990. *Programs in Aid of the Poor*, 6th ed. Baltimore: Johns Hopkins University Press.

Marmor, T. R., and J. L. Mashaw. 1990. Canada's Health Insurance and Ours: The Real Lessons, the Big Choices. *American Prospect* 1 (Fall): 18–29.

Morone, J. A., and A. B. Dunham. 1986. Slouching toward National Health Insurance. *Bulletin of the New York Academy of Medicine* 62 (6): 646–62.

Pollack, R., and P. Torda. 1991. The Pragmatic Road toward National Health Insurance. *American Prospect* 2 (Summer): 92–100.

Rohter, L. 1993. In Florida, Family Bill Wins Converts. *New York Times*, 5 February, p. A14.

Russo, M. 1991. Single-Payer System Guarantees Health Care for Less. *Christian Science Monitor*, 10 September, p. 18.

Sullivan, J. F. 1992. Judge Stays Rate Ruling for Hospitals. *New York Times*, 5 June, p. B1.

Swartz, K. 1990. Why Requiring Employers to Provide Health Insurance Is a Bad Idea. *Journal of Health Politics, Policy and Law* 15 (4): 779–92.

White House. 1992. *The President's Comprehensive Health Reform Program*. Washington, DC: White House.

Woolhandler, S., and D. Himmelstein. 1991. The Deteriorating Administrative Efficiency of the U.S. Health Care System. *New England Journal of Medicine* 324 (18): 1253–58.

Zedlewski, S. R., G. P. Acs, and C. W. Winterbottom. 1992. Play-or-Pay Employer Mandates: Potential Effects. *Health Affairs* 11 (1): 62–83.

Thanks to Michael Dukakis of Northeastern University and James Morone for their comments on a draft of this article.

Part 4
The People

Is Health Care Different?
Popular Support of Federal Health and
Social Policies

Mark Schlesinger and Taeku Lee

Abstract Over the past several years there has been a striking increase in policy-makers' attention to health care reform. This paper explores whether there has been a corresponding shift in popular attitudes and identifies factors that may have changed these attitudes. The first part of the analysis relies on survey data collected between 1975 and 1989 to estimate a set of regression models, relating support for federal involvement in health care, antipoverty programs, and general domestic policies to a set of sociodemographic characteristics. Relative to other federal policies, support for health initiatives grew over this period. During this same period, long-standing differences in support between rich and poor, old and young, educated and uneducated, all narrowed for health care, though they did not for other types of federal policies. The second part of this study explores motivations that might account for these patterns. We identify a half dozen ways in which health care may be viewed as "different," that is, more or less appropriate for federal action. Analysis of survey data from 1987 suggests that there are relatively small differences in the attitudes and perceptions that motivate support for federal health initiatives, relative to federal domestic policies in general. However, there are more striking differences between health programs and more overtly redistributive policies. Compared to redistributive federal programs, support for federal health initiatives are (a) less identified with racial minorities or economically disadvantaged groups, (b) less constrained by notions of individual responsibility, (c) more closely associated with concerns about equal opportunity in American society, and (d) somewhat more constrained by choices between federal and local government. These patterns persist whether or not respondents are politically active and whether they report themselves to be liberal or conservative. We suggest that the growing support for federal intervention in health care, relative to other social policies, is in part an inadvertent by-product of ideological positions popularized during the Reagan and Bush administrations. We draw from these results some predictions about the course of the ongoing debate over federal health policies.

The prospects for an expanded federal role in health insurance have fired the imaginations and ambitions of American politicians. The change over the past five years has been striking. In the early and mid-1980s, the potential for greater government involvement in the health care system was dismissed as politically unrealistic (Navarro 1987). By the early 1990s, the political bandwagon favoring government action seemed to be fully hitched-up and pulling out from the station, with last-minute passengers desperately scrambling for seats. Dozens of national health insurance proposals have been introduced in Congress since 1990, and more are on the way. Every candidate in the 1992 presidential campaign felt compelled to offer some sort of plan, though most had given the issue little previous attention.

Interest at the state level has been no less intense. Over the past five years, Massachusetts, Vermont, Florida, Oregon, and Minnesota have enacted laws to universalize health insurance. Though none of these provisions has been as yet implemented, comparable legislation has been introduced in a number of other state legislatures in the Northeast, Midwest, and Pacific Coast regions. This enthusiasm has been fired by reports that American voters are extremely dissatisfied with current arrangements for financing health care, are willing to consider alternatives, and are interested in having government lead them in that search (Blendon et al. 1990; Blendon and Donelan 1990; Shapiro and Young 1989).

This apparently dramatic shift in the prevailing political winds has encouraged many observers to conclude that federal action is imminent. In describing the prospects for national health care reform, the editor of the *Journal of the American Medical Association* recently wrote, "Surely we in this rich and successful country can manage to provide basic medical care because it is the right thing to do, and the time has come. A long-term crying need has developed into a national moral imperative. . . . An aura of inevitability is upon us" (Lundberg 1991: 2566).

The reading of auras, however, is always a chancy business. Are the political prospects for federal action actually this compelling? Even a brief perusal of the historical record raises some doubts. The early 1970s were a time of comparable interest in fundamental health financing reform, particularly in Washington. As Congress began its session in 1975, there were twenty-three national health insurance proposals pending before it (Coughlin 1980: 81). Popular support for a government-financed plan was high (Blendon and Donelan 1990). And that support bridged ideological boundaries, with one of the proposals before Congress carrying the endorsement of a Republican president. The same mix of concerns about costs and access to care characterized the political debates of this period (Striber and Ferber 1981; Bowler et al. 1978).

Nor were the early 1970s unique in historical perspective. The debate over national health insurance two decades ago was presaged by comparable political considerations in the late 1940s, to the extent that a writer describing the debates of the 1970s remarked that "the options being played and the thematic orchestration echo as if off a distant mountainside thirty years in the past" (Coughlin 1980: 81). National health insurance had also gained presidential support in the 1940s (Fein 1986). And it also had broad popular support, with the public evenly divided between plans that relied on privately administered insurance and those run by the government (Schlitz 1970).

In each of these episodes, there was widespread public sentiment favoring some government action, yet none followed. It will be news to none but the most politically naive that popular sentiment for government action does not in itself guarantee a response. Organized political opposition, fragmentation of authority between a Congress controlled by one party and a presidency by the other, as well as conflicting strategies for reform, have all contributed to political inertia (Fein 1986; Bowler et al. 1978; Marmor 1973). But public opinion can also have an important influence on political debates (Page and Shapiro 1992; Wright et al. 1987). One important question about current or future prospects for reform thus involves the extent to which the American public will push more or less strongly for government involvement than it has in the past.

Public support for government action in health care has fluctuated periodically over time since extensive polling began after World War II. Support for government involvement in health care rose throughout the 1950s, peaking in the early to mid-1960s; it then ebbed until about 1980, after which it began to rise once again. These patterns are found in both postelection polling (Kelley 1988; Brown 1988; Tropman 1987) or periodic random population surveys (Blendon and Donelan 1990; Shapiro and Young 1986; Coughlin 1980). The rise and fall of public support can also be seen either in the salience of health as an issue in elections (Blendon and Donelan 1989; Kelley 1988) or in solicited public opinions about the appropriate role of government in society (Brown 1988; Tropman 1987; Shapiro and Young 1986). These fluctuating levels of support for government action in health care only loosely, perhaps coincidentally, coincide with broad swings between liberal and conservative ideologies (Schlesinger 1986). Throughout this fifty-year period, while attitudes toward government involvement in health care have waxed and waned, public support for additional societal spending on health care has remained high (Blendon and Donelan 1990; Shapiro and Young 1986).

Political initiatives that are not synchronized with these ebbs and flows in public attitudes may lose legitimacy and political momentum. Declining public support for government involvement in health care, which began during the latter 1960s, may have undermined legislative efforts to enact a national health insurance plan in the early to mid-1970s (Blendon and Donelan 1990; Kelley 1988; Brown 1988; Tropman 1987). With public attention wavering, the political costs of making hard choices among competing proposals may simply have been too great (Fein 1986; Bowler et al. 1978). For similar reasons, the prospects for federal action in the 1990s thus depend both on long-term trends in public support as well as the stability of public interest in this issue.

Past studies also suggest that apparently high levels of public support for some form of government intervention in health care financing often mask substantial disagreement over the form this action should take and the extent of active federal involvement. This reflects deep-rooted differences in the public's beliefs about the appropriate role for government in American society. After reviewing some twenty years of survey data, one researcher concluded that "few issues of domestic policy have been more tenacious or controversial than that of governmental medical care. As conflicting views on this subject have continued to be deeply entrenched for many years, the issue must have close links to deep undercurrents within the U.S. value system" (Tropman 1987: 81). Historically, these differences in values have systematically divided the rich from the poor, the old from the young, and racial minorities from the white majority.

At the heart of these tensions is the long-standing American discomfort with activist government, a discomfort that has increasingly become a "crisis of confidence" in federal institutions (Rochefort and Boyer 1988). Over the past thirty years there has been a dramatic decline in Americans' perceptions of the efficacy and equity of the federal government (Tropman 1987; Sundquist 1986). If they are now to support federal action to reform health care financing, they must be willing to view interventions in health care on somewhat different terms than they do interventions into other aspects of society.

There is some evidence that health care may be different in this sense. Americans have long appeared more willing to accept a government role in this arena (Coughlin 1980). They more strongly favor additional spending on health care than on any other government-financed service, with the exception of education (Smith 1987). Even in the most influential early years of the Reagan administration, the vast majority of Americans favored increasing government regulation of both the prices and the delivery of health services (Shapiro and Young 1986). A recent review of American attitudes toward the "welfare state" concluded that "Americans' support for medical care is virtually on par with Social Security [the gold standard of electoral politics] as an entitlement" (Shapiro and Young 1989: 78–79).

But the picture that can be drawn from public opinion data is a complicated one. While favoring some government intervention, Americans grow uncomfortable at the prospect of too much involvement. For example, a 1990 survey indicated that three-quarters of those who favored a role for the federal government in promoting access to health care did *not* have great confidence that "the federal government is well-suited to run programs that affect the health and welfare of all Americans" (Blue Cross/Blue Shield 1990: 6).

To make a case that current public agitation will in fact lead to federal action thus involves addressing questions about whether the current health reform debate is "different" in two senses: different from comparable debates that resulted in political stalemate in the past and different from current debates over the role of the federal government in other areas, where differences of opinion about the legitimacy of federal involvement have stymied federal action.

Past research on public opinion related to health care has done little to address these questions. The literature treats attitudes toward health policy with little reference to attitudes about other social policy. It can thus say nothing about any distinguishing aspects of how health care reform fits into the public agenda. Nor does this past literature consider the differences in attitudes among Americans facing different social or economic circumstances. In a largely fruitless quest to characterize *the* American opinion on health reform, the research misses the social cleavages that have undermined efforts to establish collective support for federal action in all aspects of social policy.

Ironically, as political interest in health financing reform has increased in recent years, the relevance of studies of public opinion has diminished. Research in this arena has degenerated into an intellectual skirmish between opponents and proponents of government action (Rochefort and Boyer 1988). On one side are academics and politicians who see in the polls a mandate for change. On the other side are representatives of the business community and particularly the health insurance industry, who see in the polls (in addition to the threat to their livelihood) only inconsistent statements, poorly worded questions, and delusions of a free lunch (i.e., new government programs that require no substantial taxes) (Blendon et al. 1990; Jajich-Toth and Roper 1990; Blue Cross/Blue Shield 1990; Gabel et al. 1989). Squabbles of this sort over the "meaning" of survey data have their own historical precedents. For example, during the political debates of the 1940s over national health insurance, polling data were used strategically by both opponents and proponents of government action. "Each side in the public debate was attracted by the types of questions that validated its assumptions" (Schlitz 1970: 132). Although selective invocation of public attitudes thus has a certain historic pedigree, most contemporary articles on public opinion about health reform reveal more about the ideological biases or self-interest of the debaters than about the nature of American public opinion or its relationship to public policy.

This paper has been formulated to avoid these pitfalls and expand our understanding of the dynamics of public attitudes toward federal health policy. We do this by exploring the various ways in which public attitudes toward government's role in health care may be different from opinions about other forms of social policy. Using data collected in the General Social Survey (GSS) in 1975, 1983, 1987, and 1989, we track the changing sociodemographic determinants of support for government action in health care, relative to other social concerns. The findings from a set of multivariate regression models suggest that government's role in health care is viewed as different, both in terms of how much support exists for federal action, as well as how that support varies across boundaries of age, race, and socioeconomic class. To better understand why Americans value health care differently, we develop hypotheses about how health care may be viewed as different, in terms of individual self-interest, a concern for others, or norms of distributional equity. We test these hypotheses using data from the 1987 GSS. We show that the attitudes and perceptions undergirding support for health care initiatives are different, particularly from government policies that are more explicitly redistributive. The paper concludes with a discussion of the implications of our findings for ongoing debates in health policy, as well as for thinking about the role of health policy in the context of the broader welfare state.

Who Supports Government Interventions in Health and Social Policy? Changing Sociodemographic Determinants, 1975–1989

We begin by identifying who supports and who opposes an active federal role in health care reform. This involves addressing several questions: How do those who support such policies differ from those who oppose them? How do these patterns of public support for health care compare to those for other aspects of social policy? How are these differences changing over time? Past research has identified a number of characteristics that predispose Americans to favor or oppose a federal government active in social policy, or what is sometimes referred to as the "welfare state." This literature establishes an empirical baseline for this study.

Sociodemographic Influences on Support of the Welfare State

Past research has identified the personal characteristics associated with support for welfare programs, employment guarantees, guaranteed minimum incomes, ceilings on earnings, and programs targeted to the disadvantaged. In general, these studies document what is often referred to as the "self-interest" hypothesis—that people support public programs more strongly if they think that they might personally have to rely on those programs. Because individuals have very different perceptions of their need for assistance, there are sharp differences in support between upper- and lower-income households, as well as between whites and blacks (Shingles 1989; Brown 1988; Tropman 1987; Kluegel and Smith 1986; Hochschild 1981; Coughlin 1980).[1] These distinctions are sometimes referred to as "social cleavages" in support for activist government. They appear to be quite stable over time (Brown 1988). Indeed, some analysts have concluded that "there is no unequivocal evidence that these political cleavages have changed substantially since the first national surveys of the 1930s and 1940s" (Shapiro and Young 1989: 65).

Although support for government interventions is sharply divided along economic lines, other aspects of socioeconomic status produce less consistent patterns. Several researchers have found that measures of social

1. In general, past studies have identified only blacks as a distinct racial minority. They often assume that the support measured for blacks extends to other disenfranchised groups, such as Hispanics, though they do so on the basis of rather limited evidence (Coughlin 1980). For a more extensive review of the political attitudes of Hispanics, see Caplan 1987.

status such as advanced education or prestigious occupation are also negatively related to support for redistributive government policies (Tropman
1987; Hochschild 1981; Coughlin 1980). But others have found the opposite to be true (Shingles 1989) or have found that education is negatively
related to support for some interventions, but positively related to others
(Kluegel and Smith 1986). Relationships to age and sex are also somewhat inconsistent, though generally younger Americans and women appear to be most supportive of redistributive policies (Shapiro and Young
1989; Brown 1988; Tropman 1987; Kluegel and Smith 1986; Hochschild
1981).[2] Here too, different interpretations of these demographic patterns
abound. Some analysts see them as reflecting differences in the capacity
of individuals to care for others. Other analysts contend that young people
and women face greater personal uncertainty about their economic well-
being and thus support redistributive policies out of a sort of probabilistic
self-interest. Marital status appears to have little influence on support for
government welfare policies, though married people are somewhat more
supportive of programs targeted to racial minorities (Tropman 1987).

Differences between urban and rural residents are generally small
(Tropman 1987) but are more pronounced for policies likely to have concentrated urban benefits (Shapiro and Young 1989). Early studies found
substantial regional differences in support for welfare (AFDC) programs,
with the greatest opposition in southern and mountain states (Wohlenberg 1976). However, subsequent studies with more sophisticated regression models found no comparable regional differences (Tropman 1987;
Kluegel and Smith 1986). This suggests that the apparent geographic
differences were an indirect consequence of regional variation in demo-
graphics and economic conditions.

The empirical research on support for government action in health care
is more limited in scope and even less consistent in findings. Several
studies report that both income and education are correlated with attitudes
toward government's role in health care. But some conclude that this relationship is positive (Tropman 1987), others that it is negative (Brown
1988; Striber and Ferber 1981), still others that it is nonlinear, with the
greatest opposition to government involvement coming from the middle
class (Coughlin 1980). The gender of respondents, as well as whether

2. Since most of these findings are based on studies using multivariate regression models,
some of the inconsistencies emerge because different sets of variables are used in the regressions in different studies. Timing may also be an issue as well. It appears that the gap between
men's and women's attitudes toward welfare policies may be gradually expanding over time
(Brown 1988).

they live in an urban or a rural community, has been found important in some studies and not in others (Tropman 1987; Striber and Ferber 1981). Past studies do agree that age and race matter significantly—older Americans and white Americans are relatively less supportive of government health initiatives (Brown 1988; Tropman 1987; Striber and Ferber 1981). Regional factors also appear to have an influence, with the greatest support for government involvement coming from the Northeast (Striber and Ferber 1981). This remains true, controlling for other sociodemographic factors.

In sum, the research on attitudes toward government's role in health care at least hints that government may be viewed differently in this arena. Some of the social cleavages appear to be smaller for health care. But because studies of attitudes toward health policy were conducted with different respondents and different methods than the studies of attitudes toward other government programs, and because the results in health are inconsistent, any unique characteristics of health policy and public opinion remain largely a matter of speculation.

Modeling Public Support for Government's Role in Health and Other Social Policies

To more reliably assess the correlates of support for government intervention, we draw on data capturing each of these sociodemographic characteristics. The data used here were collected as part of the General Social Survey, a national survey conducted annually since 1972.[3] Although there have been many other surveys that have measured public attitudes toward social policies, drawing data from a single source eliminates problems of changes in the wording or sequencing of questions among different survey instruments. This is particularly important when comparing responses over time, since the effects of differences in wording or question order can easily confound attempts to assess changes in attitudes (Blendon and Donelan 1990; Rochefort and Boyer 1988; Tropman 1987).

Data for this part of the study are drawn from surveys administered in 1975, 1983, 1987, and 1989.[4] The latest data available when we began

3. The GSS is conducted for the National Data Program for the Social Sciences at the National Opinion Research Center at the University of Chicago.
4. Each of these surveys draws a sample of English-speaking adults (eighteen years or older), living in noninstitutional settings in the United States. Block quota sampling was used for half the 1975 sample, full probability sampling for the other half and for all other years of the survey. Sample sizes were 1,490 in 1975, 1,599 in 1983, 1,819 in 1987, and 1,537 in 1989. (The 1987

this analysis were from 1989. The first year to include questions measuring public support of government's role in the health care system was 1975. The two years have the advantage of capturing public opinion in the midst of the two most recent episodes of support for national health care initiatives. As noted earlier, 1975 represented the peak year for national health insurance initiatives introduced to Congress (though it was somewhat past the peak in favorable public opinion). Public opinion in 1989 should reflect the influence of health care in the 1988 elections, as well as ongoing trends in public opinion favoring substantial health care reform (Blendon and Donelan 1990).

The intermediate years were included to measure the course of ongoing trends in public opinion. We expect that changes between 1975 and 1983 will reflect in part the "Reagan revolution," that is, the distinct shift in prevailing political philosophy away from active federal involvement in American society. There is considerable debate about whether these changes in political vogue were much related to changes in popular sentiments. Some academics see this time as a fundamental shift in American values, leading the public to accept fewer people as "deserving" of public assistance (Brown 1988; Kelley 1988). The timing of attitudinal changes suggests that the Reagan election was a result rather than a cause of these changes, as growing public disenchantment with welfare programs was evident by the mid-1970s. Polls suggest that the public became somewhat *more* supportive of welfare spending after Reagan's election (Blendon and Donelan 1990; Shapiro and Young 1989). Although this shift in prevailing attitudes is fairly clear, it has been argued that it had little effect on or connection with public opinion about health care (Navarro 1987). However, polls do suggest that in the early 1980s, there was a distinct shift in public support away from tax-financed and government-administered health insurance programs (Shapiro and Young 1986).[5] To the extent that these political changes in the early 1980s either influenced or reflected popular sentiments, this should be most prominent during the first Reagan administration, before the impact of budget cutting produced a counter-

---

survey included an oversample of black respondents. Excluding this oversample, the survey had 1,466 respondents. Including or excluding this oversample had no measurable impact on the results reported in the text.)

5. For example, when asked to choose between health insurance schemes administered by either government or private insurance companies, 46 percent in 1978 selected the government-run plan. Asked the same question in 1984, only 37 percent preferred government administration (Shapiro and Young 1986: 423). Between 1980 and 1982, support for a national health insurance scheme that required a tax increase declined from 41 percent to 34 percent (Shapiro and Young 1986: 424).

Table 1 Sociodemographic Characteristics: Means and Standard Deviations of Independent Variables

Variables	Number of Observations	Means	Standard Deviations
Age Groups			
30 to 44	6,417	0.31	0.46
45 to 64	6,417	0.27	0.44
65 and Above	6,417	0.18	0.38
Male	6,445	0.43	0.50
Race/Ethnicity			
Black	6,445	0.16	0.37
Hispanic	4,887	0.04	0.20
Education Level (Years)	6,443	12.27	3.17
Now Married	6,445	0.58	0.49
Has Young Children	6,417	0.19	0.39
Ever Divorced	6,445	0.25	0.44
Income Quartiles			
Lowest	5,905	0.24	0.43
Second Lowest	5,905	0.27	0.43
Second Highest	5,905	0.26	0.44
Unemployed	6,445	0.047	0.21
Community Type			
Rural	6,445	0.14	0.34
Large Metropolitan	6,445	0.23	0.42
Trends over Time			
Observations in 1983	6,445	0.25	0.43
Observations in 1987	6,445	0.28	0.45
Observations in 1989	6,445	0.24	0.43

vailing sentiment to preserve or rebuild the social safety net (Gottschalk and Gottschalk 1988).

Independent Variables: Sociodemographic Characteristics. To identify the various sociodemographic factors that shape support for government programs, we have included in the regression models a set of variables measuring respondents' economic, social, and demographic characteristics. (Means and standard deviations for these variables are presented in Table 1.) The research cited above suggests that popular support for government initiatives will be a function of income,[6] education, age, sex, race, marital status, type of community (urban or rural), and geographic region of the country.[7] Because past research suggests that age and income may involve nonlinear relationships with attitudes, we have grouped respondents into four categories with each variable. Unlike past studies, which have simply distinguished between urban and rural communities, we divide communities into three categories: rural, moderate-sized localities, and large metropolitan areas. Although poverty is certainly not limited to large cities, it is more concentrated and visible in those settings. Residents of such communities may therefore be more supportive of remedial government policies.

In addition to these previously used variables, we introduce here several additional measures. Past studies, which relied primarily on data from the 1970s and early 1980s, have given little attention to the rapidly growing Hispanic population. The highly heterogeneous nature of this population makes it difficult to predict how it will behave politically. Past studies suggest, however, that Cubans are on average unsupportive of government, Mexican Americans slightly more supportive, and Puerto Ricans far more supportive than average (Caplan 1987). The sample sizes in the GSS data require that we pool all Hispanic respondents into a single category, obscuring this heterogeneity. But the growing importance of this population justifies even an imperfect measure of their attitudes towards social welfare policies. We measure Hispanic status here by whether respondents report that their families immigrated from Latin America, Central America (including Cuba), or Mexico.

Past research has also failed to distinguish between transitory and permanent shifts in income. The most common cause of short-term income fluctuations is unemployment. Unemployment could affect attitudes toward government social policies in either of two ways. On one hand, if the unemployed expect to regain their former socioeconomic status when reemployed in the near future, they may retain the income-related values common to their expected income group. These "low-income" respondents would thus be less supportive of government intervention than one would otherwise predict, based simply on their current household income.

6. One might expect that our inability to measure wealth, in addition to income, might seriously bias our results. However, Kluegel and Smith (1986) found that once one controls for income, reported wealth (a notoriously difficult factor to measure on surveys) was not significantly related to support for social welfare policies.

7. Respondents are grouped into the nine standard census regions: New England, Mid-Atlantic, East North Central, West North Central, South America, East South Central, West South Central, Mountain, and Pacific.

On the other hand, the experience of unemployment may convince people that their economic circumstances are uncertain and their well-being is at risk. This could lead them to favor a broader government role than would otherwise be predicted by their income (Goodin and Dryzek 1987). We measure here whether the respondent or the respondent's spouse is currently unemployed.

Marital status as used in past studies imperfectly measures the extent to which people believe that they can rely on their household to provide a social safety net in miniature. Past studies do suggest that some Americans oppose government action because they prefer family-derived aid in times of need (American Association of Retired Persons 1987). But whatever their preferences, people will oppose government action only if the family is a reliable alternative source of support. We predict that those who are or who have been previously divorced will be less willing to rely on family aid. Those who have young children, and thus greater potential needs, may also be less willing to assume that family support will in itself prove sufficient. We thus include measures of whether a respondent is currently or previously divorced, as well as whether there are young children in the household.

The initial regressions presented in Table 2 pool together data from four survey years. To measure trends in prevailing attitudes toward government, controlling for changes in sociodemographic factors, we include a dummy variable for each of the last three years, 1983, 1987, and 1989. The coefficients on these variables capture the change in support for government action, compared to their level in 1975.

Dependent Variables: Support for Government Initiatives. In this section of the paper, we focus on popular attitudes toward three types of government initiatives—into health care, into general domestic policies, and into policies intended specifically to help the poor. Since 1975, the GSS has periodically included a question in each of these areas. The question for health care read: "In general, some people think that it is the responsibility of the government in Washington to see to it that people have help in paying for doctors and hospital bills. Others think that these matters are not the responsibility of the federal government and that people should take care of these things themselves." Respondents were asked to place themselves on a five-point scale, one extreme "strongly agreeing" with the first statement, the other extreme agreeing with the second. The question on general domestic policy similarly juxtaposed two sentiments, the first stating that the federal government is doing "too many things that

Table 2 Sociodemographic Determinants of Support for Social Policies
(Percentage Difference in Support Associated with Each Characteristic)

Sociodemographic Characteristics of Respondents	Support for Health Policy	Support for General Domestic Policies	Support for Programs for the Poor
		Dependent Variables	
Age Group[a]			
30 to 44	−0.5	−5.8[b]	−2.8[c]
45 to 64	−3.7[b]	−10.7[b]	−4.4[b]
65 and Above	−5.0[b]	−16.2[b]	−13.6[b]
Sex	1.6	−5.7[b]	−2.6[b]
Race/Ethnicity[a]			
Black	10.3[b]	20.3[b]	18.4[b]
Hispanic	−1.8	14.0[b]	14.4[b]
Education[a]	−4.6[b]	−14.0[b]	−9.4[b]
Now Married	−0.4	−1.8	−0.1
Has Young Children	0.4	−0.5	0.7
Ever Divorced	1.3	1.7	0.1
Income Quartile[a]			
Lowest	10.8[b]	11.3[b]	14.1[b]
Second Lowest	5.4[b]	5.6[b]	5.8[b]
Second Highest	3.3[b]	5.5[b]	4.5[b]
Employment Instability[a]	8.9[b]	5.8[c]	5.4[b]
Community[a]			
Rural	−6.2[b]	−3.3	0.1
Large Metropolitan	3.6[b]	5.2[b]	3.0[b]
Trend over Time[a]			
Support in 1983	−2.8[c]	−10.9[b]	−3.3[b]
Support in 1987	1.6	−3.8[b]	−2.8[c]
Support in 1989	5.0[b]	−2.7	−0.7

a. The percentages given for the dependent variables refer to the differences in support found between respondents in the listed sociodemographic categories and others, as follows:
  1. Age group: listed groups compared to 18–29 age group
  2. Sex: male compared to female
  3. Race/ethnicity: compared to white non-Hispanics
  4. Education: eighth-grade compared to college graduate
  5. Income quartile: compared to highest quartile
  6. Employment instability: unemployed compared to employed
  7. Community: compared to moderate-size urban area
  8. Time trend: compared to support in 1975
b. Difference statistically significant at the 5 percent confidence level.
c. Difference statistically significant at the 10 percent confidence level.

should be left to individuals and private businesses," the second that government "should do even more to solve our country's problems." The question on poverty policy juxtaposed the statement that "Washington should do everything possible to improve the standard of living of all poor Americans" with one that suggests that this is not government's responsibility and that "each person should take care of himself."

Each of these variables was recoded so that a higher value on the scale indicated stronger support for government action.[8] We will refer to these as measures of "government involvement." As of 1975, the first year in which these data were collected, popular sentiments slightly favored government involvement in health care. Forty-nine percent of all respondents who answered the question agreed with the statement that help with medical bills was a responsibility of the federal government. This compared to 40 percent who believed it a federal responsibility to help all poor Americans and 38 percent who felt that the federal government should do more to solve the country's problems. There were, however, few differences in terms of those who took the extreme position of individual self-responsibility. Thirteen percent felt that individuals should be solely responsible for medical expenses; the same percentage felt that individuals should deal on their own with problems of poverty. Eighteen percent thought that the federal government should not intervene in the "country's problems" in general.

Public support for an expanded government role in health care is not the same as willingness to pay for that involvement. Recent surveys suggest that as many as a third of those who favored government action in health care are unwilling to pay any more taxes to finance this action (Blendon and Donelan 1990; Gabel et al. 1989).[9] Favorable public opinion may thus say more about good intentions than realistic support for government action.

Unfortunately, none of the questions about support for government activity on the General Social Survey incorporated any statements about costs or taxes. There is, however, a way in which a recognition of costs can be indirectly measured. Respondents are asked on another part of the survey whether they think that America should be spending more or less

8. Various nonresponsive categories—"don't know," "no answer," "not applicable"—were all recoded as "missing."

9. Though some commentators bemoan what they see as a growing American delusion about getting a "free lunch," this pattern of support is not new. In the 1940s, roughly two-thirds of all Americans favored having medical care paid for through the Social Security system. But between a quarter and a third of this support vanished if the respondents were told they would have to pay additional taxes to make this happen (Coughlin 1980).

than it does today on a variety of social problems and programs. This includes spending on medical care, welfare programs, and a variety of domestic policy areas. By combining their responses to these questions with those on support for government involvement, we can measure respondents' willingness to see government act *and* to see the country spend more in this area. To this end, we constructed combined variables for health care (e.g., spending on medical care), aid to the poor (e.g., spending on welfare), and general domestic policy (e.g., an index of spending on education, the environment, roads, and urban development).[10] We will refer to these as the "government spending" variables.

For both government involvement and government spending variables, we estimated regression models using pooled data from the four surveys (including in the regressions dummy variables for each individual year). These were estimated using ordinary least squares. In general, the findings are quite similar for both sets of dependent variables. We report here primarily the results for the government involvement variables, though we will identify those variables for which attitudes including spending were significantly different from those focusing only on government action.

Evidence from the Sociodemographic Regression Models

The results from the regression models of support for government's role in health care, poverty reduction, and general domestic policies are presented in Table 2. We will discuss first the results aggregated across all four years, then describe how these patterns have changed over time.

Aggregate Sociodemographic Patterns of Support. The same patterns of social cleavages that have long characterized Americans' attitudes toward welfare appear also to be important in shaping their attitudes about government involvement in health care. As you move up the income quartiles, you see a steady reduction in support for government action to help pay medical bills, though the sharpest break occurs between the lowest and second-lowest quartiles. This pattern is similar for general domestic initiatives as well as programs targeted to the poor, though the income-related differences in support are largest for the latter. These economic

10. These indices were constructed additively. Those who score high on this index thus support additional spending in the area *and* favor government intervention. Those who score low oppose both spending and intervention. In each area, support for additional spending and support for government action were rescaled so that they had the same variance.

divides in public opinion are reinforced by nonfinancial forms of social status. Controlling for income, better-educated Americans are significantly less supportive of government action than are other respondents. This was, however, somewhat less true for health care than for other types of domestic policy.

Short-term economic factors appear independently to influence attitudes toward government policy. Respondents who either are unemployed or have an unemployed spouse are significantly more likely to support government interventions, particularly those involving the financing of health care. Consequently, those who lose their jobs are more likely to support active government for two separate reasons. First, unemployment is associated with lower income, and this leads to greater support for government. Second, because the process of losing a job in itself appears to threaten perceptions of economic security, it encourages people to turn to government to provide some form of "insurance" against this risk.[11]

Long-standing cleavages also persist along racial lines. Blacks are significantly more supportive of all government roles than otherwise comparable whites. Hispanics share blacks' support of programs for the poor and of general domestic initiatives, though the difference between Hispanics and whites is smaller than the difference between blacks and whites. It is noteworthy, however, that minorities' support of government involvement in health care is relatively less strong than in other policy areas. Blacks are more supportive than whites, but only two-thirds as much as for antipoverty programs. Hispanics are no more supportive of government actions in health care than are non-Hispanic whites.

Past studies suggest that older voters are least supportive of activist government (Shapiro and Young 1989). This pattern was replicated here, with one important difference. While elderly Americans are less supportive of government involvement in health care than are younger respondents, these age-related differences are less pronounced than they are for other types of government intervention. The difference in support between those over sixty-five and those under thirty was only one-third the size for health as for either general domestic programs or antipoverty programs. Thus, relatively speaking, older people are less reluctant to support gov-

11. The unemployment variables were most strongly associated with support for government in 1983, when the country was in the midst of a recession. During such periods, those who are unemployed are more likely to blame their plight on macroeconomic circumstance than on their individual failings. Past research suggests that when this is the case, Americans are more ready to seek solutions in government (Kluegel and Smith 1986). Conversely, when unemployment is low, being unemployed may be more readily attributed to personal inadequacies and thus not seen as much of a social responsibility.

ernment action in health care than elsewhere. One might attribute this to their favorable experience with the Medicare program, demonstrating for them a government health program that "works." [12] Alternatively, the salience of health care as a public need may be greater for older people, who are more likely to be in ill health.

A similar pattern exists for other demographic variables. In general, men are less likely than women to support government interventions, but this difference is less pronounced for health care than for other areas of government involvement. Married respondents are less likely to support government actions but less opposed to health initiatives (these latter differences were too small to be statistically significant).[13] Other characteristics of the household—past or current divorce, having young children—appear to have little influence on attitudes toward government interventions.

Location is related to attitudes about government in two distinct ways. There are pronounced differences in attitudes between urban and rural settings. As anticipated, residents of large metropolitan areas, who are most likely to be exposed to concentrated social distress, are most supportive of all forms of government intervention. Rural dwellers are the least supportive, particularly of health care programs. Those living in moderate-size communities have distinctive attitudes toward government that are intermediate between residents of large urban centers and those living in rural areas.

The second sense in which location matters involves the region in the country in which one lives. Past research found that spending on welfare programs was accepted to a far greater extent in the Northeast and Midwest than in the South and Southwest (Wohlenberg 1976). The regressions presented here suggest that the same regional patterns exist in support for health programs and general domestic spending. There are, however, some distinct regional patterns associated with particular types of government action. For example, Pacific Coast and southwestern states—historically, regions that have not supported welfare spending—are more favorably inclined toward health initiatives.

---

12. Favorable impressions of the Medicare program continue to be quite prevalent, despite ongoing controversies over what benefits should be covered and how it should be financed (American Association for Retired Persons 1987).

13. In the regressions using government spending as the dependent variables, these marital effects were statistically significant.

Trends over Time in the Level and Correlates of Support. Past research has reported that public attitudes toward government action became more negative in the mid-1970s (Shapiro et al. 1987; Tropman 1987) but more recently have grown more supportive, particularly for health care policies (Blendon and Donelan 1990). These claims have been challenged, largely on the grounds that question wording and context changed over time (Jajich-Toth and Roper 1990). Our analyses, based on standardized question wording and survey format, suggest that these changes are real, but that they have been unevenly distributed among different sociodemographic groups.

There have clearly been shifts in support for government action, unrelated to the changing economic and social circumstances in which Americans live. As can be observed from the year-designating variables in Table 2, support for all government initiatives declined between 1975 and 1983. Support for health care and antipoverty programs fell by about the same amount during this period. Support for general domestic interventions dropped much more sharply, with three times the decline measured for the other two types of interventions. By 1987, the decline in all three areas had been reversed, but only for health care had popular support for government regained (and slightly exceeded) its 1975 level. Indeed, by 1989, support for government efforts to help the poor or to engage in other forms of domestic policy still lagged below support in 1975. Thus, only for health care have Americans become distinctly more supportive of government in the late 1980s than in the mid-1970s, controlling for other ongoing changes in their economic well-being and social characteristics.

Measuring trends using these dummy variables captures only some of the potentially important shifts in attitudes over the past fifteen years. The sociodemographic factors that shape attitudes toward government may also have had different influences in 1989 than they did in 1975. To explore these changing relationships, we reestimated the regressions presented in Table 2 separately for each of the four years. Space limitations preclude presenting these results in full, but we briefly note here some of the more striking results. (Complete results are available from the authors.)

Several of the relationships described above remained quite stable between 1975 and 1989. These include racial and ethnic differences in support for government, as well as differences between those living in urban and rural areas. In contrast, there were a number of significant changes associated with the socioeconomic and age-related cleavages that have long divided Americans' attitudes toward social policy.

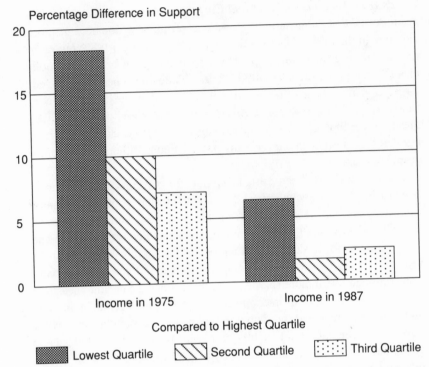

Percentage Difference in Support

Compared to Highest Quartile

▓ Lowest Quartile   ⧄ Second Quartile   ⬚ Third Quartile

Figure 1 Support for Federal Health Initiatives by Income Quartile, 1975 and 1987

In 1975, when political debates over national health insurance were by some measures reaching their peak, there were sharp differences in support of government between the rich and the poor, as well as between the old and the young (see Figures 1 and 2). Those in the highest income quartile were 20 percent less supportive of government health interventions than those in the lowest quartile. Those over the age of sixty-five were 15 percent less supportive than those under thirty. (Those most strongly opposed to government in 1975 were between forty-five and sixty-four years of age—they were 30 percent less supportive than were young adults.) These cleavages in support mirrored those for other domestic programs, though the income-related differences were sharper for health initiatives and the age-related differences less pronounced.

By the late 1980s, although there were still statistically significant differences in support for government by age and income, the gaps had closed substantially. This was particularly true for health care. The difference in support between upper- and lower-income quartiles, for ex-

Percentage Difference in Support

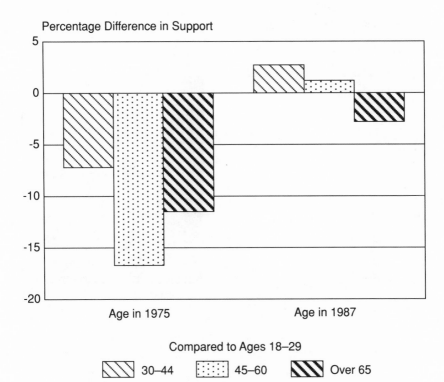

Figure 2 Support for Government Health Initiatives by Age Group, 1975 and 1987

ample, was by 1987 one-third the size it had been in 1975 (Figure 1). The "generation gap" in attitudes toward federal health policy showed comparable shrinkage (Figure 2). There were also declines in the socio-economic cleavages for antipoverty and general domestic programs, but these were less pronounced than for health care. By the late 1980s, health initiatives had become the least divisive form of federal government initiative in terms of sociodemographic conflicts and programs toward the poor the most divisive.

The narrowing of these long-prevailing social cleavages for health care occurred in two distinct phases over the past fifteen years. During the first half of this period, Americans' attitudes toward federal health initiatives became more uniformly negative than they had been in the past. But in the latter half of the 1980s, attitudes became generally more supportive, with no reemergence of the distinctions that had previously existed between old and young, rich and poor.

The second distinct change between 1975 and 1983 was reflected in

Percentage Difference in Support

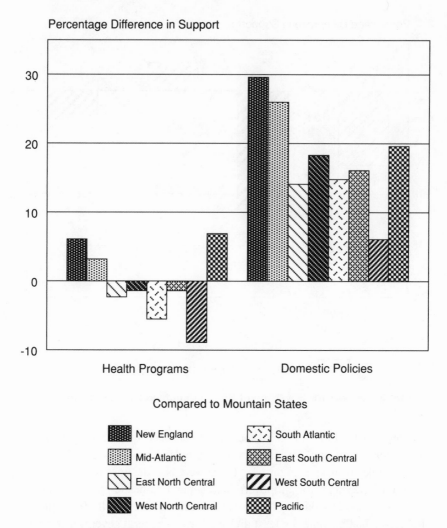

Figure 3 Regional Variation in Support for Government Initiatives, 1975

regional patterns of support for government action. In 1975, there were significant regional differences in support for government action in both health and general domestic policy (though somewhat smaller differences for programs targeted to low-income recipients). These are graphically portrayed in Figure 3. The regions that have been historically more "liberal" and supportive of government action display that greater support in response to these questions.

In the years between 1975 and 1983, however, a change occurred in this regional distribution of attitudes (Figure 4). Traditionally liberal re-

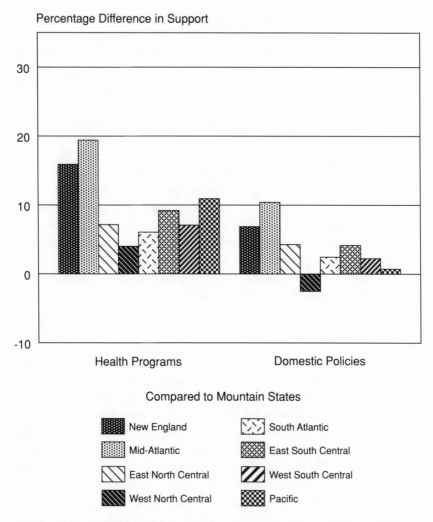

Figure 4 Regional Variation in Support for Government Initiatives, 1983

gions lost their distinctive support for general domestic policies, showing greater conformity with national norms.[14] For health care, in contrast, historical regional differences persisted. Health care was certainly not exempt from antigovernment rhetoric during this period—witness the

14. States in the Mountain region were used as a standard of comparison. The differences in the text are not simply the result of attitudes in this region converging to the national mean. Attitudes in the Mountain region were actually growing more antigovernment during this period. Even if this region is removed, the variance among regions in support for government action in general domestic policies is considerably (to a statistically significant degree) greater in 1975 than in 1983.

secular decline in support for government reflected in the year-designating variables in Table 2. But the public did seemingly perceive something different about government's role in this sector. This difference may have allowed traditionally liberal regions to maintain their relatively greater support for active government in health care even while they were abandoning it in other aspects of domestic policy.

In the latter 1980s, the historic patterns in regional support for government began to reemerge for general domestic policies, so that once more these were more like they had been in 1975 and more like health care continued to be throughout this period. At the same time, support for government health care programs spread beyond traditionally liberal parts of the country. Regions such as the Midwest, which had not been historically supportive of federal action in health care, became much more so by 1989. This may have reflected persistently high rates of unemployment in this region; as demonstrated earlier, unemployment appears to generate support for government action due to an area's loss of income and due to an increased sense of economic insecurity.

How Is Health Different?

Sociodemographic Patterns. The results presented here suggest that government's role in health care is viewed by the public as different in two ways. The first reflects differences in the level of support for government. In 1975, health care was the area for which government initiatives received the greatest popular support. Over the past fifteen years, that gap has continued to widen, particularly between health and general domestic interventions. These changes reflected shifts in the willingness to support government in health care per se, not changing economic or social conditions facing Americans or changes in the demographic composition of the American population.

A second set of differences involves who supports particular types of government action. Older Americans are relatively more supportive of a government presence in health care than of other types of policy, while blacks, Hispanics, and rural dwellers are less supportive. Although males, those who are married, and those who are better-educated are less supportive of all government actions, they are less opposed to action involving health care than to other types of interventions.

Health policy is thus less affected by the "cleavages" that have long prevailed in American public opinion about social policy. Differences in support between whites and blacks, as well as whites and Hispanics, are smaller for health care than for other types of government policy. Differences in support related to income and age, though they still persist, have become significantly smaller for health care over the past fifteen years. All told, American public opinion appears to be closer to consensus involving government's role in health care than in other aspects of domestic policy. (The sole exception involves regional differences, which remain as large or larger for health care than for other types of domestic policy.) Whether this growing consensus affects policy-making depends on how public attitudes are translated into public policy.

Sociodemographic Differences and Political Participation. Declining rates of political involvement plague contemporary American democracy. If the politically passive majority holds attitudes and perceptions very different from those who are politically active, the factors that we have identified as important here may be translated in an incomplete or biased manner into policy-making. If politically active Americans hold values very different from the general public in these issues, mass opinion provides a misleading picture of actual political decision making.

Indeed, one explanation commonly given for the failure to translate broad public support for goals, such as guaranteed employment, into effective programs cites the lack of support among the most politically influential constituents. Both education and income are correlated with political awareness and participation. Social cleavages in support for government may thus undermine political pressure for active government interventions. One important question is whether the smaller cleavages documented here for health policy recast the relationship between political participation and support for government action in this area.

Detailed data on political participation are available only from the 1987 GSS. For purposes of this analysis, we identify the politically active in two ways. The first involves an index of political participation. This was constructed from respondents' reports that they had either attended political rallies, worked on a political campaign, or attempted to influence how other people voted. Forty-five percent of the sample had engaged in at least one of these activities and was thus labeled politically active. The second measure involves political contributions. Respondents were asked whether they had contributed money to a political party, candidate, or cause in the previous three to four years. Twenty-two percent had made such a contribution. Our measures of political participation thus fall in between the distinctions that are often used by political scientists, who distinguish the 50 to 60 percent who regularly vote and the 5 to 10 percent who are referred to as the "political elite." Politically active individuals, defined by either of our measures, can be expected to exert more influence on the political process and thus have their opinions more forcefully translated into political action. (Those endorsing Will Rogers's claim that America has the best government that money can buy might give greater emphasis to the second of these measures.)

Because political involvement is positively correlated with income, education, as well as age, and because all these characteristics are negatively related to support for activist government, one would expect that those who are politically active would on average be less supportive of government. Data from the 1987 GSS confirm this (Tables 3 and 4). Three-quarters of those who participate and 70 percent of those who made political contributions support government involvement in health care. This compares to 82 percent among nonparticipants and noncontributors. For other types of government policies, support drops from a sizable majority among those not active to a minority among the politically active. The "participation gap" tends to be larger for policy areas other than health. Consequently, among the politically active health holds an even stronger priority, relative to other social policies, than it does among the population as a whole.

But if health policy does look different in this sense, it is a rather modest difference. There is still a decline in support for government among the politically active. It should be recognized, however, that data from 1987 may understate the consequences of ongoing trends. If socioeconomic cleavages have continued to narrow for health care since that time, the most politically active may be more supportive of government action in health care in the early 1990s than in the later 1980s. (Our analyses comparing 1989 and 1987 do not show a significant decline in either income- or education-related differences in support, but a two-year gap may have been too small to measure continued trends.)

Differences in the extent of support for government between those who are and those who are not politically active may only be one part of the story. It may be the case that the better-educated, more financially secure Americans have entirely different motives for supporting government action than do their less fortunate counterparts. If so, the political dynamics underlying their support may be very different. To explore this issue, we now consider the motives for favoring government intervention, comparing motives for health programs to other areas of social policy.

Table 3 Political Participation and Support for Government
Interventions, 1987

Type of Initiative	Percentage Supporting Initiative	
	Political Participants	Nonparticipants
Health Care Policies	75.4	82.0[a]
General Domestic Policies	45.8	57.3[a]
Redistributive Policies Targeted to the Poor	45.9	58.0[a]

Note. Attitudes toward government involvement were measured with an odd-valued scale. For these analyses, those answering at the midpoint for each type of government initiative were excluded. "Supporters" were those with responses above the midpoint on the scale, "opponents" those below the midpoint.

a. Difference between participants and nonparticipants statistically significant at a 1 percent confidence level.

Table 4 Political Contributions and Support for
Government Interventions, 1987

Type of Initiative	Percentage Supporting Initiative	
	Political Contributors	Noncontributors
Health Care Policies	69.7	81.6[a]
General Domestic Policies	42.0	54.7[a]
Redistributive Policies Targeted to the Poor	39.3	56.5[a]

Note. Attitudes toward government involvement were measured with an odd-valued scale. For these analyses, those answering at the midpoint for each type of government initiative were excluded. "Supporters" were those with responses above the midpoint on the scale, "opponents" those below the midpoint.

a. Difference between contributors and noncontributors statistically significant at a 1 percent confidence level.

The Perceptions and Attitudes Shaping Support
for Health and Social Policy

The analysis in this section, both conceptual and empirical, is predicated on a particular notion of how people assess the appropriateness of different roles for government. From this perspective, the public judges each potential government action in terms of a set of discrete factors or motives (as opposed to a broad and internally consistent ideology). These factors reflect how they believe that government policies will affect their own self-interest, how policies influence the well-being of others about whom they are concerned, as well as how policies conform to their notions of a just society. Although in practice these factors undoubtedly interact, we will treat them as separable. This simplifies both our discussion and the subsequent empirical models. (Readers should be aware, however, that this approach may lead us to overlook some synergies among the different motives for government intervention, an issue to which we will return in the final section of the paper.)

We begin by identifying a set of factors that may encourage people to support activist government, both in health care and in other areas. We then consider how the particular characteristics of health care may affect how people judge the appropriateness or effectiveness of government action. This leads to hypotheses about how federal health policy differs from other social policies. These hypotheses are tested using data from the General Social Survey from 1987.

Reasons for Supporting Activist Government

Citizens support government interventions into the economic and social order for a variety of reasons. They may expect to personally benefit from government action. They may expect that others, whose well-being they value, will benefit. Finally, they may support government action because they believe that it will create a more just distribution of income, social status, goods, or services. We briefly explore each of these motivations, as they apply to government policies in general and to health policy in particular.

Expected Direct Benefits and Costs. Most models of public support for policy (particularly those from the "rational choice" school) assume that individuals assess potential policies primarily in terms of the costs and benefits that they will personally experience. For example, a recent review of public attitudes toward the welfare state concluded that "part of the differences in preferences among Americans can be attributed to self-interest, mainly those general differences associated with economic status and race, and particular cases such as high levels of support among urban residents for aid to cities" (Shapiro and Young 1989: 67).

From this perspective, one would expect that individuals' support for government interventions should be positively related to the probability that they will directly benefit from the program and negatively related to the extent that they expect to finance its costs (Pescosolido et al. 1986). Because many federal policies directly or indirectly redistribute from high- to low-income groups, this would explain our findings that higher-income groups were least supportive of government initiatives.

But empirical research by political scientists and social psychologists suggests that self-interest defined in this manner can explain only a modest portion of the variation in public support for government (Citrin and Green 1990; Sears and Funk 1990; Kluegel and Smith 1986). Expected costs appear to be more consistently related to support than are expected benefits. Support for various social programs declines markedly the more they are seen to cost and the more burdened people feel by prevailing taxes (Shapiro and Young 1989; Melville and Doble 1988). The distribution of benefits has a less clearly measurable influence. Apart from spending on public schools—where having a school-age child appears to be strongly related to support for spending on public education (Hamilton and Cohen 1974)—the short-term benefits people can expect to receive from government programs are only weakly linked to support for the program (Sears and Funk 1990).

Similar patterns apply to public support for government involvement in health care (Pescosolido et al. 1986; Striber and Ferber 1981). Support appears to be quite sensitive to the costs (e.g., additional taxes) that people expect to pay (Blendon and Donelan 1990). But support is less clearly linked to immediate benefits. For example, support for national health insurance proposals appears to be unrelated to individuals' satisfaction with their own current insurance (Striber and Ferber 1981). Similarly, the elderly are less supportive of improving benefits under Medicare than are younger age groups (American Association of Retired Persons 1987).

The apparently weaker link between expected benefits and support for government actions may reflect an overly narrow definition of direct benefit. Most past research measures direct benefits by whether an individual would currently qualify for participation in a program. But this overlooks the role that such programs may play as a buffer against risk, as a safeguard against future misfortune (Goodin and Dryzek 1987). For example, individuals' current insurance coverage may matter less than the coverage they expect to have in the future—recent research suggests that the majority of those who are uninsured at any one time will in fact have health insurance coverage within the year. Conversely, those who currently have coverage may feel at risk for losing coverage.

The role of public programs as a buffer against risk leads to a much broader sense of self-interest. "Virtually no one appears to be completely immune to the possibility of experiencing a large reduction in income.

Accordingly, non-poor individuals might be willing to support income re-distribution programs if they felt they or their relatives might need them at some point during their life" (Ponza et al. 1988: 450). This may overstate the case, since most people will discount threats to their financial security that are long-term. Nonetheless, even short-term insecurity may greatly expand the base of self-interested support for a program. This motive is consistent with our observation of a positive link between unemployment and support for government, controlling for income.

External Identification. A second motivation for supporting government intervention derives from a person's identification with those who will be direct beneficiaries. This identification can be either positive or negative. In other words, one may support government programs because one cares about the well-being of the recipients or oppose programs because one sees them as competitors or undeserving of aid. Past research has identified three major forms of external identification: altruism, perceived social threats, and racial labeling.

Altruism as a motive for government action: Since Tocqueville, the United States has been characterized as a country in which people band together to aid those in need. Although political philosophers use the term *altruism* to refer only to those acts of beneficence that do not involve any potential for personal reward, we will use the term in its broader and more common sense of any concern for or willingness to assist others. Altruistic motives reflect a sense of empathy or shared community with those in need (Batson and Oleson 1991). People may turn to government to deliver that assistance if private philanthropy is seen as inadequate, demeaning, or otherwise undesirable (Dougherty 1988; Walzer 1983). This can occur if there are substantial economies of scale in providing assistance on a national basis, if private philanthropists are inconsistent in their response to cases of need, or if too many people act as "free riders," relying on others to pay for the philanthropy from which they derive psychic benefits (Buchanan 1984).

Altruistic rationales for government action can be traced back to Adam Smith (Goodin and Dryzek 1987). Contemporary social welfare programs are often justified in terms of "compassion" (Shapiro and Young 1989; Greenstone 1988). Altruistic motives may be stronger for those who are in better financial circumstances. Most Americans believe that those who are better-off financially have a greater obligation to help others. In a survey conducted by the Independent Sector in 1988, for example, 60 percent of respondents agreed with the statement that "people with higher incomes

should give a larger percentage of their incomes to charity." Seventy percent of those with annual incomes in excess of $100,000 endorsed this
statement (Hodgkinson and Weitzman 1988: 65).

Some political philosophers question whether altruism can provide a
strong and sustainable motive for government action. They contend that
an empathetic motive depends on a personal bond, or at least some mutual
awareness, between giver and recipient. A nation as large as the United
States is seen as too big, too impersonal for altruistic bonds to be very
strong.

> It is one thing to care for those particular individuals, known and be-
> loved to us, that constitute our own families. Extending such senti-
> ments from those who share our genes to all those who merely happen
> to share the same coloured passport is another thing altogether. . . .
> [T]his theory is unlikely to be true at the level it needs to be to explain
> such generalized benevolence as is practiced through the welfare state.
> (Goodin and Dryzek 1987: 39)

Even if altruism can initially motivate support for a program, there
are some doubts about whether that support can be sustained over time.
Altruism, some philosophers have argued, is by nature voluntary; altru-
ists derive their psychic benefits from having chosen to help others. In
this view, federal programs financed by compulsory taxation are the antithesis of voluntary action. Being forced to pay may in fact undermine
and eventually extinguish altruistic motivations (Moon 1988; Dougherty
1988; Goodin 1988).

Support for government's role in health care has been described as
embodying these same tensions around the role and limits of altruistic
motivations. Health problems, it is argued, induce a powerful empathetic
response, closely linked by most Americans' notions of a close-knit community (Beauchamp 1988; Walzer 1983). This is reflected in the extraordinary amount of health-related philanthropy in the United States (Hodgkinson and Weitzman 1988). Yet government programs to promote health
care, cast in the form of insurance, allow for no personal action between
those who pay and those who benefit. "The benefit paid by health insurance is to a certain extent a form of unilateral transfer. . . . [T]hose whose
benefits are disproportionately high are usually not known to other payers;
they are strangers" (Rushing 1986: 152–53). If interpersonal recognition
is important for sustained altruism, these motives are likely to play a
small role in support for government's role in promoting access to health
services.

Threat and social control as motives for government action: People may also support government action as a means to diffuse social tensions, to discourage the disadvantaged from disrupting the established social order (Pescosolido et al. 1986; Kluegel and Smith 1986). To the fervent libertarian, government action that takes property from one person and redistributes it to another can be justified only if it prevents a more substantial threat to property rights. Hayek, for example, favored social welfare programs "only in the interest of those who require protection against acts of desperation on the part of the needy" (1960: 286). As the tenor of Hayek's language suggests, compassion and empathy play little role in this motive. As a result, it may persist even when the beneficiaries are unknown to those who pay for the program. Indeed, this motive may be strongest under those circumstances, since those who are unknown may appear the most threatening.

Reducing societal tension has provided a motivation for social welfare programs since the time of Bismarck (Rimlinger 1971). But little is known about the extent to which this has motivated support for government programs in this country. Although Americans are less inclined than their European counterparts to cast political issues in terms of class conflict (Democrats' recent appeals to the middle class being a notable exception), the history of national health financing reform suggests that concern about societal threats played at least some role. A historian, recounting the debates over national health insurance prior to World War I, concluded that "in simple terms, members of the middle class were afraid that unless they did something significant to correct economically caused health problems among the poor, their own security and social position would be threatened. . . . Social insurance for illness appeared to be a way in which this problem could be solved" (Hirschfield 1970: 11).

Although little is known about more contemporary motives of this type, recent surveys do suggest that many Americans believe that reducing disparities in well-being diminishes social tensions. Over half the respondents to a survey conducted in 1980, for example, agreed with the statement that "more equality of incomes would avoid conflicts between people at different levels" (Kluegel and Smith 1986: 106).

Racial identification as a motive for government action: More than in most industrialized nations, the politics of social policy in America has been shaped by cleavages related to race and ethnicity (Carmines and Stimson 1989; Shapiro and Young 1989). This is especially true for redistributive programs. Because blacks and Hispanics are more likely to live in poverty than whites, they disproportionately benefit from means-tested programs such as AFDC, Medicaid, or food stamps. But these programs are racially identified to a far greater extent than is warranted by the facts. For example, Americans significantly overestimate the proportion of welfare beneficiaries who are black (Kluegel and Smith 1986).

Although hard evidence on this racial labeling is scarce, many believe that it is growing over time. Some attribute this to the politics of the Reagan administration, believing that problems of poverty were explicitly labeled as problems of racial minorities to reduce popular support for remedial actions (Greenstone 1988). However, racial polarization around social policies was clearly evident in the mid-1970s and was an undertone in the 1964 presidential campaign (Weir et al. 1988). In the "tax revolts" of the 1970s, state funding for programs used disproportionately by racial minorities suffered the most severe cutbacks (Sears and Citrin 1982). There were at the same time increasing tensions within the Democratic party, particularly between working-class and middle-class voters, in their support for policies that clearly benefited racial minorities (Shingles 1989; Brown 1988).

Racial identification could in principle either increase or decrease support for government programs. To the extent that a program is seen to benefit a minority group disproportionately, it is likely to lose support from white voters of modest means, who are threatened by the increased standard of living and social status of minority groups (Shingles 1989). On the other hand, it may increase support from those who feel that minority groups are particularly deserving of government assistance, perhaps because they have faced discrimination in the past (Dougherty 1988; Kluegel and Smith 1986).

Although the late 1980s saw increased attention to disparities in access and health outcomes between white and various minority groups, little is known about the extent to which various government health programs are racially identified. Programs such as Medicaid, for example, disproportionately benefit African Americans and Hispanics (Schlesinger 1987). Yet policymakers rarely cast Medicaid in these terms (though there is some evidence that they see federal funding of community health centers as embodying racially targeted benefits [Keiser 1987]). Virtually nothing is known about racial identification of health programs by the general public.

Norms of Social Justice. The third set of motivations for supporting government actions relates to various notions of social justice. The complexity of beliefs about justice and morality makes it difficult to describe concisely the various factors shaping public attitudes. At the risk of over-simplification, we describe here three sets of norms that we believe define the major perspectives on social justice in the United States. We then consider how they might provide a rationale for government action.

Compared to most industrialized countries, the United States appears to have more varied norms of societal justice (Shapiro and Young 1989; Tornblom and Foa 1983). Nonetheless, for most goods, services, and forms of social status, Americans will most consistently favor a market-oriented allocation as equitable. This is sometimes termed "economic individualism" and is sufficiently common that it has been referred to as the "dominant ideology" of American culture (Kluegel and Smith 1986). This perspective draws its moral salience from several presumed characteristics of the market: freedom of contract (Dougherty 1988; Hochschild 1981), equal opportunity of participation (Daniels 1985), and a belief that the market rewards individuals in proportion to the contribution they make to society (Kluegel and Smith 1986; Hochschild 1981). This ideology thus rests on both procedural and outcome-related notions of justice.

Two other norms provide the primary challenges to market-based allocations: norms of need and norms of equality. Need-based allocations are determined by individuals' characteristics, as opposed to their choices or contributions (Baybrooke 1987). Equality of outcome, in contrast, establishes standards for outcomes that do not vary from one individual to the next, although how individuals are treated may differ if their circumstances are different (Rae 1981).

In many aspects of society, including the distribution of income and social status, most Americans view market-based allocations as equitable. But as many as a third would allocate income primarily on the basis of need; fewer than 5 percent favor strict equality (Kluegel and Smith 1986: 106).[15] Although one could thus in principle divide people according to the norm that they favor most highly, relatively few Americans hold ideologically pure positions. Instead, they favor some combination of norms that are balanced against one another. Following a series of experiments designed to elicit how people think about justice, one set of researchers concluded that "individuals treat choices between principles as marginal decisions. Principles are much like economic goods inasmuch as individuals are willing to trade off between them" (Frohlich et al. 1987). For example, although earnings are thought to be just if they are based

---

15. About a third would support greater equalization of income than exists today, even though they oppose complete equalization (Kluegel and Smith 1986: 106).

primarily on productivity, many Americans also believe that some individuals should earn more because their needs are greater (Kluegel and Smith 1986; Alves and Rossi 1978).

The relative weight given to each norm depends in part on the nature of the good or service being allocated. Jobs, income, and social status are thought to be fairly distributed if their allocation is based primarily on productivity and social contribution (Kluegel and Smith 1986; Tornblom and Foa 1983; Alves and Rossi 1978). In contrast, certain socially valued services such as education are thought to be most fairly allocated based on need (Hochschild 1981; Tornblom and Foa 1983). Americans become most egalitarian when thinking about the distribution of political freedoms (Kluegel and Smith 1986; Hochschild 1981).

At different points in American history, different norms were given precedence in assessing equitable distributions of health care. A hundred years ago, market-based allocations were the preferred norm (Starr 1982). After the turn of the century, health care was increasingly viewed in terms of need, an emphasis that persisted through the 1960s (Boulding 1973). More recently, that perspective has been challenged by a return of the norm of market-based equity (Relman 1992). Market-based norms increasingly dominate policymakers' thinking about the health care system, though it remains unclear whether they have been accepted by the general public.

Justifications for Government Involvement. We have identified here three sets of motives for supporting government intervention. Individuals will differ in the relative importance that they place on each motive. Those that are felt more strongly potentially act as stronger catalysts or inhibiters for government action. But they legitimate government action only when combined with three sorts of perceptions.

The first perception involves the relative well-being of the individual or group relevant for that motive. For example, if voters are primarily self-interested, their support for particular government programs will depend on their assessment of their own well-being. Conversely, if they are motivated by altruism or norms of justice involving need, their support for government will depend on how "needy" they believe the groups are who would benefit from government action.[16]

16. Altruistically motivated voters may also be influenced by their perceptions of their own financial well-being, since, as noted in the text, most Americans believe that those who are better-off have a greater moral obligation to help those who are needy.

A second type of perception involves how societal institutions are seen to function. For most Americans, the presumptive benefits of the free market depend on its truly being free—that is, that all individuals have an equal opportunity to participate and to prosper through hard work. If, however, opportunities are seen to be circumscribed for particular groups, there will be greater support for remedial action, even if those groups are not necessarily seen as needy. Historically, concerns of this sort have encouraged Americans to favor nearly universal programs of assistance for higher education, in the form of both government-guaranteed loans and government subsidies to state universities (Smith 1987).

The third set of perceptions involves the public's assessment of whether the federal government is capable of remedying societal problems. Many Americans see government as relatively ineffective, due to either bureaucratic inefficiencies or domination by powerful political interest groups (Tropman 1987). They may therefore acquiesce to situations that they consider unjust or not in their best interests, simply because they feel that it is beyond the power of government to effect remedies (Hochschild 1981).

The legitimacy of government action thus rests on the combined influence of a set of motives and a set of complementary perceptions about the extent of societal problems as well as the efficacy of government in addressing those problems. We consider now how these various considerations may be seen differently for health policy than for other forms of social policy.

Some Distinct Reasons for Supporting Government Action in Health Care

Although infrequently a topic for empirical research, political scientists and philosophers have often speculated about how government action might be more or less legitimate in health care than in other aspects of American society. A number have concluded that there are no moral grounds for assuming that the distribution of health care should be treated any differently from the distribution of education, employment, income, housing, food, or legal services (Gutmann 1988; Wildavsky 1977; Fried 1976). Even if attitudes associated with health care were conceptually distinguishable, they may in practice be little different because health programs are linked in the public's mind to other government policies. For example, due to its historical association with Aid to Families with Dependent Children, Medicaid may have as much stigma as a "welfare" program as does AFDC (Blendon and Donelan 1990). Because Medicare shares financing arrangements with Social Security, it may be viewed as a social insurance program protecting elders' financial status as much as a health care program (Congressional Budget Office 1991).

But empirical research suggests that health care is seen as different by the American public. In our previous analysis of the sociodemographic determinants of support for government, we observed diverging trends in support between health and other policies over the past fifteen years. We saw that social cleavages in support of government action were narrower for health care than for other aspects of public policy. We observed distinct regional fluctuations in the support for an active government role in health care. Differences have also been observed in other surveys. Americans are far more likely to claim that health care is a basic "right" of all citizens than are other social needs. More than 80 percent believe that adequate health care is a right (as opposed to a "privilege that persons should have to earn") (Shapiro and Young 1986). Fewer than two-thirds of all Americans supported the same claim for an adequate retirement income (Smith 1987).

Over the past decade, political philosophers have devoted considerable effort to interpreting what Americans might think they mean by these claims about health care rights (Callahan 1990; Dougherty 1988; Daniels 1985; Buchanan 1984; Moskop 1983; Childress 1979; Beauchamp and Faden 1979; Bell 1979; Brown 1978). These discussions have illustrated a variety of ways in which health care might be viewed as different, in ethical and practical terms, from other socially valued goods. They highlight the extent to which the continued proclamations of rights reflect the serious concern that Americans give to issues related to health care. "To twentieth-century Americans, the language of rights seems a most natural way to articulate and emphasize those demands that claimants regard as important moral demands" (Dougherty 1988: 23).

It is not, then, the statement of rights per se that makes health care importantly different, but rather the beliefs about what health care means for individual and social well-being that motivate such statements. Drawing on our framework for understanding why people support government action, we can identify a half dozen potentially relevant characteristics about the distribution of health care, health care needs, and health care financing that could alter American attitudes toward government's role in this area. We identify each of these below. They become a set of hypotheses that we test in the next section of the paper.

How Might Health Care Be Different from Other Services? The literature suggests three principal distinctions between health care and other
socially valued goods and services. These are that (1) individuals are less
likely to be held personally accountable for bad outcomes related to health
care, so that government action is not seen as undermining individual
responsibility; (2) health needs are seen as different from other needs;
and (3) health and health care play a vital instrumental role in furthering other valued political and economic freedoms, so that health care is
closely linked in public perceptions with norms of equal opportunity. In
addition, we propose three further possible differences. First, the fiscal redistribution associated with government health policies may be perceived
differently—seen as more legitimate—than with other government programs. Second, those who are relatively well-off may be able to identify
more closely with those who are unable to get adequate health care than
they are with those who cannot find a job or who face other problems. To
the extent that altruism depends on identification, this would make altruism a stronger motive for supporting government action in health care.
Third, the interpersonal relationships that are a part of health care may
make people more wary about overly bureaucratic intrusions associated
with government, in a way that they would not be concerned for welfare
programs or other initiatives.

*Limited individual responsibility for problems with health and access
to medical care*: Americans tend to view unequal distributions as inequitable only if individuals are not held at fault for their own misfortune. To
the extent that inequalities are attributed to individual failings, they are
viewed as more acceptable or at least a less just reason for government
remedy. "Some antipathy toward the poor and hence toward welfare may
be 'natural,' inherent in the dominant-ideology belief in individualism—
which holds the poor responsible for their own position through their
blameworthy personal characteristics" (Kluegel and Smith 1986: 153).
Conversely, if bad outcomes are seen as outside an individual's control,
government remedies may be accepted even by those who emphasize a
need for individual responsibility.

Compared to other types of personal distress, sickness and disability
have historically been viewed as less a matter of individual failing. There
is a randomness to many illnesses, the result of an unfortunate genetic
endowment or unwitting exposure to infectious agents. Other diseases
may be created by some larger institutional entity outside an individual's
control. This would include illnesses that were iatrogenic or were a consequence of unhealthy working conditions or a polluted environment. Even

during relatively libertarian periods in American history, there has been widespread support for the notion that government should protect the public from these sorts of external threats to their health (Dougherty 1988; Beauchamp and Faden 1979; White 1971).

Throughout the 1960s and the first half of the 1970s, prevailing opinion held victims of illness or disability as largely blameless for one or the other of these reasons. Rarely was it asked if people "deserved" to be ill.[17] Writing at the end of the latter decade, one author concluded that "Western cultural notions about illness include a strong belief that the sick person is not responsible for his own condition. Illness is seen as a calamity that befalls an individual for no discernible reason or, at least, for reasons unrelated to the individual's behavior" (Stone 1979: 511). Yet even as this statement was being written, the perspective it described was being challenged. By the late 1970s, there was a growing sentiment that perhaps some people should be held responsible for their ill health, particularly if they increased their risk of illness through unhealthy life styles or dangerous habits (Childress 1979; Brown 1978).

From this perspective, there were undeserving sick people in the same sense that Americans had long suspected that there were undeserving poor people. Although this claim has since faced its own questions, it had an important influence on public policies during the 1980s (Stone 1987; Dougherty 1988). For example, in a survey conducted in 1990, federal officials and congressional staff strongly agreed with the acceptability of charging higher insurance premiums for whose who had "unhealthy lifestyles" (Taylor and Leitman 1991). Notions of personal responsibility have thus intruded into health policy. This undermined the claim that unequal distributions of health outcomes were necessarily inequitable. It weakened the rationale for government action based solely on unequal health outcomes.

But during the 1980s an alternative perspective emerged, suggesting that health-related distributions were inequitable for different reasons. This argument focused not on the distribution of health outcomes, but on the distribution of health insurance, and thus of financial access to the health care system. It identified three ways in which the allocation of health insurance may violate American norms of distributional equity.

Most Americans obtain their health insurance through the workplace. It is thus an "earned benefit" in the same sense as income. One would

17. There were, of course, some exceptions, most notably involving sexually transmitted diseases.

expect that it would be allocated as any other reward, to provide an incentive for increased productivity (Dougherty 1988). Inequalities would thus be perfectly compatible with what we have termed the dominant ideology, so long as they represent differences in what people have fairly earned through their own efforts.

Inequities seem apparent, however, when one examines the role of public policy in promoting employer-based insurance. The tax code subsidizes this arrangement by not counting employers' contributions to health insurance coverage as taxable income. Those with higher income tend to have access to more comprehensive policies, with larger employer payments and hence larger tax subsidies (Moon 1990). This conflicts with norms of both the dominant ideology and need. Those in better-paying jobs are getting more than they have earned, while those with greater needs are getting relatively less.

Moreover, not all Americans have equal access to employer-based coverage and its associated subsidies. Millions of Americans working at respectable (albeit low-paying) jobs are not offered health insurance by their employer (Pepper Commission 1990). Although they could in principle switch jobs to find one that offers insurance, there are whole industries (involving smaller firms or self-employed individuals) where this may not be practical. Moreover, those who do switch may not be covered for previously existing conditions. These inequities conflict with prevailing notions of equal opportunity, since many Americans have no realistic chance to purchase insurance (Pepper Commission 1990).

Government action in health care may therefore appear more legitimate either because health needs are less under individual control or because labor markets are not fairly rewarding productivity with increased health benefits. To the extent that health status is viewed as beyond a person's individual control, one would expect that those who see life's opportunities as more random, as more dictated by chance, will be particularly supportive of government action in health care. To the extent that the labor markets are seen to distribute health care benefits unfairly, perceptions about the overall fairness of labor markets will do less to reduce support for government action involving health care than for other forms of government intervention.

The peculiar nature of health care needs: Whether health care needs are somehow distinct, in either a moral or a practical sense, from other needs has been the subject of considerable academic debate over the past fifteen years. On one hand, it is argued that health care needs are somehow more basic and fundamental than other needs, because they are closely linked to the fundamental need for individual survival (Walzer 1983). They have also been argued to be more readily and objectively measured than other aspects of "need." This makes it easier to design need-based programs for health care and has led to a proliferation of health tests as a means of qualifying for other public benefits (Stern 1983; Stone 1979).

On the other hand, there are those who believe that health care needs are different primarily because they represent such a problematic and impractical concept. There is a prevailing sense that what many Americans characterize as health care needs are essentially unlimited, because the norms of being "healthy" are always relative to other members of society, though genetic differences and personal habits make it impossible to make some as healthy as others (Callahan 1990). From this it is argued that health care needs are a "bottomless pit," a phrase that appears to be sufficiently catchy that it is reiterated in almost every discussion of this topic (Callahan 1990; Baybrooke 1987; Stern 1983; Moskop 1983).

A second problematic aspect of health care needs is their link to technology. It is sometimes argued that as new techniques and procedures become technically feasible, they are automatically assumed by the public to be needed (Callahan 1990; Brown 1978). Consequently, needs are never stable. Nor, in the absence of controls on research and development, can they be met without continually increasing the amount of money spent on health care. Under these conditions, the whole concept of need may "break down" when applied to medical care. "Not only does the concept of needs not help policy-making to find solutions to this problem; any social policy adopted to cope with it must struggle against the weight of the concept of needs" (Baybrooke 1987: 293).

In a 1990 survey, three-quarters of the public agreed that "even if we spent twice as much on health care, it wouldn't be enough to provide all the care that people would like to have" (Blue Cross/Blue Shield 1990: 13). Although needs are not equivalent to the things "people would like to have," this perception suggests that the public may be wary of the notion of need because of its potential for significantly expanded costs.

The extent and impact of need-based motives for government intervention in medical care thus depend on whether the more positive or negative perception of need most shapes public thinking. To the extent that needs are seen as more basic, fundamental, or readily applied to health care programs, people most concerned with the norm of need should support health care interventions more strongly than other forms of social policy. If health needs are seen as unlimited or especially ill defined, those concerned most about norms of need will be least supportive of government intervention in health care.

The instrumental nature of health care benefits: Health care benefits have been argued to be distinct because health is a necessary condition for other values that Americans hold dear. One line of argument links health to political freedoms (Moon 1988). Before the close of the eighteenth century, claims were made in Congress that health care in itself was an "inalienable right" (Brown 1978). Citizens who are impaired, it was argued, cannot exercise their rights of political participation. They thus have their most basic rights compromised, rights which Americans believe should be equally available to all (Hochschild 1981).

A second line of argument plays off the principle of equal opportunity. From this perspective, health care is a prerequisite for free economic participation (Buchanan 1984; Brown 1978). The dominant ideology of market-based desert can thus be moral only if people remain sufficiently healthy that they have access to market-based rewards. And health care thus assumes the same moral importance as does equality of opportunity. "I urge the fair equality of opportunity principle as an appropriate principle to govern macro decisions about the design of our health-care system. Such a principle defines, from the perspective of justice, what the moral *function* of the health-care system must be—to help guarantee fair equality of opportunity" (Daniels 1985: 41). In this broad sense, access to health care becomes a prerequisite for a just society, that is, a society of equal opportunity, in much the same sense as education (Dougherty 1988; Goodin 1988; Greenstone 1988).

Although health care may be no more a prerequisite to political freedom or economic participation than adequate nutrition or shelter (given the difficulty of registering to vote or applying for a job without a permanent address), Americans who are most concerned about equal opportunity may give greater priority to health care than some other forms of government intervention. Similarly, those who believe that current opportunities are not equal may be particularly supportive of government health programs to remedy these inequities.

Diffused and unpredictable benefits from government interventions in health care: One of the less-studied differences between health and other forms of social policy involves the nature of the redistribution associated with government action. Most government policies are redistributive in relatively clear ways, either from rich to poor, or from working-age to the young and the old. Because blacks and Hispanics have on average lower incomes than Anglos, there is a relatively clear redistribution toward these groups as well. Consequently, support for government interventions depends in large part on how Americans perceive and value the well-being of these recipient groups.

Health care interventions are also redistributive. In part, these redistributions follow the same patterns as do those from other government programs, benefiting most those groups that are currently disadvantaged in economic terms. For example, the tax credits advocated by the Bush administration would have redistributed some $20 billion annually to low- and lower-middle-income citizens. Income-related redistributions of health benefits also have the greatest benefits for minority groups. As of the late 1980s, 20 percent of blacks and 30 percent of Hispanics had no health insurance coverage, compared to 12 percent for non-Hispanic whites (Health Insurance Association of America 1991: 24–25). Proposals for reforming health care finance would transfer billions of dollars each year to these groups (Schlesinger 1987).

In some important ways, however, redistribution under health programs is different from other government programs. Health insurance, whether public or private, always involves substantial redistributions from the healthy to the sick. Because people of any income, race, or age may fear the costs and consequences of ill health, these can be thought of as random redistribution. Random transfers may offset and obscure the more predictable redistributions along racial and economic lines.

In addition, because access to health benefits depends on one's employment situation, even relatively well-off individuals may be at risk for loss of insurance (and hence federal tax subsidies) if they work for a small employer. Since 33 million Americans (and 7.3 million of those uninsured) work for firms with twenty-five or fewer employees, the potential benefits of government intervention may be quite broadly anticipated (Pepper Commission 1990). In a 1982 survey conducted by ABC News and the *Washington Post*, more than 20 percent of working-age respondents with above-average incomes reported that their health care benefits were at least "somewhat a problem." [18] Recent surveys suggest that these concerns among the better-off may have doubled over the past decade (Blendon and Szalay 1992).

In addition to the direct benefits of government assistance, a broader federal role could be seen to reduce health care costs. Concerns about costs have become widespread. The Pepper Commission report (1990) asserted, for example, that "explosive increases in health care costs are beginning to jeopardize access to care even for adequately insured Americans" (p. 38). This is reflected in prevailing public opinion. In a 1987 poll conducted by Yankelovich, 59 percent of Americans with annual in-

---

18. Based on original polling data, reanalyzed by the authors.

comes of $75,000 and above reported that they were concerned or very concerned about future medical costs.[19]

Evidence from Canada and Europe suggests that as government becomes responsible for paying for a broader segment of the insured population, it is better able to control costs (Reinhardt 1990; Merlis 1990). To the extent that this claim is accepted by the public, broader federal participation may be seen as reducing overall health care costs. This directly benefits individuals as taxpayers, reducing the burdens of supporting Medicare and Medicaid. It may also indirectly reduce costs for the privately insured, allaying widespread concerns.

Both the direct and indirect returns on government involvement in health care lead to more diffused benefits than other forms of government intervention. This has several possible implications for the distribution of public support. To the extent that random redistribution masks redistribution along economic and ethnic lines, external identification may be less important a motivation for health policy than for other forms of social policy. Concern for the poor and for racial minorities and threats of social conflict become less salient influences. To the extent that nonpoor Americans feel threatened with a loss of insurance coverage, self-interested motivations will be less closely linked with personal financial well-being. To the extent that an expanded government role is seen to reduce health care costs and the taxes required to finance Medicare and Medicaid, people who already feel burdened by taxes may be more accepting of government interventions in health care than in other areas.

Altruism and empathy: Although the diffusion of benefits from government health programs may reduce the importance of some forms of external identification, other types of identification may increase. Altruistic motives are a case in point. One important source of altruism is an empathic link with those being assisted (Batson and Oleson 1991). The prevalence of illness and the spreading fears of losing one's insurance coverage should make it relatively easy for most Americans to identify with those who have unmet health care needs (Buchanan 1984; Sass 1983; Beauchamp and Faden 1979). By contrast, many Americans have difficulty identifying with and achieving empathy for the homeless or the jobless.

If these suppositions are valid, altruism will prove a more important rationale for government involvement in health care than in other areas.

---

19. This compared to 87 percent of those with income under $15,000. Calculated from original survey data, reanalyzed by the authors.

Those who are most altruistic should thus be relatively more supportive of government health programs. In addition, because most Americans believe that beneficence should be greater among those who are financially better-off, one may actually find a *positive* relationship between financial well-being and support for government action in health care.

The interactive character of health care services: Health care is clearly different from programs such as AFDC or Social Security in another sense. Much of what Americans value in health care depends on the quality of the interaction between patient and medical professional (Dougherty 1988; Rushing 1986). Virtually all Americans place great importance on being able to select a provider with whom they feel compatible (Blue Cross/Blue Shield 1990: 21).

For this reason, government involvement in health care faces a hurdle that is not faced with cash benefit programs. People must be convinced that government involvement will not significantly alter the aspects of medical care with which they are currently quite satisfied (Gabel et al. 1989). Historically, one of the most consistently raised objections to government involvement in health care has been the claim that it would unduly "standardize" either the nature of health care or the range of health care insurance coverages (Dougherty 1988; Sass 1983; Siegler 1979).

Those who fear "standardization" of medicine under federal auspices may prefer more locally controlled arrangements, which offer greater potential for adapting the health care system to variations in local needs. There are two possible options: retaining employer control over health benefits or vesting this control with local governments. Because worksite benefits reflect the negotiation of interests between employers and employees, some observers see these arrangements as creating a social structure that assesses and responds to the needs of employee groups (Rushing 1986; Sapolsky et al. 1981).

Even if the public accepted government supplanting the employer's role, it might prefer that the health care system not be controlled at the federal level. It may believe that it has more control over local government, which could better reflect local variations in preferences or health needs. A desire for local autonomy has been a consistent tension in popular acceptance of federal programs since World War II (Coughlin 1980). A preference for local control was a significant part of the philosophy underlying the development of neighborhood health centers during the 1960s (Sardell 1988) and the health care planning programs established during the 1970s (Morone 1981).

One would thus anticipate that attitudes toward federal government involvement would be sensitive to three popular perceptions. The first involves the extent to which people are satisfied with their current health care arrangements. The more satisfied they are, the more they might feel they have to lose if federal interventions go awry (Gabel et al. 1989). The second attitude involves satisfaction with the role of business. The more they see current workplace practices as fair, the more they may be concerned about the disruption created by a broader federal role in health care. Similarly, the more people see local government as effectively serving the public, the more they may balk at federal involvement. To the extent that health care involves practices that the public wishes not to have standardized, perceptions of the fairness of more local settings for administering benefits may have a larger effect on support for federal involvement in health care than in other aspects of social policy.

Health-related Differences as Testable Hypotheses. We have identified here six factors that make the distribution of health care potentially different from the distribution of income or other socially valued services. There is, to date, no empirical research that documents whether these perceptions shape public attitudes about the just distribution of health care or the appropriate types of health policy.

These differences can thus be conceived as hypotheses about the link between public perceptions and support for public policy, as they apply specifically to health care. To the extent that members of the public perceive each difference to be relevant and important, they will alter their support for government action. Each different aspect carries several implications about how support for government action in health care would vary with individual circumstances.

Note that in several cases, there is not a one-to-one link between a presumed feature of health care and predicted changes in support for government. In the case of health needs, this is because it is unclear if need-based motives will have more or less salience for health care. The more clearly that needs can be defined for health care, relative to other social priorities, the more the notion of needs will be emphasized in considering the appropriate role of the federal government. But if health care needs are seen as ill defined, greater perceived needs would have less of an influence on the acceptance of a greater federal role.

In the case of an individual's financial well-being, two different aspects of health care both suggest that financial well-being will be less negatively related to support for government action in health care than in other areas. If benefits are more broadly diffused, self-interest will be less directly linked to financial well-being. Even those who are relatively well-off financially may favor a broader role for government if they anticipate that this role might reduce their personal costs or risks. Altruism may also reduce the negative relationship between financial well-being and support for government action. The presumption that those who are better-off should be more beneficent could thus lead respondents who were better-off actually to be more supportive of government than their counterparts with more limited financial resources. Because both of these factors suggest similar changes for the coefficients on the financial self-interest variables, we cannot completely disentangle them in the empirical results that follow.

Does Public Support for Health Policy Draw on Different Attitudes and Perceptions?

We have identified an array of perceptions and attitudes that may influence public support for government action in health care. No survey has measured these factors in a manner that allows us to test directly all the hypotheses formulated in the last section. However, the 1987 version of the General Social Survey did contain a special supplement which collected information about Americans' perceptions of social equity. Although these questions were for the most part not about health care per se, responses from this survey can be used to formulate some more indirect tests of the relationship between public opinion and support for federal initiatives.

These indirect measures require some justification. They relate a particular attitude about social equity or perception about how society functions to the respondent's willingness to support federal action in health care or other areas. This is an *indirect* measure; respondents were not asked if they supported federal health initiatives *because* of some value or some perception, only whether they held that value and whether they supported government initiatives. From the statistical models that we estimate below, one can thus infer a relationship from the correlation in responses.

Inferences of this sort run the risk of inappropriately asserting a causal relationship. Respondents may favor a particular value and favor government interventions not because they connect the two but because there is some unmeasured third factor that is correlated with them both. But indirect measures also have some advantages over directly asking Americans why they favor particular policies. Past studies of public attitudes toward government programs suggest that many respondents cannot clearly identify or articulate a rationale for favoring a program, even though their support can be consistently linked to particular circumstances or motives (Page and Shapiro 1992; Hamilton and Cohen 1974). The approach used here does not presume a conscious connection, only a systematically observable pattern in responses.

Because these estimates are based on a survey designed for other purposes, some of our measures are only crude approximations of the relevant attitudes or perceptions. To offset in part the limitations of any one measure, we will, where possible, use multiple measures for each hypothesized relationship. Thus, the test of each hypothesis involves examining whether the combination of several measures is related in differing ways or in differing degrees to various government policies.

The Specification of Independent Variables

We describe below the explanatory variables used in the regressions. These are presented according to the hypothesis for which they are relevant, with the hypotheses covered in the order in which they were presented in the previous section of the paper.

Reduced Personal Responsibility for Health-related Outcomes. We hypothesized that if individuals were held less responsible for bad outcomes related to health care, then support for government involvement would be more responsive to perceptions that life was risky and would be less limited by concerns that some Americans had not "earned" the right to government assistance.

There are two types of generic risks with which people may be concerned (Dougherty 1988). The first is related to genetic endowments, which political philosophers refer to as the "natural lottery" (Rawls 1971). Perceptions of this type of risk are measured here by an index of respondents' assessments of the extent to which they believe that doing well economically depends on one's race, sex, religion, or natural abilities. The higher the index, the more respondents believe that economic well-being depends on these factors largely established at birth. Only 6 percent of the sample considered these factors highly important. A second type of risk involves more contemporary threats to economic security. Contemporaneous risks are measured by the extent to which current well-being is thought to depend on luck. Again, about 6 percent of the sample saw luck as importantly determining economic well-being. If this hypothesis is correct, then respondents who see life as risky should be more supportive of government intervention in health care.

Americans' discomfort with broad eligibility for government benefits is closely linked to the belief that some people don't deserve assistance because they have not worked sufficiently hard on their own behalf (Katz 1986; Kluegel and Smith 1986; Hochschild 1981). This attitude presumes that hard work is in fact rewarded. We measure this assumption directly by an index of responses to two questions that attribute economic well-being to hard work. Respondents who feel that hard work is rewarded should be less supportive of government programs. To the extent that problems associated with health or health care access are treated differently in this regard, this perception should have a smaller negative correlation with support for government health initiatives than for other public policies.

The Differing Nature of Need for Health Care. Some of the unique aspects of health needs may make the concept of need more relevant for the support of health policy; others may make need-related factors less salient. Unfortunately, the 1987 GSS does not ask respondents about the need for health care per se, only about more general notions of the "neediness" of the public and of the federal government's responsibility in meeting those needs. Our analysis presumes that if need plays a larger role in the support of health policy, this will be reflected in stronger correlations between general perceptions of need and support for health interventions.

Respondents were asked whether they thought the "lot of the average man" was getting better or worse over time. Two-thirds reported that it was getting worse. We assume that this indicates that people have greater unmet needs. Support for policies that are particularly responsive to need should be more strongly influenced by this perception. A willingness to have the federal government address needs is measured by respondents' endorsement of the statement that the federal government should "provide a decent standard of living for the unemployed." The unemployed are clearly in need: because they are not directly contributing to society through work, this provides a measure of acceptance of government assistance for those who are not "earning" those benefits. Just over half the sample agreed that the federal government should meet these needs.

The Instrumental Nature of Health Care. Government involvement in health care may be legitimized by a belief that health is a prerequisite for equal opportunity. One would thus expect that respondents who were more concerned about equal opportunity would be relatively more supportive of government action in health care. More specifically, respondents should favor greater government intervention in health care the more they perceive there to be unequal opportunity in the current system and the more they think that it is a federal responsibility to equalize opportunities for the average American.

To assess the extent to which respondents believed that Americans currently have equal opportunities, we examined their responses to questions asked about a variety of factors that they felt were associated with "doing well" in America. Among these were parents' income and education. The more parental background matters, the less equal opportunity can actually be realized. Twenty percent of the respondents felt that parental background was an important determinant of a person's economic opportunities. This group sees opportunities as clearly unequal. To the extent that government policies could reduce these inequities, this group should favor remedial government interventions. Support for federal action in this role is measured by whether respondents agreed that the federal government should aid low-income students who wished to go to college. Education has long been linked to norms of equal opportunity in American culture (Smith 1987). Three-quarters of the sample favored this role for government. To the extent that health policies are legitimized by a concern for equal opportunity, one would expect this group to be most supportive of federal health initiatives.

Diffused Benefits and Redistribution from Government Health Initiatives.
To the extent that the expected benefits of government health interventions extend beyond disadvantaged groups, support for health policies should be less related to a respondent's personal financial well-being and less identified with concerns about particular disadvantaged groups.

Respondents' financial well-being is measured by three variables. Subjective perceptions of financial well-being depend on two types of comparisons: people compare their own financial status to the standard of living that they perceive others to have, as well as to their own standard of living in previous years (Kluegel and Smith 1986; Hochschild 1981). We measure here both these comparisons. Respondents on the 1987 GSS were asked to assess their current standard of living "compared to American families in general" and relative to their financial well-being "during the last few years." Nineteen percent of the sample reported themselves to be better-off than the average American; 40 percent reported that their standard of living had improved over the past several years.

As noted earlier, even those who are relatively well-off may support government programs as a buffer against the risk of bad outcomes in the future. This motive should be strongest among those whose financial situation is most insecure and those who are most risk-averse. Controlling for respondents' perception of their current well-being, relative to other American families, those whose financial status has changed in recent years will likely feel less secure, since they were recently in a more difficult situation. They might therefore be more supportive of protective government programs. Risk aversion is measured by respondents' preference for job security as a characteristic of employment. Those who score highest on this variable—roughly one in five respondents—are likely to be the most risk-averse and the most supportive of government actions to buffer risks.

To the extent that self-interest motivates support for public policies, there should be greater support the worse off respondents perceive themselves to be, and the more they are averse to risk. The diffusion of benefits from health interventions should reduce the extent to which self-interest is correlated with either of these factors.

Self-interested responses also depend on the expected burden of the taxes to pay for new government initiatives. Willingness to pay additional taxes can be assessed in terms of how "burdened" taxpayers feel by their current taxes (Shapiro and Young 1989). Those who feel more burdened can be expected to resist new federal programs, whatever their distribution of benefits. In the 1987 GSS, respondents were asked whether their current federal income tax was "too high," "about right," or "too low." Not surprisingly, relatively few respondents felt that they paid too few taxes; almost two-thirds complained that they were overly taxed. To the extent that federal interventions in health care are seen as a means of controlling costs, greater intervention may actually reduce tax burdens by controlling the costs of Medicare and Medicaid. Given these perceptions, the negative relationship between burden and support for federal programs should be reduced or eliminated for health initiatives.

External identification is measured by three variables. The first two are associated with identification with low-income groups, the third with racial minorities. Identification with the poor can be either positive or negative. In other words, one can support social programs for the benefit of the poor either because one is concerned about their well-being or because one fears their unrest. The first of these motives is measured by whether respondents agreed that "differences in income in America are too large." Those who responded positively (slightly more than half the sample) are arguably most concerned about the economically disadvantaged.

Concern about social threat is measured by the extent to which respondents perceive a potential for class-based conflict in American society. The survey asks about four possible intergroup conflicts "in American society today": between the rich and the poor, the employed and the unemployed, the middle class and the working class, and urban residents and those who live in rural areas. The index of social threat used here combines responses for the first two types of conflict. Judged by this measure, roughly half the public fears some form of economically linked societal tension.

A third external identification involves race. The degree of identification with others on the basis of race, or racial affect, is also measured indirectly. Respondents were asked if they supported additional societal spending on a variety of social problems, including "improving the condition of blacks." To assess racial affect, we constructed the variable that measures the support for spending on blacks relative to support for a composite of other social problems. Those with positive scores on this variable thus are more in favor of spending to assist blacks than spending on these other problems; those with negative scores would be less inclined to target spending in this way. A third of the sample registered positive racial affect by this criterion.

In general, one would expect support for government programs to be higher the greater the concern for the economically disadvantaged, the greater the perceived threat of societal conflict, and the greater the concern for disadvantaged racial minorities. To the extent that the lateral redistributions of health programs obscure or legitimize other forms of redistribution, all these motives will be less important for health programs than for other, equally redistributive government policies.

Altruism and Health Care Problems. To the extent that altruism shapes attitudes toward public policies, those who report that they place a higher value on altruism should be most supportive of policies to assist the disadvantaged. Respondents on the survey were asked to rate the importance of a variety of values that could be taught to children as they were growing up. One of a half dozen options involved teaching children "to help others when they need help." People who placed great importance on this value—about 12 percent of the sample—are considered here to be most altruistic; those who rated it lowest are considered least altruistic.

Valued Relationships and Concern about Federal Bureaucracy. To the extent that the public's perception of high-quality health care is linked with a belief in a strong relationship between patient and provider, respondents may reject a federal role because they feel that it will overly structure or bureaucratize this relationship. Although this concern cannot be directly measured using data from the survey, several indirect measures are available. Those most satisfied with existing arrangements for health care have the most to lose from a "bureaucratized" system. This is measured here by respondents who reported confidence in the medical care system and their satisfaction with their current level of health.[20]

Those concerned about federal bureaucracy may prefer a health care system that is more locally controlled, allowing greater flexibility in the system of paying for or delivering health services. Their willingness to support federal initiatives may thus depend on their assessment of alternative institutions that might instead play that role. As noted earlier, two alternative institutional arrangements would provide more local autonomy than would federal administration: either employment-based insurance or benefits controlled by local government. One would expect that the more confidence respondents had in these institutions, the less they would support federal initiatives. For those programs where bureaucracy represented the greatest concern, the salience of these more local options should have a greater influence on support for federal involvement. In other words, those most confident in either employers or local government should show less support for federal health initiatives than for other types of federal intervention. The legitimacy of an employment-based system is measured here by an index of two variables: the confidence the respondent has in American business and the extent to which he or she agrees that "allowing business to make profits is the best way of improving everyone's standard of living." About 40 percent of all respondents had a favorable assessment of business by this measure. The legitimacy of local government is measured by the amount of trust that respondents have in their own local government. Sixty percent of respondents felt that they could trust their local government to "do what is right" most or all of the time.

We have thus identified nineteen variables with which to test the hypotheses about how support for federal health policies differs from support for other federal policies. The means and standard deviations for these variables are summarized in Table 5.

20. For those who are less healthy, the potential changes produced by government involvement become considerably more salient than those who see themselves in good health. This may encourage either a more positive or more negative stance toward federal action, depending on whether that action was perceived to improve or harm the medical care that the respondent is likely to need.

Table 5 Means and Standard Deviations of Independent Variables: Values, Attitudes, and Perceptions

Variable	Range of Response Scale	Mean	Standard Deviation
Risk, Reward, and Economic Well-Being			
Believes Well-Being Determined by Happenstance	(1–3)	1.51	0.76
Believes Well-Being Determined by Birth Traits	(4–20)	10.60	2.81
Believes Well-Being Determined by Own Effort	(2–6)	5.03	1.05
Perceived Need and Perceived Role of Government			
Believes Average Man Getting Worse Off	(1–2)	0.66	0.47
Believes Federal Government Provides Decent Standard of Living for Unemployed	(1–5)	3.15	1.07
Perceived Equal Opportunity and Role of Government			
Believes Well-Being Determined by Parents' Income or Education	(2–10)	5.86	1.72
Supports College Aid for Low-Income Youth	(1–5)	3.93	0.94
External Identifications			
Supports Aid to Blacks (Racial Affect)	(−1.5–2)	−0.27	0.72
Concerned about Societal Conflict	(2–8)	5.38	1.32
Believes Income Differences in U.S. Too Large	(1–5)	3.53	1.04
Financial Measures of Self-Interest			
Feels Burdened by Current Taxes	(1–4)	3.57	0.64
Feels Well-off Relative to Other Americans	(1–5)	2.84	0.83
Feels Better-off Relative to Recent Past	(1–3)	2.20	0.74
Values Secure Job (Risk Aversion)	(1–5)	2.39	1.20
Altruism/Concern for Others			
Believes It Important to Teach Children to Care for Others	(1–5)	3.23	1.03
Provider Relationship and Concern about Bureaucracy			
Confident in Health Care System	(1–3)	1.54	0.60
Satisfied with Own Health	(1–7)	5.46	1.47
Confident in Business Community	(2–8)	5.45	1.30
Trusts Local Government	(1–4)	2.59	0.79

Dependent variables and regression techniques: To assess the impact of these attitudes, perceptions and values on health and social policy, we regressed the variables described above on our set of government involvement and government spending variables. These regression models identify the extent to which direct self-interest, external identification, and norms of social justice are related to support for government involvement in health care, general domestic programs, and programs targeted to the poor.[21]

The 1987 version of the General Social Survey also contained a fourth measure of government involvement not available in earlier years. This assessed support for policies redistributing income. As with the other questions on government involvement, respondents were asked to choose between two statements, in this case whether "government should do something to reduce income differences between rich and poor" as opposed to "government should not concern itself with income differences." In 1987, just under half the respondents favored government initiatives to redistribute income. Twenty-three percent were strongly in favor of such policies.

We have included this fourth dependent variable to assess how attitudes and perceptions affect popular support for explicitly redistributive programs. Because redistribution by nature involves government taxing some parties to pay others, it seems most appropriate to compare support for redistributive policies to the government spending variables, since these variables measure support for spending more on a problem in addition to support for government involvement. In both cases, respondents are supporting government actions that are costly—if not to them personally, then to some other members of society.

Our empirical comparisons thus involve estimating four regression models: one for federal action in health care, one for general federal domestic programs, one for federal programs to help the poor, and one for redistributive federal policies. Respondents' support for federal action in each of these four areas may alter their attitudes about federal initiatives in the other three areas. This potential interaction introduces both conceptual and statistical complications to the task of determining if Americans treat federal involvement in health care as different from involvement in other policy areas. The four types of policies may act as either substitutes for or complements to one another. Policy areas may be viewed as substitutes when resources are seen as limited. For example, those who favor federal programs for the poor may be less inclined to support health interventions, because they fear that the latter would drain tax dol-

21. As mentioned in footnote 4, the 1987 GSS involved an oversampling of black Americans. To ensure that the regressions model representative patterns in American opinion, one can either exclude this oversample or else include a variable to control for whether the respondent was black. The regressions were estimated using both approaches, with virtually no differences in results. The findings reported in the text are from the full sample, with a dummy variable measuring the race of the respondent. (The coefficient on this dummy variable is not reported in the text.)

lars away from antipoverty programs. Conversely, support for programs may be complementary. This would be true if one program is seen to promote indirectly the same outcomes as another type of policy. For example, there may be some respondents who want the federal government to improve access to health care but who are not directly concerned about the distribution of income. Nonetheless, they may favor federal programs that redistribute income because they anticipate that redistribution will increase the financial resources for low-income Americans, who will then be better able to purchase health services.

In statistical terms, support for the four types of policies is simultaneously determined. As a result, particular attitudes or perceptions may be associated with support for specific policy areas through an indirect linkage. Let us return to the example introduced above and assume that respondents favor federal action to improve access to health care in part because they believe it to be government's role to promote equal opportunity and see health as an important prerequisite for taking advantage of opportunities. In a regression model, support for programs promoting equal opportunity would be positively associated with support for health interventions. Let us assume also that support for redistributive policies is unrelated to perceptions about equal opportunity. Nonetheless, if respondents favor redistributive programs because they think that they will indirectly increase access to health care, then those who are most concerned about equal opportunity will, all else being equal, be more supportive of redistributive policies. In the regression model for redistributive programs, the coefficient on the variable measuring support for equal opportunity would again be positive.

There are therefore two ways in which an attitude or perception may be linked to support for federal action in a particular area. The first case, which we will refer to here as a "direct" linkage, involves respondents' associating some attitude or perception with support for a particular aspect of federal policy. In the second case, which we term an "indirect" linkage, particular attitudes or perceptions are related to support for a federal policy because that policy is seen as instrumental in furthering some other social goal.

To separate out these various ways in which attitudes and perceptions may be linked to support for particular public policies, it is necessary to estimate simultaneously the complete system of four equations.[22] The

22. To do this, the equation must be identified. Separate variables must be introduced that are related to support for each of the four aspects of policy but unrelated to the other three. For health initiatives, these unique variables are the measures of satisfaction with health and confi-

"structural equations" associated with these estimates measure both the direct influence of attitudes on support for each of the four policy areas and the extent to which support for any one policy area is positively or negatively related to support for the other three areas. From these structural equations one can then calculate "reduced form" equations that combine both the direct and indirect influences of attitudes and perceptions on each of the four types of federal policy. We will initially present the reduced form results. These are appropriate for answering questions about how changes in particular attitudes or perceptions can be expected to change support for particular policies. We will then consider how these relationships differ if we measure instead only the direct linkages. These are appropriate for questions involving differences in how Americans think about each of these four policy interventions. The structural equations also provide measures of the interactions in support among the four types of policy.

Results from the Attitude Regressions

Estimating this four-equation system, we can explain about 40 percent of the variation in public attitudes toward a federal role in these four policy areas. The results from these regression estimates are presented in Table 6. The variables are grouped according to the hypotheses about how health may be different from other policy areas. Because the explanatory dependent variables largely involve subjective scales of differing magnitude, the size of the coefficients on these regressions is not particularly meaningful. To provide a more useful interpretation of the relative magnitudes of these effects, we report the estimated change in support for health and social policies associated with moving from the low to the high extreme on each of these scales.

What Attitudes and Perceptions Affect Support for Federal Health Initiatives? The results from the reduced form regressions suggest that support for federal improvements of access to health care is linked to four separate factors: a concern about needs, a concern about equal opportunity, a moderate amount of external identification, as well as a faith in insti-

dence in the medical care system, described previously in the text. For antipoverty programs, the additional variables include several measures of what respondents believe are the causes of poverty. For redistributive programs, the additional variables are measures of why respondents think that inequality persists in American society. Finally, for general domestic policies, the additional variables measure respondents' confidence and trust in various branches of the federal government.

Table 6 Attitudes, Perceptions, and Norms That Shape Support for Social Policies (Percentage Difference in Support for Health and General Domestic Policies Associated with Each Characteristic)

Attitudes, Norms, and Perceptions of Respondents	Dependent Variables			
	Support for Health Policy	Support for General Domestic Policy	Support for Programs That Support the Poor	Support for Redistribution from Rich to Poor
Belief in Individual Responsibility for Outcomes				
Believes Well-Being Shaped by Happenstance	1.1	1.1	1.1	4.1
Believes Well-Being Shaped by Traits at Birth	6.6	−1.8	−7.8	9.8
Believes Well-Being Determined by Hard Work	1.1	1.5	−10.1[a]	−6.3
Ethical Basis for Responding to Others' Needs				
Believes Average Person Getting Worse Off	2.1	0.3	6.5[a]	11.2[a]
Believes Standard of Living Should Be Guaranteed for Unemployed	15.5[a]	13.7[a]	19.6[a]	23.2[a]
Belief in Policy as Prerequisite for Equal Opportunity, as Indicated By				
Belief That Well-Being Is Shaped by Parents' Education/Wealth	8.1[a]	6.1[a]	8.3[a]	1.1
Support for College Aid for Low-Income Youth	20.5[a]	15.5[a]	27.6[a]	21.2[a]
Support for Redistribution, as Indicated By				
Concern about Societal Conflict	4.7	4.2	3.2	16.7[a]
Belief That Income Differences in U.S. Are Too Large	5.2[a]	3.1	11.9[a]	30.4[a]
Support for Aid to Blacks (Racial Affect)	−2.6	0.8	6.5	23.4[a]
Perception of Self-Interest				
Feeling Well-off Relative to Other Americans	−3.6[b]	−2.6	1.8	1.0
Feeling Better-off Than in Past Few Years	3.6	5.9[a]	2.1	−2.9
Feeling Burdened by Taxes	−0.7	−6.0[a]	−8.1[b]	13.7[a]
Preference for Secure Job (Risk Aversion)	1.3	4.8[a]	2.1	12.0[a]

Table 6 Continued

Attitudes, Norms, and Perceptions of Respondents	Dependent Variables			
	Support for Health Policy	Support for General Domestic Policy	Support for Programs That Support the Poor	Support for Redistribution from Rich to Poor
Altruistic Concerns				
Perceives Importance of Altruism	7.6[a]	5.4[a]	12.8[a]	11.6[a]
Institutional Concerns and Concern about Bureaucracy				
Confidence in Health Care System	−3.2			
Satisfaction with Own Health	−0.2			
Confidence in Business Community	−8.7[a]	−5.4[a]	−9.4[a]	−25.8[a]
Trust in Local Government	−5.8[a]	−2.0	1.3	−1.1

Note. The percentages given for the dependent variables refer to the differences found between those at the upper and lower bounds of the attitude scales.
a. Statistically significant at a 5 percent confidence level.
b. Statistically significant at a 10 percent confidence level.

tutions that represent alternatives to federal administration (see the first column in Table 6).

Norms of need and equal opportunity both legitimize government intervention in health care. The more strongly that respondents believe that the federal government is seen as responsible for meeting needs (as exemplified by the needs of the unemployed), the greater the support for federal action to promote access to health care. The more that family background is thought to limit equal opportunity and the more that the federal government is thought to have a role in promoting opportunity (as measured by federal college aid), the greater the support for government involvement in health care. The relative size of these relationships suggests that federal initiatives in health are somewhat more responsive to norms of opportunity than concerns about need.

External identification has only a modest influence on support for federal health initiatives. Respondents who place greater emphasis on altruism are more supportive of federal programs to promote access to health care. Those who think that the income gap between rich and poor is too large are also more likely to support federal health initiatives. But neither the threat of class conflict nor a concern for racial minorities appears to be related to support for this type of federal intervention.

The fourth significant relationship involves assessments of public and private institutions. Respondents who have greater faith in business or local government are less likely to support federal initiatives in health care. This suggests that these other institutions are seen as real or potential substitutes for federal involvement.

The factors that are *not* associated with support for federal health programs also present an interesting pattern. Perceptions about whether the labor market rewards workers' efforts are unrelated to support. Those who feel that people can earn more if they simply work harder are no less willing to have government assist with health care problems than are people who feel that the labor market is less equitable. Similarly, the extent to which a person's well-being is determined by random events, either at birth or currently, appears to have little relationship to support for federal health initiatives.

Nor do measures of financial self-interest appear to have much influence. Support for federal health initiatives is unrelated to respondents' perception of relative financial well-being as well as to their perceived tax burden. Measures of financial insecurity (e.g., recent changes in financial status) and risk aversion are also unrelated to support for programs to increase access to health services.

How Is Health Care Different from Other Social Policies? Following our analysis of the direct and indirect linkages between attitudes and support for federal action, there are two broad ways in which health care may be different. The first involves differences in the interactions in support among the four policy areas. The second involves differences in how particular attitudes and perceptions shape support for federal intervention.

Interactions in support among the four types of federal policy: From the structural equations we can estimate the size and direction of the interactions in support among the four policy areas. The estimated coefficients from the structural equations are presented in the Appendix; the interaction among the policy areas is summarized in Table 7. Attitudes toward health interventions appear to be different in two ways. Support for federal health initiatives is only weakly influenced by attitudes toward other forms of federal policy. Most strikingly, support for health initiatives does not depend on acceptance of a broad role for the federal government in domestic policies generally. (Compare this to support for antipoverty programs; when support for a broad federal domestic role declines by 10 percent, support for antipoverty programs declines almost as sharply.) Conversely, support for an active federal role that increases access to

Table 7 Interactions in Support among Four Types
of Federal Initiatives, 1987

A 10 Percent Increase in Popular Support for This Type of Initiative	Is Associated with the Following Change In			
	Health Programs	Anti-poverty Programs	General Domestic Policies	Income Redistri-bution
Health Care Programs		8.6% increase[a]	6.7% decrease	13% increase[a]
Antipoverty Programs	4.6% increase[a]		6.9% increase[b]	1.7% increase
General Domestic Policies	2.3% decrease	8.6% increase[a]		7.9% decrease
Redistributive Policies	1% increase	1.7% increase	0.1% decrease	

a. Relationship statistically significant at a 5 percent confidence level.
b. Relationship statistically significant at a 10 percent confidence level.

health care appears to increase support substantially for several other policies. Ten percent greater acceptance of health interventions is associated with an 8.6 percent increase in support for antipoverty programs and a 13 percent increase in support for income redistribution. Concern about health care thus appears to legitimize a range of other federal policies. (Note, however, that it does not increase acceptance of a broad general domestic role for the federal government.)

An additional set of differences can be identified by comparing the attitudes and perceptions that motivate support for federal health initiatives to those that encourage support for other federal policies. Earlier in this paper, we described several ways in which health policies might be considered different from other social policies. These hypotheses can be tested by comparing either the reduced form or the structural equations. As noted above, each is appropriate for answering a slightly different question about the terms under which health care policies are viewed as different from other social policies. In practice, the two sets of results are quite similar. We focus our discussion on the reduced form results.

Comparing predictors of support for federal health policies to predictors of support for a general federal role in domestic issues, there appear to be remarkably few differences. However, comparing support for health policies to more overtly redistributive federal initiatives (programs for the poor or programs to redistribute income) leads to sharper distinctions.

Health initiatives compared to general domestic policies: Several distinctions do appear between support for federal health and general domestic policies (compare the first two columns in Table 6). As anticipated, financial measures of self-interest are less directly related to support for health policies than for general domestic policies. Respondents who felt more burdened by taxes were more likely to oppose a broader general federal role in American society. But they were no more likely to oppose health initiatives. Those who were most risk-averse (and who therefore might favor a greater role for government to buffer against risk) were more supportive of a general federal role. Risk aversion was unrelated to support for health interventions. Those whose financial status had recently changed (and who thus might feel more insecure) are more supportive of both health and a general federal activism, but support for health initiatives is considerably less sensitive to this perception.

The other differences in patterns of support, though all in the directions hypothesized, were smaller and were statistically significant only at a 10 percent confidence level. Greater trust in business and local government reduced support for federal actions of all types, but more so for health than for general domestic policies. A perception that outcomes were determined largely by a natural lottery (that is, by characteristics at birth) motivated support for health policies more than for general domestic policies. Support for health initiatives appears to be somewhat more responsive to perceptions about equal opportunity.

Though these differences all exist, with the exception of those related to self-interest, the distinctions are modest in scale. One is left with the primary conclusion that the factors encouraging public support for federal health policies are not much different from those that legitimize activist government in general.

Health initiatives compared to redistributive policies: One reaches quite different conclusions, however, comparing health to more overtly redistributive policies. (Compare the first, third, and fourth columns in Table 6.) The two examples included here are programs directed to the poor and policies that redistribute income. The regression results support three of the hypotheses presented earlier and offer mixed support for two others. The remaining hypotheses receive little support.

The first of the hypotheses supported by these results involves individual responsibility for personal well-being. Support for federal involvement in health care appears less sensitive to notions of self-responsibility than is support for redistributive programs. The perception that people who work hard are rewarded economically significantly reduces support for redistributive programs but does not do so for federal health initiatives.

The second striking difference involves external identification. Support for redistributive programs is much more strongly linked to external identification with the economically disadvantaged and racial minorities. The greater the concern for the well-being of blacks, for example, the more support is shifted away from health programs toward redistributive programs and policies. Support for both health initiatives and redistributive programs is positively related to perceptions that there is too large a gap between the rich and the poor, but the relationship is two to six times larger for redistributive policies. Negative identification—perceived societal threats—motivates support for overtly redistributive policies but has little influence on health policies.

The third hypothesis supported by these results involves the association between health and equal opportunity. Compared to redistributive policies, support for health initiatives is more sensitive to perceptions that opportunities are currently unequal or that the federal government should play a role in promoting equal opportunity. These differences are clearest when one controls for the interaction among policy areas, measured through the structural equations. (See the Appendix.) These differences, however, are relatively small in magnitude.

Two hypotheses received mixed support. The first involves the other societal institutions that might serve as alternatives to federal administration of health interventions. Support for federal health initiatives does appear to be more linked to perceived confidence in local government. Those who have the most confidence in local government are less supportive of federal health initiatives; there is no comparable influence for redistributive programs. But the same is not true for perceived confidence in the business community. Support for redistributive policies declines *more* sharply than does support for health interventions among those who have confidence in business.

The self-interest hypothesis also receives mixed support. As hypothesized, support for federal health initiatives is less sensitive to concerns about tax burden than is support for federal programs for the poor. But support for redistributive programs is actually higher among those who feel most burdened by taxes (perhaps based on the belief that their current burdens would assure that they are the beneficiaries of any future redistribution). Support for access-promoting health policies appears to be less motivated by risk aversion than is support for income redistribution. But measures of financial insecurity, proxied by recent changes in financial well-being, are no more related to support for redistributive policies than for health initiatives.

Several hypotheses receive little support from these results. Support for federal health programs appears to be no more responsive than are redistributive policies to altruistic motives or concerns about the needy. These attitudes and perceptions encourage support for both types of policies about equally. Those who believe that the conditions facing the average American are worsening over time—are most concerned about needs—are relatively more supportive of redistributive policies than of health initiatives. But again, both these differences are sufficiently small to be statistically insignificant.

Discussion and Conclusion: Translating Public Opinion into Policy

The regression analyses presented in this paper suggest that health policy is demonstrably different from other types of social policy. Three distinct differences emerged. First, there is a higher level of popular support for government action in health care, and this support is distributed among the population differently than for other types of policies. More specifically, the gaps in support between rich and poor, educated and uneducated, old and young that exist for most federal policies are significantly reduced for health initiatives. Second, support for health policies is less correlated with support for other federal roles. In particular, support for a federal role in health care does not depend on general support for an activist federal role in American society. Third, the reasons people have for favoring government action in health care appear to be different. This is particularly true when compared to overtly redistributive programs. Although many of the measures of attitudes and perceptions that were used here were not ideally designed for identifying the ways in which health policy might be viewed as different, systematic differences did emerge. Some implications of these findings are discussed below.

Methodological Caveats and Refinements

One should, however, view these findings in light of several caveats. First, data were not available to measure directly a number of the values that can importantly influence public policy. Most notably, we lacked direct measures of the relative importance of various norms of justice. Although we believe that the indirect measures used here provide a plausible assessment and that they are unbiased when comparing across different types of government interventions, it is possible that mismeasured values affected the results of the last set of regressions. These results should be treated as only a first step in defining and measuring this complex set of relationships.

Second, survey responses about the appropriateness of government policies are notoriously sensitive to the wording of questions (Smith 1987). This is as true for health care as elsewhere (Blendon and Donelan 1990; Rochefort and Boyer 1988). Although we used questions that were worded consistently over time and that were unlikely to be biased by accompanying questions, this sort of measurement error also cannot be fully discounted. Third, because the data measuring attitudes and perceptions were drawn from a single year, we have no way of determining if the relationships that were identified here persist over time.

Several other questions involve possible variations in methods. First, several of the variables that were used here as explanatory variables may actually have been endogenous—that is, may have been determined by the same personal characteristics, attitudes, and perceptions that influenced support for health initiatives and the three other forms of social policy. The two most problematic variables are those measuring support for government protections for the standard of living of the unemployed and support for government college assistance. Because each of these attitudes may themselves be influenced by self-interest, external identification, and altruism, including them in the regression equation may partially obscure the influence of these other variables. To assess this concern, the regressions were reestimated as a multistage system. The first stage included predictors of support for government policies for the unemployed and for college students. The second stage used the predicted values for these variables as explanatory measures in the regressions predicting support for health care, general domestic policies, and redistributive programs. By calculating the reduced form of these two stages, one can measure the combined influence of the other dependent variables.

There were relatively few differences between these regressions and those presented earlier. Support for health initiatives became somewhat more sensitive to concerns about need and to altruistic motivations. In neither case, however, was health more sensitive to those motivations than were the more overtly redistributive policies. The differences—or lack of differences—between health and other policy areas persist.

A second methodological issue involves the generalizability and political relevance of these relationships. We noted earlier that certain individuals—those who are best-off financially and those who are most politically active—are likely to have a larger influence on the political process than do other constituents. In an era in which conservative politics have played an important role in determining the national agenda, it may also be important to consider whether those who view themselves as politically conservative have a different set of motivations for supporting public policies than those who would label themselves as liberal. The central question is thus whether the results that we have presented apply to each of these subgroups, as well as to the sample as a whole.

To explore these issues, we divided our sample in three different ways and reestimated the regressions. The first separated respondents who were politically active (according to the definitions and measures presented earlier) from those who were not. The second divided the sample based on income. The third separated those who reported themselves to be conservative (on a seven-point scale) from those describing themselves as liberal.

To a remarkable degree, the basic pattern of relationships linking attitudes, perceptions, and support for federal policies persists across all of these subsamples. (This is consistent with previous research based on small numbers of interviews that suggests that Americans of all socioeconomic backgrounds share a common set of values, particularly involving norms of social justice [Hochschild 1981].) The differences that did exist tended, not surprisingly, to be similar for both the politically active and those with above-average income. Relative to the general attitudes in the population, there is some shift from positive to negative (e.g., societal threat) external identification as a motivation for government policy. The perceived legitimacy of local government (for health care) and the business community (for general domestic policies and programs for the poor) more strongly limited support for federal action. Concerns about need and altruism, in contrast, appeared to play less of a role legitimizing policy.

The basic structure of preferences supporting federal policies was also similar between liberals and conservatives. (This may reflect the relatively narrow range of political ideology in contemporary American society.) Conservatives were more sensitive to the perceived legitimacy of business and local government, which more strongly diminished their support for federal interventions. They were more sensitive to perceptions of need and motives of altruism than were their liberal counterparts, and less motivated by considerations of equal opportunity. Concerns about societal threats also played a larger role in motivating policy among conservative respondents.

Despite these modest differences among subgroups, the findings suggest a relatively stable pattern across socioeconomic, political, and ideological groups for the factors that enhance or diminish support for federal programs. The differences associated with health policy, particularly those compared to more redistributive programs, persist among the politically active, the economically well-off, and the politically conservative. These differences are thus likely to be salient in shaping the attitudes of policymakers, either because the policymakers will respond to these most influential constituents or because they will share their attitudes and perceptions.

Past Changes and Future Prospects for Federal Health Care Reform

To the extent that the findings presented here are reasonably stable and generalizable, they may explain some of the recent growth in public support for federal action in health care, in an era when overall confidence in the federal government remains rather limited. The "Reagan revolution" (which arguably traces to changes in public attitudes beginning in the mid-1970s) was predicated on several propositions: (a) that the market fairly rewarded individual efforts (and that government interference could therefore only make things more inequitable), (b) that the federal government had taken over the roles most appropriately played by other social institutions, and (c) that in doing so, federal taxes had become too burdensome (Weir et al. 1988). Crystallized in the 1980 presidential campaign, these contentions held sway in political debates for most of the subsequent decade. In addition to these ideological positions, the Republican party effectively used a political strategy of attributing any discontent with their policies to minority groups seeking more than their fair share of societal resources. For at least some Americans, this strategy reduced positive attitudes toward racial minorities and economically disadvantaged groups.

As we have documented here, all of these shifts in attitudes and perceptions reduce popular support for federal programs that aid the poor or that redistribute income. But none of these factors do much to undermine support for federal health initiatives. Only concerns about the size of the income gap between rich and poor have any direct influence on support for health initiatives, and they have a much smaller influence on health policies than on more overtly redistributive policies.

This last point merits special emphasis. Most proposed federal health initiatives would entail massive redistribution of resources to those least well-off. Even with the relatively modest proposals offered by candidates Bush and Clinton, low-income households would receive subsidies of tens of billions of dollars annually. Low-income black households alone would receive benefits on the order of $15 billion of redistributed dollars annually (Schlesinger 1987). This is a significantly larger redistribution than that going to black households under AFDC. Yet welfare programs are strongly racially identified, and health programs are not.

All these factors contributed to the uniquely strong popular support for federal health initiatives, and these trends in support were evident well before the flurry of interest shown by policymakers over the past two years. Nor do these differences in attitudes depend on the perception that health care costs have grown so large that they demand federal action. Recent fears about costs have undoubtedly added to the depth of public concern about health, but the distinctive role of health policy reflects other considerations as well.

Many of these findings suggest that support for a larger federal role in health care will continue to grow in the near future. The presidential campaign of 1992 was dominated by concerns about the economy. As long as these concerns persist, they will fuel popular support for federal health care initiatives. Unemployment, disenchantment with the business community, and individuals' concerns about their personal financial well-being all increase during economic slumps. And each of these factors also increases support for federal involvement in health care, both in absolute terms and relative to other domestic policies. In a year in which public opinion polls indicated that the economy was foremost in the minds of prospective voters, it is thus not surprising that health was ranked in these same polls as a second most influential issue. (This also explains in part why health played such a small role during the relatively prosperous economic conditions of 1988, though health care costs and gaps in private insurance were every bit as evident as they are today.)

The specific reforms that can best capture public support, however, will depend in part on how policymakers frame particular issues and cast different reform proposals. Our findings may also shed some light on these prospects. Consider two examples.

The first involves the characterization of health care as a societal investment. Virtually every proposal that has been introduced to Congress has been cast in these terms. The Pepper Commission report (1990), for example, described gradually "building universal coverage" and spoke of the long-term costs of an inadequate investment strategy. "Some say we cannot afford universal coverage. The Commission believes that a decision *not* to make this investment would cost the country incomparably more: the disintegration of our health care system and the waste of our most precious resource, the health and human potential of our people" (pp. 9–10).

Describing health care reform in these terms is tempting. Characterizing health care initiatives as an investment alludes to the promise of long-term benefits to society. These might convince voters to accept larger short-term costs. Describing health care as an investment builds upon philosophers' claims that health and health care are essential prerequisites for equal economic opportunity. Equal opportunity is perhaps the most broadly held and deeply felt norm in contemporary American society (Kluegel and Smith 1986). And our results suggest that support for health initiatives is linked, more than for other social policies, to concerns about equal opportunity. Since norms of opportunity have motivated other societal investments, such as public support for higher education, this would also seem an effective strategy for health care (Smith 1987).

However, a concern for equal opportunity does not necessarily translate into thinking about health care as an investment, particularly a long-term investment. Americans may view health as a prerequisite for opportunity in a more immediate sense, and thus expect health care spending to have more immediate returns. To explore this issue, we attempted to determine which types of societal spending were favored by those who supported more spending on health care. The rationale is that if people think about health care as a long-term investment, those who support more spending on health care should also favor other long-term investments, such as education or the environment. Conversely, if health care is expected to have short-term returns, those who favor greater spending on health care should also favor greater spending in other areas with short-term payoffs.

The 1987 GSS asked respondents about their support for greater societal spending in fifteen different areas. These included areas with short-term benefits (e.g., crime control, welfare programs, or Social Security cash benefits) as well as those with long-term benefits (e.g., education or the environment). A factor analysis was used to determine how people tended to group together their support for different types of spending.[23] One factor could be best described as spending that was perceived as an investment. This included spending on education, the environment, mass transit, and highways. Support for spending on health care was only slightly correlated with this factor. Health care was instead grouped with

23. The factors were estimated using a maximum likelihood technique. The results described in the text are invariant to whether the factors were analyzed using either orthogonal or oblique rotations.

spending on Social Security and other programs with short-term "pay-offs." This suggests that health spending is in fact not associated with long-term societal investments.

These findings do not imply that health care could not be recast into a form of investment in American thinking. Such a shift might well be politically advantageous. But this perspective on health care does not apparently exist today, so that simply describing health care as an investment is not likely to tap into a natural reservoir of popular support.

A second issue in the implementation of federal health care reforms involves the relationship between government-sponsored benefits and methods of paying for those benefits. This connection has received relatively little attention. Not surprisingly, most politicians have focused attention on the benefits offered by their plans and been vague about financing those benefits. Some analysts of American public opinion, however, have made claims about how health care reform should be financed. A recent review of public opinion surveys, for example, recommended that "any new program of universal health care should rely on taxes other than the progressive income tax for its chief financing" (Blendon and Donelan 1990). This assessment was based largely on the popular rejection and political repeal of the Medicare catastrophic amendments in 1989. Their failure was linked to income tax financing that was part of the amendments. They were seen as a harbinger of prospects for broader reform of the health care system.

But there are a number of reasons to believe that this rejection of progressive taxation is a serious misreading of American public opinion. The Medicare amendments did not lose popular support because of their financing arrangements. A 1990 survey found that 58 percent of all Americans (and more than half of all elders) supported the proposal that "Medicare premiums should be based on income." Only about a quarter of all respondents were opposed to this reform (Schlesinger and Kronebusch 1991). The rejection of the Medicare catastrophic amendments occurred not because taxes were viewed as inequitable, but because the benefits were seen as inadequate by elders, whether or not they expected to pay any taxes to support the coverage (Rice et al. 1990). More generally, our analyses suggest that there are several potential positive linkages between health care reform and progressive mechanisms for financing those reforms. Those who support health care appear to do so in part because they believe there to be too large a gap between the rich and the poor in American society. A financing mechanism that directly addresses this gap should thus reinforce support. Moreover, support for health care initiatives appears to legitimize greater support for income redistribution. Thus health-related benefits that are tied to a particular tax make progressive financing more acceptable to the American public (see Table 7).

Because the data used in this paper represented only crude measures of the attitudes, perceptions, and levels of support that we attempted to measure, these interpretations of the past and forecasts for the future must be viewed as rather speculative. More careful study is required of what Americans think they are getting when they demand federal action in the health care arena.

However sophisticated the analyses, though, one cannot and should not read too much into simple reports of popular opinion. Based on naive projections of public opinion, the United States should have adopted national health insurance a half century ago. But this is less a caution against examining public opinion than it is a caveat against an overly simplistic approach to that task. We have attempted to demonstrate here that many of the more interesting questions involve looking, not at the level of public support for different proposals—standard operating procedure in this area—but at differences in support: over time, across policy areas, among different groups of respondents. It is these differences that offer perhaps the greatest insights into how Americans think about government's role in health care as well as how these attitudes and perceptions subsequently translate into public policy.

Appendix Attitudes, Perceptions, and Norms That Shape Support for Social Policies (Three-stage Least Squares Regression Models)

				Dependent Variables				
	Support for Health Policy		Support for General Domestic Policies		Support for Programs for the Poor		Support for Redistribution from Rich to Poor	
Attitudes, Norms, and Perceptions of Respondents	Coefficient	T-Statistic	Coefficient	T-Statistic	Coefficient	T-Statistic	Coefficient	T-Statistic
Support for Other Policies								
Health Care Programs			−0.84	0.82	0.76	2.35	0.89	1.96
Antipoverty Programs	0.52	2.66	0.98	1.89			0.13	0.41
General Domestic Policies	−0.19	0.76			0.60	2.93	−0.43	1.08
Income Redistribution	0.15	0.56	−0.01	0.02	0.22	0.30		
Individual Responsibility for Outcomes								
Believes Well-Being Shaped by Happenstance	0.02	0.35	0.07	0.65	−0.06	0.91	0.04	0.46
Believes Well-Being Shaped by Traits at Birth	0.03	1.27	0.03	0.63	−0.04	1.65	0.01	0.21
Believes Well-Being Determined by Hard Work	0.12	2.30	0.17	1.38	−0.15	2.50	−0.07	0.82
Ethical Basis for Responding to Others' Needs								
Believes Average Man Getting Worse Off	−0.11	0.77	−0.20	0.76	0.11	0.64	0.30	1.83
Believes Standard of Living Should Be Guaranteed for Unemployed	0.13	1.66	0.21	1.05	−0.15	1.76	0.07	0.68

Belief in Policy as Prerequisite for Equal Opportunity, as Indicated By

Belief That Well-Being Is Shaped by Parents' Education/Wealth	0.06	2.17	−0.07	0.82	−0.04	0.93	−0.06	1.17
Support for College Aid for Low-Income Youth	0.12	1.57	0.18	0.94	−0.12	1.37	0.03	0.27
Support for Redistribution, as Indicated By								
Concern about Societal Conflict	0.05	1.16	0.08	0.80	−0.08	1.70	0.04	0.66
Belief That Income Differences in U.S. Are Too Large	−0.05	0.57	−0.01	0.09	−0.002	0.02	0.25	3.48
Support for Aid to Blacks (Racial Affect)	−0.17	1.72	−0.13	0.59	0.05	0.37	0.38	3.26
Perception of Self-Interest								
Feeling Well-off Relative to Other Americans	−0.10	−1.65	−0.14	1.05	0.11	1.67	0.06	0.61
Feeling Better-off Than in Past Few Years	0.17	2.15	0.29	1.66	−0.19	2.01	−0.22	0.82
Feeling Burdened by Taxes	0.01	0.05	−0.02	0.13	−0.05	0.53	0.11	0.92
Preference for Secure Job (Risk Aversion)	0.02	0.39	0.08	0.85	−0.08	1.42	0.12	1.85
Altruistic Concerns								
Perceives Importance of Altruism	0.02	0.52	0.02	0.26	−0.002	0.04	0.002	0.03
Institutional Concerns and Concern about Bureaucracy								
Confidence in Health Care System	0.02	0.57						
Satisfaction with Own Health	0.00	0.01						
Confidence in Business Community	−0.04	0.76	−0.86	0.66	0.08	1.42	−0.10	1.45
Trust in Local Government	−0.09	1.51	−0.18	1.52	0.13	1.87	0.02	0.21

References

Alves, Wayne, and Peter Rossi. 1978. Who Should Get What? Fairness Judgments of the Distribution of Income. *American Journal of Sociology* 84 (3): 541–64.

American Association of Retired Persons. 1987. *Intergenerational Tensions: Real or Imagined?* Washington, DC: American Association of Retired Persons.

Batson, C. Daniel, and Kathryn Oleson. 1991. Current Status of the Empathy-Altruism Hypothesis. In *Prosocial Behavior*, ed. Margaret Clark. Newbury Park, CA: Sage.

Baybrooke, David. 1987. *Meeting Needs*. Princeton, NJ: Princeton University Press.

Beauchamp, Dan. 1988. *The Health of the Republic: Epidemics, Medicine and Moralism as Challenges to Democracy*. Philadelphia: Temple University Press.

Beauchamp, Tom, and Ruth Faden. 1979. The Right to Health and the Right to Health Care. *Journal of Medicine and Philosophy* 4 (2): 118–31.

Bell, Nora. 1979. The Scarcity of Medical Resources: Are There Rights to Health Care? *Journal of Medicine and Philosophy* 4 (2): 158–69.

Blendon, Robert, and Karen Donelan. 1989. The 1988 Election: How Important Was Health? *Health Affairs* 8 (3): 6–15.

———. 1990. The Public and the Emerging Debate over National Health Insurance. *New England Journal of Medicine* 323 (3): 208–12.

Blendon, Robert, Robert Leitman, Ian Morrison, and Karen Donelan. 1990. Satisfaction with Health Systems in Ten Nations. *Health Affairs* 9 (2): 185–92.

Blendon, Robert, and Ulrike Szalay. 1992. Americans and Their Health Care. Boston, MA: Harvard University School of Public Health.

Blue Cross/Blue Shield. 1990. *Second Opinions: America's Voices and Views on Health Care*. Chicago: Blue Cross/Blue Shield Association.

Boulding, Kenneth. 1973. The Concept of Need for Health Services. In *Economic Aspects of Health Care*, ed. John McKinlay. New York: Prodist.

Bowler, Kenneth, Robert Kudrle, and Theodore Marmor. 1978. The Political Economy of National Health Insurance: Policy Analysis and Political Evaluation. In *Toward a National Health Policy*, ed. Kenneth Friedman and Stuart Rakoff. Lexington, MA: Lexington Books.

Brown, Lawrence. 1978. The Scope and Limits of Equality as a Normative Guide to Federal Health Care Policy. *Public Policy* 26 (4): 481–532.

Brown, Michael. 1988. The Segmented Welfare System: Distributive Conflict and Retrenchment in the United States, 1968–84. In *Remaking the Welfare State: Retrenchment and Social Policy in America and Europe*, ed. Michael Brown. Philadelphia: Temple University Press.

Buchanan, Allen. 1984. The Right to a Decent Minimum of Health Care. *Philosophy and Public Affairs* 13:55–78.

Callahan, Daniel. 1990. *What Kind of Life?* New York: Simon and Schuster.

Caplan, Barbara. 1987. Linking Cultural Characteristics to Political Opinions. In *Ignored Voices: Public Opinion Polls and the Latino Community*, ed. Rodolfo de la Garza. Austin, TX: Center for Mexican American Studies Publications, University of Texas Press.

Carmines, Edward, and James Stimson. 1989. *Issue Evolution: Race and the Transformation of American Politics*. Princeton, NJ: Princeton University Press.

Childress, James. 1979. A Right to Health Care. *Journal of Medicine and Philosophy* 4 (2): 132–47.

Citrin, Jack, and Donald Green. 1990. The Self-Interest Motive in American Public Opinion. In *Research in Micropolitics: A Research Annual*, ed. Samuel Long. Greenwich, CT: JAI.

Congressional Budget Office. 1991. *Policy Choices for Long-Term Care*. Washington, DC: Congressional Budget Office.

Coughlin, Richard. 1980. *Ideology, Public Opinion and Welfare Policy: Attitudes toward Taxes and Spending in Industrialized Societies*. Berkeley: University of California, Institute of International Studies.

Daniels, Norm. 1985. *Just Health Care*. London: Cambridge University Press.

Dougherty, Charles. 1988. *American Health Care: Realities, Rights and Reforms*. New York: Oxford University Press.

Fein, Rashi. 1986. *Medical Care, Medical Costs*. Cambridge, MA: Harvard University Press.

Fried, Charles. 1976. Equality and Rights in Medical Care. *Hastings Center Report* 6 (February): 29–34.

Frohlich, Norman, Joe Oppenheimer, and Cheryl Eavey. 1987. Laboratory Results on Rawl's Distributive Justice. *British Journal of Political Science* 17:1–21.

Gabel, John, Howard Cohen, and Stephen Fink. 1989. Americans' Views on Health Care: Foolish Inconsistencies? *Health Affairs* 8 (1): 103–18.

Gallup Organization. 1992. *Public Attitudes on National Health Insurance, 1992*. Washington, DC: Employee Benefit Research Institute.

General Social Survey. 1975, 1983, 1987, 1989. Surveys conducted for the National Data Program for the Social Sciences at the National Opinion Research Center, University of Chicago.

Goodin, Robert. 1988. *Reasons for Welfare: The Political Theory of the Welfare State*. Princeton, NJ: Princeton University Press.

Goodin, Robert, and John Dryzek. 1987. Risk-sharing and Social Justice: The Motivational Foundations of the Post-War Welfare State. In *Not Only the Poor*, ed. J. LeGrand and R. Goodin. London: Allen and Unwin.

Gottschalk, Barbara, and Peter Gottschalk. 1988. The Reagan Retrenchment in Historical Context. In *Remaking the Welfare State: Retrenchment and Social Policy in America and Europe*, ed. Michael Brown. Philadelphia: Temple University Press.

Greenstone, J. David. 1988. The Decline and Revival of the American Welfare State: Moral Criteria and Instrumental Reasoning in Critical Elections. In *Remaking the Welfare State: Retrenchment and Social Policy in America and Europe*, ed. Michael Brown. Philadelphia: Temple University Press.

Gutmann, Amy. 1988. Introduction. In *Democracy and the Welfare State*, ed. Amy Gutmann. Princeton, NJ: Princeton University Press.

Hamilton, Howard, and Sylvan Cohen. 1974. *Policy Making by Plebiscite: School Referenda*. Lexington, MA: Lexington Books.

Hayek, F. 1960. *The Constitution of Liberty*. London: Routledge and Kegan Paul.

Health Insurance Association of America. 1991. *Source Book of Health Insurance Data*. Washington, DC: Health Insurance Association of America.

Hirschfield, Daniel. 1970. *The Lost Reform: The Campaign for Compulsory Health Insurance in the United States from 1932 to 1945*. Cambridge, MA: Harvard University Press.

Hochschild, Jennifer. 1981. *What's Fair? American Beliefs about Distributive Justice*. Cambridge, MA: Harvard University Press.

Hodgkinson, Virginia, and Murray Weitzman. 1988. *Giving and Volunteering in the United States: Findings from a National Survey*. Washington, DC: Independent Sector.

Jajich-Toth, Cindy, and Burns Roper. 1990. Americans' Views on Health Care: A Study in Contradictions. *Health Affairs* 9 (4): 149–57.

Katz, Michael. 1986. *In the Shadow of the Poorhouse: A Social History of Welfare in America*. New York: Basic.

Keiser, K. 1987. Congress and Black Health: Dynamics and Strategies. In *Health Care Issues in Black America*, ed. W. Jones and M. Rice. New York: Greenwood.

Kelley, Stanley. 1988. Democracy and the New Deal Party System. In *Democracy and the Welfare State*, ed. Amy Gutmann. Princeton, NJ: Princeton University Press.

Kluegel, James, and Eliot Smith. 1986. *Beliefs about Inequality: Americans' Views of What Is and What Ought to Be*. New York: Aldine de Gruyter.

Lundberg, George. 1991. National Health Care Reform: An Aura of Inevitability Is upon Us. *Journal of the American Medical Association* 265 (10): 2566–67.

Marmor, Theodore. 1973. *The Politics of Medicare*. Chicago: Aldine.

Melville, Keith, and John Doble, eds. 1988. *The Public's Perspective on Social Welfare Reform*. New York: Public Agenda Foundation.

Merlis, Mark. 1990. Controlling Health Care Costs. In *A Call for Action* (Supplement to Final Report). Washington, DC: U.S. Government Printing Office.

Moon, J. Donald. 1988. The Moral Basis of the Democratic Welfare State. In *Democracy and the Welfare State*, ed. Amy Gutmann. Princeton, NJ: Princeton University Press.

Moon, Marilyn. 1990. Limiting Favored Tax Treatment for Employee Health Insurance. In *A Call for Action* (Supplement to Final Report). Washington, DC: U.S. Government Printing Office.

Morone, James. 1981. The Real World of Representation and the HSAs. In *Health Planning in the United States: Selected Policy Issues*, vol. 2, ed. Committee on Health Planning Goals and Standards, Institute of Medicine. Washington, DC: National Academy Press.

Moskop, John. 1983. Rawlsian Justice and a Human Right to Health Care. *Journal of Medicine and Philosophy* 8 (4): 329–38.

Navarro, V. 1987. Federal Health Policies in the United States: An Alternative Explanation. *Milbank Quarterly* 65 (1): 81–111.

Page, Benjamin, and Robert Shapiro. 1992. *The Rational Public*. Chicago: University of Chicago Press.

Pepper Commission (U.S. Bipartisan Commission on Comprehensive Health Care). 1990. *A Call for Action*. Washington, DC: U.S. Government Printing Office.

Pescosolido, Bernice, Carol Boyer, and Wai Ying Tsui. 1986. Medical Care in the

Welfare State: A Cross-National Study of Public Evaluations. *Journal of Health and Social Behavior* 26 (December): 276–97.

Ponza, Michael, Greg Duncan, Mary Corcoran, and Fred Groskind. 1988. The Guns of Autumn? Age Differences in Support for Income Transfers to the Young and Old. *Public Opinion Quarterly* 52:441–66.

Rae, Douglas. 1981. *Equalities*. Cambridge, MA: Harvard University Press.

Rawls, John. 1971. *A Theory of Justice*. Cambridge, MA: Harvard University Press.

Reinhardt, Uwe. 1990. West Germany's Health-Care and Health-Insurance System: Combining Universal Access with Cost Control. In *A Call for Action* (Supplement to Final Report). Washington, DC: U.S. Government Printing Office.

Relman, Arnold. 1992. What Market Values Are Doing to Medicine. *Atlantic* (March): 99–106.

Rice, Thomas, Kathrine Desmond, and Jon Gabel. 1990. Medicare Catastrophic Coverage Act: A Post-Mortem. *Health Affairs* 9 (3): 75–87.

Rimlinger, Gaston. 1971. *Welfare Policy and Industrialization in Europe, America and Russia*. New York: John Wiley.

Rochefort, David, and Carol Boyer. 1988. Use of Public Opinion Data in Public Administration: Health Care Polls. *Public Administration Review* 48 (March/April): 649–60.

Rushing, William. 1986. *Social Functions and Economic Aspects of Health Insurance*. Boston: Kluwer-Nijhoff.

Sapolsky, Harvey, Drew Altman, Richard Greene, and Judith Moore. 1981. Corporate Attitudes toward Health Care Costs. *Milbank Memorial Fund Quarterly* 59 (Fall): 561–85.

Sardell, Alice. 1988. *The U.S. Experiment in Social Medicine: The Community Health Center Program, 1965–1986*. Pittsburgh, PA: University of Pittsburgh Press.

Sass, Hans-Martin. 1983. Justice, Beneficence or Common Sense?: The President's Commission's Report on Access to Health Care. *Journal of Medicine and Philosophy* 8 (4): 381–88.

Schlesinger, Mark. 1986. On the Limits of Expanding Health Care Reform: Chronic Care in Prepaid Settings. *Milbank Quarterly* 64 (2): 189–215.

———. 1987. Paying the Price: Medical Care, Minorities and the Newly Competitive Health Care System. *Milbank Quarterly* 65 (Supplement 2): 270–96.

Schlesinger, Mark, and Karl Kronebusch. 1991. Intergenerational Relations, Tensions and Conflict: Attitudes and Perceptions about Social Justice and Age-related Needs. Paper presented at the annual meetings of the American Gerontological Society, 21–24 November 1991.

Schlitz, Michael. 1970. *Public Attitudes toward Social Security 1935–1965*. USDHEW SSA Research Report 33. Washington, DC: Social Security Administration, Office of Research and Statistics.

Sears, David, and Jack Citrin. 1982. *Tax Revolt: Something for Nothing in California*. Cambridge, MA: Harvard University Press.

Sears, David, and Carolyn Funk. 1990. Self-Interest in Americans' Political Opinions. In *Beyond Self-Interest*, ed. Jane Mansbridge. Chicago: University of Chicago Press.

Shapiro, Robert, Kelly Patterson, Judith Russell, and John Young. 1987. The Polls—

A Report: Employment and Social Welfare. *Public Opinion Quarterly* 51:268–81.

Shapiro, Robert, and John Young. 1986. The Polls: Medical Care in the United States. *Public Opinion Quarterly* 50:418–28.

———. 1989. Public Opinion and the Welfare State: The United States in Comparative Perspective. *Political Science Quarterly* 104 (1): 59–89.

Shingles, Richard. 1989. Class, Status, and Support for Government Aid to Disadvantaged Groups. *Journal of Politics* 51 (4): 933–62.

Siegler, Mark. 1979. A Right to Health Care: Ambiguity, Professional Responsibility and Patient Liberty. *Journal of Medicine and Philosophy* 4 (2): 148–57.

Smith, Tom. 1987. The Polls—A Report: The Welfare State in Cross-National Perspective. *Public Opinion Quarterly* 51:404–21.

Starr, Paul. 1982. *The Social Transformation of American Medicine*. New York: Basic.

Stern, Lawrence. 1983. Opportunity and Health Care: Criticisms and Suggestions. *Journal of Medicine and Philosophy* 8 (4): 339–62.

Stone, Deborah. 1979. Diagnosis and the Dole: The Function of Illness in American Distributive Politics. *Journal of Health Politics, Policy and Law* 4 (3): 507–21.

———. 1987. The Resistible Rise of Preventive Medicine. In *Health Policy in Transition*, ed. Lawrence Brown. Durham, NC: Duke University Press.

Striber, Steven, and Leonard Ferber. 1981. Support for National Health Insurance. *Public Opinion Quarterly* 45:179–98.

Sundquist, James. 1986. Has America Lost Its Social Conscience—And How Will It Get It Back? *Political Science Quarterly* 101 (4): 513–33.

Taylor, Humphrey, and Robert Leitman. 1991. *Trade-Offs and Choices: Health Policy Options for the 1990s*. New York: Louis Harris.

Tornblom, Kjell, and Uriel Foa. 1983. Choice of a Distribution Principle: Crosscultural Evidence on the Effects of Resources. *Acta Sociologica* 26:161–73.

Tropman, John. 1987. *Public Policy Opinion and the Elderly, 1952–1978: A Kaleidoscope of Culture*. Westport, CT: Greenwood.

Walzer, Michael. 1983. *Spheres of Justice: A Defense of Pluralism and Equality*. New York: Basic.

Weir, Margaret, Ann Shola Orloff, and Theda Skocpol. 1988. Introduction: Understanding American Social Politics. In *The Politics of Social Policy in the United States*, ed. Margaret Weir, Ann Shola Orloff, and Theda Skocpol. Princeton, NJ: Princeton University Press.

White, Robert. 1971. *Right to Health Care: The Evolution of an Idea*. Des Moines: University of Iowa Press.

Wildavsky, Aaron. 1977. Doing Better and Feeling Worse: The Political Pathology of Health Policy. *Daedalus* 107 (1): 105–23.

Wohlenberg, Ernest. 1976. A Regional Approach to Public Attitudes and Public Assistance. *Social Service Review* (September): 491–505.

Wright, Gerald, Robert Erikson, and John McIver. 1987. Public Opinion and Political Liberalism in the American States. *American Journal of Political Science* 31: 980–1001.

The Politics
of American Ambivalence
toward Government

Lawrence R. Jacobs

Abstract This paper presents two interrelated arguments: it rethinks conventional understanding of the policy-making process and analyzes an important substantive issue regarding public opinion. The substantive issue involves the public's deep ambivalence toward government reforms: Americans are simultaneously supportive of significant reform and uneasy about expanding government involvement. The critical question is what, if any, impact this public ambivalence will have on policy deliberations. Answering this question requires an analysis of the role of public opinion in policy-making. Investigation of historic as well as contemporary health reform suggests that the impact of public opinion varies, depending on the character of both public opinion and the policy issue. The public's preferences are not especially influential when they are characterized by uncertainty or when an issue is not salient, but strong and sustained sentiment can affect agenda setting, interest group leverage over government officials, and policymakers' formulation of detailed administrative arrangements.

Americans are deeply ambivalent toward reforming government involvement in health care: they are simultaneously supportive of significant reform and uneasy about expanding the government's role. What is the political relevance of this ambivalence? Its impact is not revealed by an exclusive focus on the content and distribution of public opinion. After all, public sentiment—even when directed toward a politically charged subject—does not have an inherent political significance. Officeholders and policy specialists may well misperceive, fail to recognize, or outright defy public opinion. What must be studied, then, is not only Americans' simultaneous support and dread of government reform but also whether and how a relationship develops between these public preferences and policy-making. The critical question is, what, if any, impact will public ambivalence have on health reform deliberations?

The relationship between Americans' ambivalence and policy-making is important because it helps explain the current, peculiar mismatch between skyrocketing budgetary outlays for health care and weak governmental controls over costs. When Medicare was formulated in the early 1960s, politicians and policy specialists responded both to the public's support for expanding access to health care and its uneasiness with direct and visible government regulation of the associated costs. They significantly expanded the government's financial commitment to health care but ceded authority over budgetary decisions to private entities—insurers acting as financial intermediaries. Following the passage of Medicare in 1965, American health policy took a perverse turn: in an effort to avoid the most dreaded outcome—overt government regulation of aggregate budgets—policymakers were forced as health costs soared to rely on less visible but far more intrusive government scrutiny of providers' everyday clinical behavior. During the past three decades, providers, private purchasers, and insurers have used the public's dread of government as a shield to resist central budgetary control; they prefer regulation of clinical behavior because it is relatively less threatening to their incomes and institutional positions (Brown 1992).[1]

Enduring public ambivalence toward government, then, is the underlying source of America's impasse—its inability to expand access to essential care while administratively containing the associated costs. This paper explores the political relevance of current public attitudes for contemporary debates over health reform. The first section concentrates on public opinion per se and on the contours of Americans' current ambivalence toward government. The next section discusses the general institutional and political context for public opinion's growing role in policy-making. The final part examines the relationship between public ambivalence and contemporary health policy debates; in it, I suggest that public opinion's impact fluctuates depending on the character of both Americans' attitudes and the policy issue.

The Impasse

The Constitution's framers deliberately designed American governmental institutions to encourage division and rivalry. To offset the systemic pres-

---

1. See Morone 1990 for an alternative interpretation of policy innovation in the context of dread of government.

sure toward deadlock, modern officeholders have looked—as Theodore Lowi explains—to "mobilize the electorate in order to unify the elite" (1985: 165). Attempts to mobilize Americans behind comprehensive health reform present a special problem; both opponents and supporters of reform can legitimately draw on competing elements of public opinion.

The Public's Support of Government Reform

Today, Americans both place health reform high on their policy-making agenda and favor specific policy arrangements like universal coverage. By the 1990s, the public identified major health care reform as a top priority because they were dissatisfied with the current system and preferred— nine out of ten of them—to rebuild or fundamentally change this system (Jacobs et al. forthcoming). By December 1991, 11 percent ranked health care as the issue that mattered most to them in the upcoming presidential elections; an additional 72 percent ranked it as one of several important issues.[2] Harris Wofford's dramatic comeback victory in Pennsylvania's 1991 senatorial contest became a resounding symbol of the public's strong interest in reform.

The signal of public concern that was sent by Wofford's upset landslide was reinforced by the 1992 presidential elections. Two separate opinion surveys conducted on election night, 3 November 1992, reported that Americans ranked health care as the third most important issue facing the country, behind the economy and the budget deficit. What makes these findings striking is that the economy has been the top concern in nearly all postwar elections, with other policy issues competing for the other slots; in 1992, health care rose above often more salient issues like abortion, crime, taxes, education, and foreign policy (see polls reported in Blendon et al. 1992; Roper Center 1992b).[3] Health care's salience was especially high among Bill Clinton's supporters, who ranked the issue as their second most important concern (Blendon et al. 1992). Since the election, Americans have continued to rank health care quite high.[4]

2. The ABC/*Washington Post* survey (11–15 December 1991) asked "In the next presidential election, how important will a candidate's position on health care be in determining your vote?" One percent responded that they had no opinion, and 16 percent responded that it would not have much influence.

3. The Harris poll (Louis Harris and Associates 1992a) found that the economy and candidate character were the top two issues while the Roper poll (Roper Center 1992b) reported the economy and budget deficit receiving top billing.

4. Blendon et al. (1992) reported in December 1992 that health care was third on the public's agenda for action by the new Congress and president during their first hundred days (the economy and the deficit won the top two spots).

Not only do Americans place health reform near the top of their policy agenda, but they also hold strong, sustained preferences regarding the specific direction of policy formulation. Both direct and indirect evidence suggests that the public has clear preferences on whether to extend health insurance coverage to all Americans—regardless of age or income.

The general policy objective of establishing a national health insurance (NHI) plan covering all Americans—which would be financed through taxes—has been found by different polling organizations to attract support from 60 percent to 70 percent of respondents.[5] This level of support for a tax-financed program is ten to twenty points higher than it was a decade ago and represents a forty-year high. Moreover, Americans' preference for the Canadian health care system over their own country's stems in part from support for universal coverage: 94 percent of respondents identified this principle as an attractive feature of the Canadian system.[6] Finally, the public's support for the general principle of universalism is confirmed by a fall 1991 poll, which reported 82 percent agreeing that the government should guarantee everyone health insurance coverage (16 percent disagreed) (Princeton Survey 1991).

An important issue is left unanswered by this evidence: do Americans prefer an all-encompassing program or one that extends insurance to low-income Americans? The evidence suggests that the public leans toward the former. Polling results consistently indicate that the public's support for national health insurance is greatest when the reform promises to cover all Americans rather than target the uninsured and poor.[7]

5. In the early 1980s, the levels of support for national health insurance, financed by tax money and paying for most forms of health care, hovered around 50 percent (approximately 42 percent opposed it); by 1993, support for a national health plan moved to 64 percent and opposition dropped to 26 percent (Jacobs et al. forthcoming; Shapiro and Young 1986; Roper Center 1991). The following polls were distributed by the Roper Center: CBS/*New York Times* 1991; Louis Harris and Associates 1991a, 1991b; Yankelovich, Clancy, Shulman 1991; CBS/*New York Times* 1992.

6. Surveys in 1988, 1990, and 1991 all reported that Americans preferred the Canadian health care system over the existing system in the U.S. The wording for the three surveys was as follows: "In the Canadian system of National Health Insurance, the government pays most of the cost of health care for everyone out of taxes, and the government sets all fees charged by doctors and hospitals. Under the Canadian system, people can choose their own doctors and hospitals. On balance, would you prefer the Canadian system or the system we have here?" The following were the levels of support reported by each poll: In the 1991 survey, 68 percent favored the Canadian system, 29 percent opted for the American, and 3 percent were not sure; for 1990, the respective percentages were 45 percent, 37 percent, and 18 percent; for 1988, 61 percent, 37 percent, and 1 percent (Jajich-Toth and Roper 1990; Louis Harris and Associates 1988, 1991b). The 1990 survey asked respondents favoring the Canadian system what made it attractive. For a critique of Jajich-Toth and Roper's analysis of the 1990 survey see Blendon and Donelan 1991.

7. An August 1991 poll found that 67 percent favored providing a "national health insurance program for all Americans, even if this would require higher taxes" (28 percent were opposed

Perhaps the most convincing case, though, for public support of universalism involves the instability and erosion of middle America's insurance coverage: the issue of access has been transformed from a matter of sympathy for the down-and-out who lack insurance to a question of maintaining coverage for the stably employed. In one survey, 32 percent of respondents identified access as the second leading source of dissatisfaction with the existing health system; what is striking, though, is that the primary object of frustration was cost (identified by 56 percent) (Jajich-Toth and Roper 1990). The ranking of cost followed by access is a pattern that emerges from multiple surveys (Jacobs et al. forthcoming). This disillusionment with cost stems not so much from apprehension over abstract issues relating to governmental and business budgets as from Americans' fear that uncontrollable health expenses leave them personally vulnerable to having their access curtailed or suspended.

Support for universal coverage reflects the public's broad-based anxiety about the future and its ability to meet the everyday expenses associated with health care—the costs of premiums, of using a doctor or hospital, and of filling prescriptions. A series of surveys in 1989 and in the fall of 1991 found that a large majority of Americans—even among the insured—feared that their current insurance coverage would be reduced or eliminated and that their future health care needs would be unaffordable and inaccessible (Roper Center 1992a). These fears are firmly rooted in the experiences of millions of Americans: the numbers reporting that their insurance benefits had been reduced during the previous two years jumped from nearly one in five respondents in 1990 to one in three in 1991; employees are picking up a greater portion of their premiums and are going on strike not to raise their wages but to keep their health benefits.[8] Not surprisingly, the ranks of the uninsured are increasingly taking on the characteristics of mainstream America—they are neither poor nor unemployed. This mainstreaming of the uninsured population is likely to

---

and 5 percent were not sure). Just four months later, another poll found that when the question was framed in terms of "Americans who are not likely to be covered by health insurance," the level of support for reform dropped to 54 percent and the level of opposition rose to 42 percent (Yankelovich, Clancy, Shulman 1991; Mellman and Lazarus Public Opinion 1992). Moreover, a 1979 survey explicitly asked respondents to choose either a health insurance program that expanded coverage for the unemployed and poor or a plan that would encompass all Americans; two-thirds chose the universal program (Blendon 1988).

8. Health care is cited as the major issue for striking by 55 percent of those on picket lines. The importance of rising health costs to working America is illustrated by the fact that 69 percent of workers permanently replaced had primarily gone on strike over health care (Roper Center 1991: 5; 1992a: 87).

continue as businesses are forced by rising costs to curtail or withdraw insurance coverage (Rovner 1992; Blendon and Donelan 1990).

The widespread support for universalism is often underestimated by national policymakers. According to the *National Journal*, many in Washington fear that "universal coverage" will be perceived as a concentrated benefit, which helps only the one-fifth of Americans who are uninsured. The suspected political danger is that this concentrated payoff of reform will not offset the clear and widely shared costs associated with increased restrictions and financial charges: the four out of five who are insured will have little of substance to show for their sacrifices (Kosterlitz 1993). But polling results and changes in Americans' real-world experiences clearly suggest that universal coverage would be welcomed by middle America's insured population as a solution to the erosion both in their ability to meet future health care costs and in their job security and flexibility. Because of the fundamental changes of the past two decades, universalism would be perceived today as a widely shared (and not concentrated) benefit.

The Public's Dread of Government

The public's support for putting reform at the top of the agenda and establishing universalism coexists with an enduring uneasiness toward government. This peculiar intermingling of support and dread is the defining characteristic of American public opinion toward health reform, and it is a source of America's impasse over universalizing access while containing costs.

There are two broad indicators of the public's lingering uneasiness toward government involvement in the provision of social welfare benefits in general and health care in particular. The first broad indicator is general: analysis of public opinion in a number of policy areas suggests that uneasiness over the government's role transcends ideological or partisan identification. Democrats are much more likely than Republicans to support a tax-financed national health plan, but even liberal support is tempered by concern over the problems of bureaucracy and the practical limits to what government can accomplish.[9] Moreover, Americans' confidence and trust in government has eroded over the past several decades

9. See Feldman and Zaller 1992 for a discussion of dread of government among Americans who most strongly support social welfare programs.

(Lipset and Schneider 1983). Americans' dread of government, then, is a general trend that characterizes divergent ideological groups as well as public opinion toward different policy areas.

The second broad indicator of Americans' governmental dread involves several types of survey data specifically on health reform. Thus, a series of survey questions has asked respondents to choose between a reliance on government and a private-oriented approach; large numbers of respondents have identified the private approach.[10] An election night poll by Louis Harris (1992a) found similar results: when voters were given descriptions of Clinton's and Bush's plans (without mentioning the candidate's name), the Democrat's proposal was more popular, but the margin (52 to 41 percent) was not large.[11]

Moreover, a number of recent surveys have reported that Americans harbor quite specific fears regarding greater government involvement; they anticipate—among other things—undesirable trends regarding the cost of care, the quality of treatment, and the freedom of choice available to them.[12] On election day, Louis Harris (1992b) found that many Americans were opposed (by a 48 to 43 percent margin) to the "federal government setting a yearly dollar limit on total private and government spending for all health care" (Blendon et al. 1992).

This evidence does not indicate that Americans have written government off and remain unalterably opposed to its role in social welfare provision. The enthusiastic acceptance of Social Security and Medicare alone shatters any simplistic notion of American fidelity to genuine laissez-faire individualism. What wide-ranging opinion surveys do indicate, though,

10. Between 1990 and 1992, three surveys asked the question "Would you rather pay higher taxes and have the government be in charge of the organization and delivery of health care services, or would you rather pay more money out of your pocket directly to private doctors and hospitals, with government involvement only for people who cannot pay for their own care?" Majorities consistently preferred paying private providers over putting the government in charge. By 1992, though, the public was more ambivalent over this choice: the split narrowed from 60 to 34 percent in 1990 to 52 to 44 percent in 1992 (Jacobs et al. forthcoming).

11. The Louis Harris survey was conducted on behalf of the Henry J. Kaiser Family Foundation (Blendon et al. 1992).

12. Surveys in 1990 and 1992 indicate strong reservations about a "government-run national health insurance plan": in 1990, 31 percent feared the program would cost more, and 39 percent expected it to cost less; opinion shifted by 1992, with 42 percent anxious that it would cost more and only 25 percent anticipating it costing less. In terms of quality, the 1990 survey reported that 39 percent expected lower quality and 16 percent improved quality; the 1992 poll found similar results (37 percent and 13 percent, respectively). Finally, a majority of respondents in both surveys envisioned less freedom of choice (53 percent in 1990 and 54 percent in 1992); in both polls only 12 percent expected freedom to increase (Jajich-Toth and Roper 1990; Roper Center 1992a).

is that uneasiness toward government persists. Fears of bureaucratic red tape, of infringement on the doctor-patient relationship, and of erosion in the quality and timeliness of treatment may all appear exaggerated or unfounded to policy experts, but they nonetheless define the context in which health reform will be formulated. Administrative science—however compelling—is insufficient to overcome Americans' deep-seated and enduring ambivalence toward government.[13]

This ambivalence has implications for public opinion toward other important policy issues, such as whether to increase taxes to pay for universal access to health care. Recent political battles over taxation—both Ronald Reagan's success and George Bush's Waterloo—have firmly implanted the impression that Americans are unambiguously antitax. As Bill Gradison, who left the House of Representatives to lead the Health Insurance Association of America (HIAA), puts it: The "public view is . . . 'Fix it, but don't send me the bill' " (quoted in *National Journal* 1993). Polling results, however, do not support this interpretation of public opinion as contradictory and fiscally irresponsible—as benefit-hungry but recklessly cost-averse.

The impression that public opinion is antitax feeds on opinion surveys that report Americans are unwilling to pay more than a relatively small tax increase for an NHI plan. Numerous surveys find only about one in five respondents willing to pay more than a modest tax increase (approximately $200 per year) to make a universal health plan a reality (Blendon and Donelan 1990; Roper Center 1992a; Blendon et al. 1992).

Three distinct bodies of evidence, though, suggest that Americans' attitudes toward funding health reform are responsible, though certainly not unambiguous. First, the polling results that purport to show that Americans oppose tax increases may be an artifact of the survey questions themselves: they fail to mention possible savings incurred from avoiding future increases in insurance premiums and other costs. Not surprisingly, a January 1992 survey found that among those favoring NHI, 53 percent were willing to pay an additional $1,000 a year in taxes if they had no further health costs.[14]

Moreover, Americans' attitudes toward increasing taxes to finance a

13. See Marmor 1991 for a concise discussion of the disjuncture between the "myths" associated with national health insurance and the reality suggested by administrative practice.

14. The question was the following: "Would you be willing to pay $1,000 a year more in federal taxes for national health insurance if it meant that you would have no other costs for health insurance and health care, or not?" Ten percent were not willing to pay the additional tax, 2 percent were not sure, and 35 percent were not asked because they either opposed national health insurance or did not know if they favored or opposed it (CBS/*New York Times* 25 January 1992).

new health program are not monolithic and unchanging. Opinion surveys consistently report acceptance of increases in a range of taxes other than income taxes, such as new levies on liquor and cigarette sales as well as on health providers and insurance premiums paid by employers (Blendon and Donelan 1990; Blendon et al. 1992). Americans' tax attitudes are quite contingent not only on the type of taxation but also on the time period. During the late 1970s, when the level of inflation was high, Americans were especially resistant to taxes. But, the easing of inflation over the past decade has calmed public distress about taxation (Page and Shapiro 1992).

Finally, analysts of public opinion often assume erroneously that respondents equate the financing of new government programs with taxes. Thus, analysts (like Gradison) assume that respondents duck the hard choices over financing when they favor expanded benefits while opposing significant new tax hikes. In fact, evidence suggests that Americans look to sources other than taxes for additional funding. Opinion surveys report that the end of the Cold War has led Americans to favor funding health care reform through reallocation and, in particular, by reshuffling funds from within the health sector itself and from non-health-related areas such as the military (Blendon and Donelan 1990). Indeed, public support for increased military spending stands at historically low levels (Page and Shapiro 1992).

Public Opinion in the Policy-Making Process

What, if any, effect will Americans' ambivalence toward health reform have on policy deliberations? Public preferences—even when strong and persistent—are never merely encoded into policy, with government officials serving as latter-day scribes. Disjunctures develop between the values and preferences of elites and those of the mass public because politicians and bureaucrats misunderstand or resist public opinion.

The conventional wisdom emphasizes the restrictions that limit public opinion's causal significance. The influence of public opinion is assumed to be limited to the broad boundaries of government decisions, with elites exercising free rein to determine the "specifics" of policy-making.[15] According to this prevailing account, today's cluster of public attitudes—

15. Key (1961), Dahl (1956), and Kingdon (1984) treat public opinion as effectively irrelevant for specific policy-making. Published works that treat health policy-making as the almost exclusive work of elites include the following: Eckstein 1958, 1960; Hollingsworth 1986; Hollingsworth et al. 1990; Klein 1983; and Marmor 1973. Fox (1986), Rochefort and Boyer (1988), and Rochefort and Pezza (1991) demonstrate a greater appreciation of nonelite influences.

simultaneous support and dread of government reform—establishes the general opportunities and parameters of possible legislation. The public's ambivalence is, in effect, irrelevant to the making of specific policy, which is expected to be the nearly exclusive work of a small circle of medical professionals, labor and business groups, and other influentials.

This conventional assumption—that the public's influence on decision making is quite limited—often rests on the assumption that public opinion is an unreliable (and therefore unsuitable) partner for policy-making; its judgments are fickle, ill-considered, or simply wrong. Policymakers complain, for instance, that the public misunderstands such proposals as "play or pay" and managed competition and adopts positions that are logically inconsistent (e.g., expecting new benefits without new costs) (Kosterlitz 1993).

This paper offers a different (though not opposite) account. While public opinion cannot somehow be ratified into government policy, it can (under certain conditions) influence detailed decisions. This alternative account is based on a growing body of research that challenges conventional assumptions about the supposedly mercurial and incompetent judgments of the public at large (Page and Shapiro 1992; Popkin 1991).

One comprehensive study of public opinion trends over the past fifty years reports that Americans' policy preferences are in fact quite stable; when change does occur, it tends to follow reasonable responses to changing information and circumstances (Page and Shapiro 1992). On the occasions when the public does appear ignorant or fickle, its attitude can often be traced to events or rapid changes in circumstances and even to faulty or misleading information. For instance, the public's recent confusion over different reform proposals and its apparent reluctance to pay for new benefits echo the information presented by politicians. Politicians (including candidate Clinton) persistently took positions on health reform that were ambiguous, fickle, and misleading (e.g., promising new benefits without painful sacrifices). But, if the public does not master all policy details, it does possess—not unlike legislators and chief executives—sufficient knowledge and information to identify coherently and consistently support general principles.

The conventional wisdom is challenged not only by unsustainable assumptions about public opinion per se but also by important real-world changes in policy-making. Policymakers' ubiquitous (and expensive) commitment to polling today is symptomatic of fundamental and relatively recent institutional developments (Jacobs 1992).

In the early twentieth century, institutional norms regarding the behavior of national politicians (especially presidents) discouraged direct, responsive relations with the mass public; when policymakers did interact with the public, they were mainly interested in manipulating Americans in order to generate support for their desired policies (Jacobs 1992; Tulis 1987). Policymakers' *perspective* on the public, however, qualitatively changed during the latter half of the twentieth century. Their internal disposition and behavior became more sensitive to public opinion; this important shift was fueled by politicians' struggle for electoral advantage and institutional position (especially the battle between Congress and chief executives over controlling policy).

One result of the qualitative change in policymakers' relationship with the public was that polls were brought into the inner sanctum of government. Beginning with John Kennedy, presidents and presidential candidates established regular, routine relationships with private pollsters. For instance, to persuade Kennedy to back Medicare, Wilbur Cohen anchored his successful pitch in survey data—he assembled recent polls to "tell Kennedy and his people: this proves . . . [w]e've got public opinion" (interview by author, 1 April 1987).

Policymakers' commitment to polling reflected a new perception of the public. As a Kennedy aide explained, "The President is no longer a mysterious figure operating behind closed doors" (Salinger 1961). Rather, presidents and other policymakers have become more outward-looking and sensitive to the concerns of the general public.

The historic development of these new institutional norms is reinforced by the critical influence of competitive elections on the motivation of politicians and, by extension, bureaucrats. While the strategic importance of the public's policy preferences to a candidate are mitigated by voters' reliance on political party labels and candidate image, politicians remain sensitive toward highly salient, well-supported issues. They calculate that popular issues may attract independent voters who swing elections and that bending to mood shifts is less dangerous than courting revolt (Mayhew 1974; Shapiro and Young 1988; Jacobs and Shapiro 1991). For instance, Kennedy's and Johnson's decision to campaign for Medicare in their respective presidential campaigns reflected political pressure to respond to strong public opinion. Their victories created symbols of public support for Medicare and generated strong incentives for Congress to enact legislation—for many, it was too "hot" an issue to oppose.

More recent electoral battles have profoundly disrupted the country's political landscape and received wisdom. Both Harris Wofford and Bill Clinton were motivated by competitive elections to respond to polling results that identified popular issues like health care and to build their campaigns on advocating reform to address those issues. Their subsequent victories created clear signals of public support for health reform and motivated Democratic members of Congress, who are eager to construct a record of their party's leadership, to seriously consider major health legislation.

The Effect Public Ambivalence Has on Policy-Making

The emerging relationship between public opinion and policy-making sets the context for contemporary attitudes toward health policy—simultaneous support and dread of government reform—to influence policy deliberations. Existing research on the overall opinion-policy relationship as well as on the formulation of landmark health care legislation provides useful guides for analyzing the political relevance of contemporary public opinion toward health reform.[16] Evaluation of the American Medicare legislation of 1965 and the British National Health Service (NHS) Act of 1946 is especially useful because the story of each act has been captured in voluminous and private records, which allows the researcher to get behind the scenes and identify policymakers' motivations and intentions. The making of Medicare and the NHS suggests that Americans' current ambivalence toward health care is likely to affect two aspects of the policy-making process: the setting of policy agendas and the formulation of specific policies.

Agenda-Setting

Existing research suggests that strong, sustained public preferences can contribute to agenda setting—that is, the process by which an issue moves from the margins of policy discussions to its mainstream, where executive and legislative branch officials assign it a high priority (Jacobs 1993; Jacobs and Shapiro 1991). The original Medicare and NHS acts as well as current proposals for health care reform in America all received serious attention by policymakers and the media after the public had developed strong, stable patterns of interest in and support for major policy change.

In the case of Medicare and the NHS, evidence from polls and media coverage indicates that the issue of major health care reform became

16. Detailed analysis of public opinion's effect on the making of the Medicare and NHS acts is contained in Jacobs 1993. Rochefort and Boyer (1988) and Rochefort and Pezza (1991) also provide useful insights on public opinion's relevance to health policy; and Page and Shapiro (1992) summarize the general research on the opinion-policy relationship.

salient approximately half a dozen years before the passage of actual legislation. For instance, even before Britain's important planning document, the Beveridge Report, was completed during World War II, the issue of major health care reform was highly salient to the general population. Politicians and bureaucrats recognized this growing public interest in health reform and began to devote serious, sustained attention to the issue. After November 1942, public support for major new policy initiatives intensified, culminating in the widespread backing of "sweeping changes" in the July 1945 election. Policymakers' deliberations corresponded with the public's growing interest in major reform. The National Health Service dominated policy deliberations both within the wartime coalition of the Labour and Conservative parties (especially during 1943 and 1944) as well as within the Labour government that was swept into office in 1945.

Americans today—as suggested above—place health reform high on their policy-making agenda. By the early 1990s, a diverse group of elites agreed with the general public that health care deserved policymakers' serious attention. Even before the 1992 elections, Republican senators and President Bush had moved health reform to the top of their policy agenda. Rising public interest and Wofford's upset had convinced the Bush White House that it was politically necessary to acknowledge public concern by outlining in February 1992 the administration's health reform plan. As Senate Majority Leader George Mitchell explained at the time, the president's speech was intended to defuse the "perception that [he] doesn't care about health care" (Rovner 1992).

The Clinton administration has further elevated health reform on the policy agenda. During both his campaign and his term in office, Bill Clinton has consistently ranked health reform as among the three most important issues facing the country. Indeed, health care is arguably the White House's top priority: the administration, recognizing that presidents are handcuffed by such competing domestic institutions as Congress and by intractable economic problems that defy short-term solutions, sees health reform as one of the president's few opportunities to respond to strong public opinion and deliver a sweeping change.

In short, the public's strong concern with health care reform corresponds with the high priority that Democratic and Republican policymakers accord it. In spite of Americans' ambivalence today over the design of a new health plan, the public has strong, unambiguous feelings that health care is among the country's most pressing problems; policymakers have detected and responded to this component of public opinion.

Policy Formulation

With health reform's placement near the top of the policy-making agenda, officeholders and policy specialists have devoted sustained attention to the formulation of new policies. These policy deliberations raise two issues for analysis: the influence of interest groups and the design of specific administrative arrangements.

Interest Group Influence. Analysis of Medicare's formulation and subsequent development has typically concentrated on the positions of major interest groups, which are treated as the single best predictor of policy (Eckstein 1958, 1960; Marmor 1973, 1983: chap. 6; Hollingsworth 1986). For instance, it is generally assumed that during the period of Medicare's initial formulation and passage, representatives of doctors and hospitals wielded significant power (Harris 1966). In the context of an administratively weak government, policymakers became locked into an insulated and highly cooperative relationship with these interest groups.

More recent research on the Medicare and NHS acts yields two important new findings (Jacobs 1993). First, policy discussions were characterized by variations in the degree of interest group influence. Obviously, health care providers were incorporated in the government's deliberations, but on important issues politicians and specialists protected and used their positions of authority to reject interest group claims. The lesson for our own time, then, is that the influence of medical interest groups is not uniform: on some issues their claims will result in concessions, while on others their concerns will be rejected. The key issue, however, involves explaining the fluctuation in policymakers' relationship with medical interest groups.

The second finding coming out of recent research is that fluctuations in the political strength of medical providers are tied to policymakers' perceptions of public opinion. In particular, the relationship between levels of public opinion and the influence of an interest group was inverse: policymakers compromised with relevant sectional interests on principles that lacked strong public support and defied these groups when there was unmistakable public enthusiasm for a policy.

Indeed, reformers like Wilbur Cohen traced the defeat by the American Medical Association (AMA) of President Truman's national health insurance proposal to the AMA's success in drawing on strong public doubts concerning government—namely, the "innate frontier, capitalistic, . . . local . . . atmosphere in which socialized anything was a big bogeyman." [17] The influence of interest groups, Cohen and others concluded, was not a monolithic barrier but varied according to how well it was rooted in public understandings and preferences. The challenge for reformers (then and now) is to shape health reform carefully to reflect the enduring meanings that Americans associate with health care and government. Indeed, the strategic importance of aligning policy with public opinion is fully appreciated today by the Clinton White House as well as by groups representing providers and insurers; each set of actors has conducted extensive polling in order to formulate and anchor its position in public sentiment (Matlack 1992: 390).

The relationship between the language and decisions of politicians and experts and the patterns of public opinion is illustrated by the Medicare and NHS cases. The general pattern that emerges from these two cases provides a basis for speculating about interest group influence on future health care reform in the U.S.

Weak interest group influence: In Britain, beginning in the early 1940s, both qualitative and quantitative studies repeatedly indicated that the public supported the free and universal provision of hospital and doctor services; these principles were among the most attractive features of the Beveridge Report. Mirroring public opinion, both the coalition and Labour governments repeatedly defied medical providers' positions and endorsed these principles; as indicated in countless memoranda, minutes, and reports from the Ministry of Health and the cabinet, politicians and bureaucrats successfully made the case for universal and free care by pointing to the "great weight of public opinion."

Like the British, Americans embraced the major principles of health reform six years before Medicare legislation was passed. Echoing the public's negative perception of "welfare" and acceptance of social insurance, private surveys for Kennedy and Johnson as well as published polls indicated strong, sustained support for the adoption of Social Security's financing mechanism and its practice of covering the elderly. While Americans were comparatively unfamiliar with the government's provision of social welfare, they enthusiastically accepted the most familiar and popular form of government provision—it was, as Louis Harris repeatedly reported to Kennedy, a "popular issue . . . in every State we have surveyed" (Harris 1961). Corresponding to strong public preferences, con-

---

17. The quotation comes from an interview with Wilbur Cohen by the author, 1 April 1987. See also transcripts of the interviews, of Wilbur Cohen (8 December 1968) and with Robert Ball (5 November 1968).

gressional and administration officials repeatedly ignored interest group opposition and adopted the principles of Social Security financing and complete coverage of the aged.

In the current battle over American health care reform, representatives of health care providers, health insurers, and small businesses are quite active in protecting their particular interests. Although medical interest groups may not be as powerful as in past decades, representatives of sectional interests remain well-financed and well-organized; they will continue to be incorporated into government deliberations.

Adopting the principle of universal insurance coverage of all Americans may well spark conflict. Historically, the American Medical Association (AMA) has advocated confining governmental involvement to those in "need" and creating needs-tested programs to handle low-income Americans. The very assumption that government has a responsibility to ensure that all Americans have insurance coverage has been attacked for threatening the country's moral fiber and undermining individual and family responsibility. Indeed, one of the AMA's criticisms of Medicare was that it represented the "first step" to universal coverage. Today, disagreement continues over whether health reform should encompass all Americans regardless of employment or income status, or if it should largely focus on low-income Americans and those who are unemployed. Private insurers, specifically the Health Insurance Association of America (HIAA), were—prior to the November 1992 elections—adamantly opposed to universal insurance coverage, believing that protecting those not in need would invariably reduce their numbers and profits.

Policymakers' positions, on the other hand, correspond with public opinion, which, as discussed earlier, strongly supports universalism. Even former president Bush announced in his February 1992 speech that he was committed "above all . . . to ensuring every American universal access to affordable health insurance." Motivated by the "cold reality" of an upcoming election, he framed his plan for universal coverage to closely mirror public opinion. Rather than presenting his plan as a program for the less well-off, he emphasized that its tax incentives for the middle class would alleviate their "worry" regarding future health care costs: his plan should ease, he emphasized, "the all-too-familiar fear about what happens to their health care if they change jobs, or worse still, if they lose their jobs."

After championing universal coverage during his election campaign, Bill Clinton remains committed to universalism even in the face of budgetary constraints. His administration, like his predecessor's, has responded to broad middle-class support for universalism by emphasizing that expanding coverage would offer widely shared (rather than concentrated) benefits. For instance, Hillary Rodham Clinton has presented the administration's plan not as a special bailout of the uninsured and poor but as a benefit for "people who have been denied health insurance because of a pre-existing condition, [and] who cannot change jobs because . . . they [could] lose the insurance" (Kelly 1993). To neutralize the opposition of interest groups to universalism (and other administration policies), the White House is fully committed to mobilizing public support by maintaining Clinton's campaign apparatus (Cohen 1993; Fessler 1993). It is indicative of the new political climate and the Democrats' commitment to responding to public support for universalism that HIAA decided to reverse its earlier position and endorse the principle of expanding access to all Americans.

Major health care reform is being pressed today—by Democrats and Republicans—not out of charity but as a bulwark for the American middle class. In the past, universal coverage lacked a powerful constituency because the uninsured had low voting participation rates; today, universal coverage has a powerful new friend—voters. In short, interest group claims are not likely to be effective in limiting coverage to the needy; universalism is emerging as a bedrock principle of policy debates.

Strong interest group influence: Claims by interest groups, though, tend to wield significant influence when they involve nonsalient issues or hold out the potential to appeal to the public. For instance, during the formulation of the NHS, both the coalition and Labour governments considered the nonsalient issues of whether private practice should be preserved and whether capitation should continue as the basis for payment. In the end, even the reformist Labour cabinet compromised with relevant producer groups, citing public apathy or potential public support for interest groups' positions. Similarly, the influence of American interest groups was significant on issues that were not particularly salient to the public. In the absence, then, of Britain's extensive Friendly Societies or NHI provisions, American policymakers did not perceive—as their British counterparts did—public expectations that doctors would provide comprehensive services and that such care should be free. In this context, they acceded to sectional pressure and agreed to include deductibles and to exclude from the compulsory program medical specialists (namely, radiologists, anesthetists, pathologists, and psychiatrists).

In contemporary America, interest groups may well exercise significant influence over nonsalient issues related to the design of new government regulations. In his review of government regulations over the past three decades, Lawrence Brown (1992) indicates that major medical groups have exercised considerable influence in the absence of countervailing public demands. Because the public's "concerns and demands are amorphous, diffuse, and ill focused," members of Congress may well continue to defer to insurers and providers on regulatory design (Brown 1992: 35).

In addition, representatives of the providers and insurers may successfully press congressional moderates to narrow the scope of health reform by drawing on public ambivalence—as discussed earlier—over whether to increase taxation to fund the new plan. Thus, as HIAA claims, Americans' unwillingness to pay substantially higher taxes reveals that their support for reform is illusory: a wide-ranging reform that created a government-run health insurance system may well spark public opposition (Jajich-Toth and Roper 1990). Before the 1992 elections, the Bush administration and congressional Republicans similarly seized on public reluctance to foot a larger tax bill as the central obstacle to NHI. In an attack that may foreshadow future criticisms, Bush charged in February 1992 that a "massive tax increase is simply unacceptable, and the American people should not be asked to accept it."

The Clinton administration and many Democrats in Congress are likely to be quite sensitive to Americans' misgivings over tax increases and to their potential receptiveness to warnings from interest groups of massive new tax hikes. Perceived public misgivings over tax would discourage many politicians from openly embracing single-payer plans, which rely on higher personal and corporate taxes for funding. The Clinton administration's plan will attempt to skirt apparent public antipathy to higher personal income taxes by raising funds from other taxes, by reshuffling the federal government's budget, and by employer mandates.

The NHS and Medicare cases have two important implications which may be critical for future efforts to reform health care: the influence of interest groups varies across different policy issues, and this variability is tied to differing levels of public sentiment. On issues that are nonsalient or that could enjoy public backing, interest groups can exert significant influence. But, on matters that enjoy strong public support, even the efforts of the most well-financed and organized lobby will be ineffectual. There is enduring wisdom in Wilbur Cohen's strategy in the 1950s: "latch" health reform onto popular arrangements, because once government officials recognize its popularity they will defy even fierce interest group pressure—it is precisely for such reasons that Britain's free and universal care and America's complete coverage of the elderly were enshrined over the objections of special interests.

The political relevance, then, of Americans' current ambivalence toward government health reform—surging support amidst enduring uneasiness—is variable. Americans' backing of universalism will likely be quite influential, establishing the guiding principle for reform. The public, though, is likely to be less influential on other government decisions. In particular, elites will find Americans' preferences less relevant and more permissive on issues that the public either fails to consider important, like regulatory design, or feels genuine ambiguity over, like taxation.

Designing Administrative Arrangements. Public opinion has a second kind of influence on policy formulation—namely, on the designing of specific administrative arrangements. Existing research suggests that formulating administrative features is the work of experts: specific arrangements, for instance, over reimbursing providers are expected to result from the judgment of informed politicians and specialists.[18] It is these experts who presumably understand what will work. Thus, during Medicare's formulation policymakers might be expected to have had strong reservations (unlike their British counterparts) about whether the American government had the administrative capacity to fund or provide health care. After all, the American government is notorious for its low degree of hierarchical control and its lack of a skilled civil service comparable to that in Britain. According to this conventional wisdom, official deliberations over detailed administrative arrangements should first focus on the capacity of existing governmental organizations and, second, be determined by expert judgment concerning administrative capacity.

An important part of the Medicare story—its arrangements for reimbursing hospitals—challenges this conventional wisdom. At the outset of the Kennedy administration, officials in the Department of Health, Education, and Welfare (DHEW) and the Bureau of the Budget (BOB) launched a strong and persistent campaign for "direct Federal administration" over the disbursement and use of Medicare funds.[19] Contrary to the conventional wisdom, these officials were quite confident that the central government had the expertise to ensure quality of care for Medicare beneficiaries

18. For research that connects the formulation of the Medicare and NHS acts to the expertise of elites, see Hollingsworth 1986; Klein 1983; Eckstein 1958.

19. The consideration of direct federal administration is discussed in detail in Jacobs 1993 and is partly based on archival records. See Bell 1961; DHEW 1960a, 1960b, 1961a, 1961b, 1961c.

and to control the cost of the program. In pressing its case to the White House and President Kennedy, BOB prophetically warned that failure to establish direct and strong central state control over the reimbursement of hospitals would begin an "irreversible" process of rapid cost escalation; the predicted result was "a more costly and less satisfactory service" (DHEW 1961b, 1961c).

Here, then, is an important case of American policymakers exhibiting real confidence in the government's organizational capacity. What is critical, though, is that this expert judgment was not the focus of subsequent decisions by presidents and influential members of Congress; rather, the focus and critical influence on detailed decisions about reimbursing hospitals was policymakers' perception of public preferences and understandings. The result was administrative arrangements that dispersed DHEW's authority by using Blue Cross agencies to monitor the quality of a hospital's care and the payments it received.

The context for policymakers' deliberations over administrative arrangements was a persistent uncertainty that many Americans harbored toward government. Even with the public's acceptance of state involvement via Social Security, there was an enduring uneasiness regarding the prospect of excessive interference; as a private pollster reported to Kennedy, "Most people . . . want something done [but] have doubts about the method" (Kraft 1963).

The proposal for "direct federal administration" was resisted by administration and congressional officials because they feared it would arouse Americans' enduring uneasiness with state interference—it would fuel the perception of "state control" and the AMA's warnings about "socialized medicine." Instead, politicians and officials decided to create an "intermediary" between hospitals and the federal government—one which would decentralize reimbursement and rely on such familiar private agencies as Blue Cross. Policymakers focused on the "public relations advantages" of decentralized arrangements: the use of Blue Cross agencies would defuse "widespread and vocal concern" about "government meddling," "control," and "interference" in hospital care. In the end, officials in the mid-1960s were far more concerned with addressing the public's uneasiness toward government than with the consequences of initiating weak administrative arrangements that minimized direct government involvement and relied on private entities.

In short, the primary focus of, and influence on, the White House and members of Congress was Americans' dread of government rather than administrative experts' arguments about what would work. Conceding that new institutional arrangements would be weak, policymakers concentrated not on "what works best," but on what *mattered* and would be acceptable in terms of public preferences and understandings.

It should be stressed, however, that in contrast to public opinion toward major principles like universal access, Americans' reactions to administrative arrangements were less focused. As a result, Washington's discretion in responding to Americans' dread of government was relatively greater. Because public opinion did not focus on detailed policies, elite decision makers could exercise discretion in framing reimbursement arrangements.

In the 1990s, Americans' long-standing ambivalence toward government continues to influence policymakers and discourage them from designing administrative arrangements for controlling costs. Such major interest groups as the AMA and HIAA have unambiguously rejected the idea of expanding the government's role to provide caps or other spending targets on health care spending. Former president Bush's February 1992 health speech articulated the objection to expanding the government's role: Federal budgetary constraints would "put the government in control" and "shovel [people] into some new health-care bureaucracy." Critics of governmental constraints can credibly echo—as Bush did—Americans' fears (as captured in opinion surveys) that the new government program will lower quality, increase costs, and create longer waiting lists.

The Clinton administration, as well as congressional moderates, is likely to resist schemes like the single-payer plan because they fear that a visible, direct transfer of budgetary control from private to government hands could ignite Americans' enduring uneasiness with state interference. According to members of the president's transition team, Bill Clinton's sensitivity to the general public's "deep-seated suspicion about having the government run this" has meant "ruling [the single-payer scheme] out of the relevant debate" (Kenneth Thorpe, interview by author, 30 October 1992). To deflect reform opponents' appeals to public dread of government, the administration will likely hammer away at Ronald Reagan's theme that "government is not the answer" and emphasize its attempts to preserve the role of private insurers, patient choice, and providers' independence.

Clinton's Achilles' heel, though, is that even his relatively moderate plan must introduce fundamental change in governmental authority in order to contain health costs and establish universalism by mandating employers to provide health care coverage to their workers. Americans' deep ambivalence over government reform may well stalemate quick action on major health reform. The administration's proposals to expand government authority will provide ample ammunition to reform opponents, who are eager to exploit Americans' dread of government and divide the ranks of congressional Democrats.

Conclusion

Americans' simultaneous support and dread of government reform will likely influence contemporary health policy debates, but the impact will vary depending on the character of both the public's preferences and the policy issue. Public opinion is most influential in directing policy deliberations when it is unambiguous and strong. Americans' support for placing health reform on the agenda and enacting universalism are especially relevant to the current deliberations. Public opinion, though, is unlikely to exert a comparable influence when Americans are either uninterested or genuinely uncertain: on such nonsalient issues as whether Medicare should cover medical providers, American policymakers tend to defer to special interest groups.

The degree of public opinion's effect on policy-making, then, can vary between two extremes: the public is directive on strongly preferred principles and uninfluential on nonsalient issues. There is, though, a third relationship between public opinion and policy-making—a kind of twilight zone between the two extremes. In particular, Americans' dread of government constrains policymakers, barring the massive and visible state role that is conceivable in Britain; but the public's misgivings represent broad parameters rather than focused directives. Because the public is genuinely uncertain, it is more permissive of elites than when its preferences are definitive: within broad boundaries, elites have leeway to exercise discretion.

It is this twilight zone of constrained autonomy that gives rise to America's impasse over major reform. In the past, policymakers' excessive timidity in the face of Americans' dread of government has steered them away from central budgetary regulations. As a result, health costs soared while officeholders and policy experts remained deadlocked over establishing the necessary administrative constraints.

Avoiding deadlock requires skillful leadership, which both responds to the core preferences of an existing or latent majority and induces the public to accept new reforms in terms of its prevailing repertoire of understandings and preferences. Skillfully formulating major new reforms requires aligning or—as Wilbur Cohen explained—"latching" policy proposals onto existing public attitudes. The primary task of policy leadership, then, involves the detachment and reattachment of widely shared meanings: politicians and experts detach public attitudes from their prevailing points of reference and *reposition* them. For instance, Medicare's original advocates attempted to detach powerful symbols like Social Security, which were tied to one set of historical associations, and rearticulate them in a different direction; provider groups and their allies countered by summoning opposing meanings and preferences associated with the poor law stigma or dread of government.

Contemporary policymakers can exert this kind of leadership by drawing, for example, on existing assumptions about universalism. Wofford skillfully pursued this strategy by basing his campaign on the query: "If every criminal has a right to a lawyer, shouldn't every American have a right to a doctor?" The Clinton administration can also evoke the language and assumptions associated with private insurance and health provision; it may claim that its proposal merely facilitates or revives consumer choice and competitive bargaining among and between providers and consumers. Americans must be convinced—as one transition official explained—that reformers can "achieve their objectives within the context of our current system" (Kenneth Thorpe, interview by author, 30 October 1992).

Moreover, skillful leadership by reformers may involve redirecting public attention from the contested issue of government control to the clear and highly popular objective of universalism. Reform advocates can use the country's overwhelming acceptance of this objective to build acceptance gradually for the necessary though mistrusted means—a significant government role in capping the health budget.

What remains unclear is if American policymakers are prepared to advocate a demonstrably larger government role. During the early 1960s, BOB's argument for direct federal control over costs fell on deaf ears. While British policymakers' success in establishing social welfare programs encouraged them—as one administrator explained—to "get as much as possible" when the NHS was designed, their American counterparts adopted (after successive defeats) a conservative philosophy that emphasized incremental changes instead of bold innovations like administrative cost controls. In the three decades since Medicare's enactment, though, Washington has repeatedly failed to contain costs by relying on micromanagement of providers' clinical behavior. As a result, Congress and successive Republican administrations were forced to adopt direct budgetary regulations in the form of Medicare's prospective payment system and the resource-based relative value scale. American policy-makers, then, are on the verge of accepting—with some trepidation—the legitimacy of BOB's initial recommendation: direct federal administration of costs.

In short, public preferences and understandings are a central focus and influence on government decisions regarding interest group claims and specific changes in administrative arrangements. Ordinary people cannot master all policy details or hold beliefs that are relevant to all policy issues. But the public does develop consistent, reasonable patterns of understandings and preferences, which can and do guide government decisions.

References

ABC/*Washington Post*. 1991. Survey, 11–15 December. Roper Center for Public Opinion Research, Storrs, CT.

Ball, Robert. 1968. Interview by David McComb, 5 November. Transcript in Lyndon Baynes Johnson Library, Austin, TX.

Bell, David. 1961. Note to T. Sorensen and M. Feldman, 24 January. M. Feldman Papers, Box 27, John F. Kennedy Library, Dorchester, MA.

Blendon, Robert. 1988. The Public's View of the Future of Health Care. *Journal of the American Medical Association* 259 (2): 3587–89.

Blendon, Robert, Drew Altman, John Benson, Humphrey Taylor, Matt James, and Mark Smith. 1992. Public Opinion and Health Care. *Journal of the American Medical Association* 268 (23): 3371–75.

Blendon, Robert, and Karen Donelan. 1990. Special Report: The Public and the Emerging Debate over National Health Insurance. *New England Journal of Medicine* 323:208–12.

———. 1991. Interpreting Public Opinion Surveys. *Health Affairs* 10 (2): 166–69.

Brown, Lawrence D. 1992. Political Evolution of Federal Health Care Regulation. *Health Affairs* 11 (4): 17–37.

Bush, George. Health policy speech. *Congressional Quarterly*, 8 February, p. 305.

CBS/*New York Times*. 1991. Poll, 3 June. Roper Center for Public Opinion Research, Storrs, CT.

———. 1992. Poll, 25 January. Roper Center for Public Opinion Research, Storrs, CT.

Cohen, Richard. 1993. Two Heavyweights in Clinton's Corner. *National Journal*, 9 January, p. 92.

Cohen, Wilbur. 1968. Interview by David McComb, 8 December. Lyndon Baynes Johnson Library, Austin, TX.

Dahl, Robert. 1956. *A Preface to Democratic Theory*. Chicago: University of Chicago Press.

DHEW (U.S. Department of Health, Education, and Welfare). 1960a. Issues to Be Resolved. Draft by M. Pond, 22 December. DHEW Microfilm Roll 24, John F. Kennedy Library, Dorchester, MA.

———. 1960b. Proposed Specifications for Medical Insurance Benefits. 16 December. DHEW Microfilm Roll 24, John F. Kennedy Library, Dorchester, MA.

———. 1961a. Reasons Pro and Con the Use of Private Health Insurance Agencies in the Administration of a Health Insurance Program: For Meeting with Secretary-Designate, 1/5/61. 4 January. DHEW Microfilm Roll 24, John F. Kennedy Library, Dorchester, MA.

———. 1961b. Health Insurance Benefits. Attached to covering slip from R. Ball to S. Saperstein. 16 January. DHEW Microfilm Roll 24, John F. Kennedy Library, Dorchester, MA.

———. 1961c. Memorandum to director of the Bureau of the Budget from the Labor and Welfare Division, 22 January. DHEW Microfilm Roll 24 and M. Feldman Papers, Box 27, John F. Kennedy Library, Dorchester, MA.

———. 1961d. Summary of Health Insurance Proposals. Attached to letter to Senator Anderson's assistant from W. Cohen, 8 February. DHEW Microfilm Roll 24, John F. Kennedy Library, Dorchester, MA.

Eckstein, Harry. 1958. *The English Health Service*. Cambridge, MA: Harvard University Press.

———. 1960. *Pressure Group Politics: The Case of the British Medical Association*. London: Allen and Unwin.

Feldman, Stanley, and John Zaller. 1992. The Political Culture of Ambivalence: Ideological Responses to the Welfare State. *American Journal of Political Science* 36:268–307.

Fessler, Pamela. 1993. Anticipation for Clinton Builds, but Delays Breed Anxiety. *Congressional Quarterly*, 16 January, pp. 105–9.

Fox, Daniel. 1986. *Health Policies, Health Politics: The British and American Experience, 1911–1965*. Princeton, NJ: Princeton University Press.

Ginsberg, Benjamin. 1986. *The Captive Public*. New York: Basic.

Harris, Louis. 1961. A Study of the Primary Outlook in South Carolina. Robert Fitzgerald Kennedy Papers, John F. Kennedy Library, Dorchester, MA.

Harris, Richard. 1966. *A Sacred Trust*. New York: New American Library.

Hollingsworth, J. Rogers. 1986. *A Political Economy of Medicine: Great Britain and the United States*. Baltimore, MD: Johns Hopkins University Press.

Hollingsworth, J. Rogers, Jerald Hage, and Robert Hanneman. 1990. *State Intervention in Medical Care: Consequences for Britain, France, Sweden and the U.S., 1890–1970*. Ithaca, NY: Cornell University Press.

Jacobs, Lawrence. 1992. The Recoil Effect: Public Opinion and Policy Making in the U.S. and Britain. *Comparative Politics* 24 (2): 199–217.

———. 1993. *The Health of Nations: Public Opinion and the Making of American and British Health Policy*. Ithaca, NY: Cornell University Press.

Jacobs, Lawrence, and Robert Shapiro. 1991. Democracy, Leadership, and the Private Polls of Kennedy and Johnson. Paper presented at the annual meeting of the American Political Science Association, Washington, DC, 30 August–1 September.

Jacobs, Lawrence, Robert Shapiro, and Eli Schulman. Forthcoming. Poll Trends: Medical Care in the United States. *Public Opinion Quarterly*.

Jajich-Toth, Cindy, and Burns W. Roper. 1990. Americans' Views on Health Care: A Study in Contradictions. *Health Affairs* 9 (4): 149–57.

Kelly, Michael. 1993. Hillary Clinton Takes to Hill in Vivid Display of Influence. *New York Times*, 5 February, p. 1.

Key, V. O. 1961. *Public Opinion and American Democracy*. New York: Knopf.

Kingdon, John. 1984. *Agendas, Alternatives, and Public Policies*. Boston: Little, Brown.

Klein, Rudolf. 1983. *The Politics of the National Health Service*. London: Longman.

Kosterlitz, Julie. 1993. Dangerous Diagnosis. *National Journal*, 16 January, pp. 127–30.

Kraft, John. 1963. A Study of Attitudes in North Dakota. M. Feldman Papers, Box 104, John F. Kennedy Library, Dorchester, MA.

Lipset, Martin Seymour, and William Schneider. 1983. *The Confidence Gap: Business, Labor, and Government in the Public Mind*. New York: Free Press.

Louis Harris and Associates. 1988. Survey, 10 November. Roper Center for Public Opinion Research, Storrs, CT.

———. 1991a. Survey, 13 November. Roper Center for Public Opinion Research, Storrs, CT.

———. 1991b. Survey, 18 November. Roper Center for Public Opinion Research, Storrs, CT.

———. 1992a. Survey, 2 November. Roper Center for Public Opinion Research, Storrs, CT.

———. 1992b. Survey, 3 November. Roper Center for Public Opinion Research, Storrs, CT.

———. 1992b. Survey, 3 November. Roper Center for Public Opinion Research.

Lowi, Theodore. 1985. *The Personal President: Power Invested, Promise Unfulfilled*. Ithaca, NY: Cornell University Press.

Marmor, Theodore. 1973. *The Politics of Medicare*. Chicago: Aldine.

———. 1983. *Political Analysis and American Medical Care*. New York: Cambridge University Press.

———. 1991. Misleading Notions. *Health Management Quarterly* 13 (4): 18–24.

Marmor, Theodore, Jerry Mashaw, and Philip Harvey. 1990. *America's Misunderstood Welfare State: Persistent Myths, Enduring Realities*. New York: Basic.

Matlack, Carol. 1992. Staking Out Turf. *National Journal*, 15 February, p. 390.

Mayhew, David. 1974. *Congress: The Electoral Connection*. New Haven, CT: Yale University Press.

Mellman and Lazarus Public Opinion. 1992. Survey, 5 January. Roper Center for Public Opinion Research, Storrs, CT.

Morone, James. 1990. *The Democratic Wish: Popular Participation and the Limits of American Government*. New York: Basic.

National Journal. 1993. Why Bill Gradison's Heading Downtown. 30 January, p. 290.

Page, Benjamin, and Robert Shapiro. 1992. *The Rational Public*. Chicago: University of Chicago Press.

Poen, Monte M. 1979. *Harry S. Truman versus the Medical Lobby: The Genius of Medicare*. Columbia: University of Missouri Press.

Popkin, Samuel. 1991. *The Reasoning Voter: Communication and Persuasion in Presidential Campaigns*. Chicago: University of Chicago Press.

Princeton Survey (Princeton Survey Research Associates). 1991. Poll, 13 November. Roper Center for Public Opinion Research, Storrs, CT.

Rochefort, David, and Paul Pezza. 1991. Public Opinion and Health Policy. In *Health Politics and Policy*, ed. T. Litman and L. Robins. Albany, NY: Delmar.

Roper Center. 1991. *American Enterprise* 2 (March/April). Roper Center for Public Opinion Research, Storrs, CT.

———. 1992a. *American Enterprise* 3 (March/April). Roper Center for Public Opinion Research, Storrs, CT.

———. 1992b. Poll, 3 November. Roper Center for Public Opinion Research, Storrs, CT.

Rovner, Julie. 1992. Bush's Plan Short on Details, Long on Ambition, Critics. *Congressional Quarterly*, 8 February, p. 305–9.

Salinger, Pierre. 1961. Memorandum to T. Sorensen. Salinger Papers, John F. Kennedy Library, Dorchester, MA.

Shapiro, Robert, and John Young. 1986. The Polls: Medical Care in the United States. *Public Opinion Quarterly* 50:418–28.

———. 1988. Public Opinion toward Social Welfare Issues: The United State in Comparative Perspective. In *Research in Micropolitics*, vol. 3., ed. Samuel Long. Greenwich, CT: JAI.

Tulis, Jeffrey. 1987. *The Rhetorical Presidency*. Princeton, NJ: Princeton University Press.

Yankelovich, Clancy, Shulman. 1991. Survey, 27 August. Roper Center for Public Opinion Research, Storrs, CT.

I would like to acknowledge the insightful comments of Theodore Marmor, Theda Skocpol, and especially James Morone and Robert Y. Shapiro.

Part 5
Federalism

American States and Canadian Provinces: A Comparative Analysis of Health Care Spending

Kenneth E. Thorpe

Abstract Most comparisons of the relative effectiveness of cost containment in the Canadian and U.S. health systems trace Canada's greater success to its single-payer approach. However, these studies ignore the substantial variation that exists in hospital and personal health care spending among both the American states and the provinces and territories of Canada. Four American states have adopted all-payer hospital rate setting; one other uses competitive bidding. All five show rates of growth in per capita hospital spending comparable to (and in some cases, lower than) the Canadian jurisdictions. Hospital spending, as a percentage of state gross domestic product (GDP), declined or remained constant in four of the five states. In four out of the five, growth in per capita spending on personal care, as a percentage of GDP, remained or fell below the national average. By contrast, in Canada, per capita spending on both hospitals and personal health care increased as a percentage of GDP in ten out of eleven jurisdictions. In each of the U.S. states, government played a central role in structuring the terms of payment and thus strengthened the hand of purchasers over providers. This strategy, rather than specifically a single-payer or universal health insurance approach, seems to be the key to limiting the growth in health costs to the growth in state or national income.

Health spending and the uninsured continue to dominate the American health policy debate. Though the issues are not new, a number of factors have raised the intensity of the debate:

- A prolonged recession, in which average payroll has risen 4 to 5 percent per year, while health insurance premiums have risen at three times this rate

- The apparent failure of managed care to "sufficiently" control the growth in health spending within the private sector (though managed care appears to generate lower growth than conventional plans, the savings only amount to a one-time reduction of approximately 10 percent [Thorpe 1992])
- Intensified efforts by the Medicare program to control the growth in health spending, reflecting budgetary strains and the financial status of the Medicare trust fund, and concern in the private sector that it will have to finance any savings resulting from Medicare's new cost controls

With the apparent failure of domestic initiatives to control costs, the search for solutions has focused increasingly on international approaches. Canada's single-payer approach to cost containment and its system of universal coverage have received growing attention. In contrast to people living in the United States, all Canadians receive a defined set of benefits financed largely through federal and provincial taxes. Canadians rely on a single payer and a single public health plan to deliver services. Private insurance is available, but only for services not specifically provided under the Canadian Health Act.

Numerous studies have compared the cost containment performance of the Canadian and U.S. systems (Evans et al. 1991). Nearly all agree that the Canadian single-payer approach has produced a lower spending growth than the American multiple-payer system. In many of these studies, Canada's relative success is traced to both universal coverage (thought by some to be a prerequisite) and the single payer. The inability of the U.S. delivery system to generate a similar rate of growth in spending is commonly traced to its fragmented financing and payment system. According to the studies, fragmentation encourages cost shifting, which undermines the system's ability to control aggregate spending.

Though these studies have contributed greatly to our understanding of the potential advantages of the Canadian approach, some shortcomings with the research are evident. In particular, by examining national averages in each country, the studies ignore the substantial variation that exists among the American states and Canadian provinces. The focus on national results in each country overlooks the fundamental fact that, to a large degree, health spending within each country is influenced by decisions made in each state or province. Several American states, for instance, have adopted innovative statewide approaches: four states have adopted all-payer hospital rate setting; Rochester, New York, has determined hospital payments by a comprehensive revenue cap for several years; and Medi-Cal in California relies on selective contracting to limit hospital revenues. In the Canadian system, the federal government contributes a per capita allotment related to growth in gross national product; ultimate responsibility for aggregate provincial spending relies on decisions made within each province.

In this article, I focus on two related questions. First, how much variation in cost growth exists within each country? Second, how do the U.S. states that have implemented innovative programs to control costs compare to the Canadian provinces? The question underlying my analysis is whether a single payer is both a necessary and a sufficient condition for cost containment. As I hope to show, the answer is no: cost containment can be pursued within either a multipayer or a single-payer financing system.

Growth in health care spending ultimately reflects the relative bargaining strengths of purchasers and providers (Peltzman 1976). The institutional setting in which purchasers attempt to limit growth in expenditures (i.e., provider income) is one measure of political power. For instance, jurisdictions that develop a single set of payment rules through a centralized (public) decision-making process are more successful in limiting the growth in health spending compared to those using less structured approaches. Centralization, or coordination, reflects the relatively greater political bargaining power of purchasers, facilitating the development and promulgation of uniform payment rates. Centralized rules can be developed either for a single payer (as in Canada) or for multiple payers (as in the U.S. rate-setting states, Germany, Japan, and France).

Methods

I examine the cost containment experience of five states that have adopted innovative cost containment strategies: New York, Maryland, New Jersey, Massachusetts, and California. I compare the rate of per capita spending in these states to each of the ten Canadian provinces. This comparison makes it possible to examine variations both within and among jurisdictions. Two types of health care spending are examined: per capita hospital and per capita total personal expenditures. To account for differences in general economic growth within each jurisdiction, I also index spending within each state or province to gross domestic product (GDP).

My analysis examines the growth of spending in each state and province between 1978 and 1987. The part of the analysis that relates spending to gross domestic product focuses on the period from 1980 to 1986. I use this more limited time frame because none of the experiments in the five U.S. states was in operation prior to 1977. These five U.S. states were selected because each state either assumed a major role in directly setting hospital and other payment rates or (as in the case of California) assisted in restructuring the state health care market to promote managed care and price competition. The cost containment approaches are outlined below.

State-level comparisons of health spending are difficult because the data are limited. For four U.S. states, I rely on estimated personal health spending provided by Lewin/ICF (Families USA 1990). These data provide state-level estimates for 1980 and 1990. I estimate spending in each state during 1986 and 1987 by assuming that the average annual growth in health spending is similar between 1980 and 1990 and between 1980 and 1987. Data on hospital revenue were provided by the Health Care Financing Administration (unpublished worksheet 1992). I also examined hospital expenditure data within each state as reported by the American Hospital Association's yearly *Hospital Statistics* series, but the data lay outside the terms of my analysis. Data for each Canadian province were derived from Health and Welfare Canada (1991).

All-Payer Rate Setting and Competitive Bidding

During the late 1970s and early 1980s, New York, Massachusetts, New Jersey, and Maryland adopted all-payer hospital rate-setting programs. In doing so, they centralized control over inpatient hospital payments, either directly at the state level (in the case of New York) or through a state rate-setting board (as in the case of Maryland). With large payment differentials among payers eliminated, an auxiliary mechanism was required to finance uncompensated care. Each state, therefore, developed an uncompensated care pool, designed to spread the burden of financing such care among all payers. In some cases, the regulatory controls expanded beyond inpatient hospital care (as they did in the Rochester, New York, area) and included strict certificate-of-need laws and tight control over Medicaid payments.

Though California appeared equally dedicated to controlling costs, the state pursued an alternative policy: selective contracting. This required the state of California to assume a leadership role in restructuring the California health insurance market to promote competition. With respect to Medi-Cal, its Medicaid program, it selectively contracted with hospitals, using a competitive bidding process. By definition, some hospitals would not receive a Medi-Cal contract. This competitive bidding approach also spawned a new era of competitive, managed care health plans within the private sector.

Though the rate-setting states and California adopted dramatically different approaches to cost containment, both strategies had a common characteristic: the central role assumed by the state in structuring the terms of payment. The regulatory strategy of the eastern states involved coordinating payment rates across multiple health plans; though several sources of insurance remained, these states assumed primary control over the rates of inpatient hospital payment. In many respects, the nature of this control is similar to, though less comprehensive than, that exercised by each of the ten Canadian provinces. Both competitive bidding and all-payer rate-setting controls increased the bargaining power of purchasers relative to providers.

In addition to a separate examination of these five U.S. states, I also examine cost containment in each of the Canadian provinces. Under the Canadian system, the federal government provides a per capita allocation to each province. Changes in this allocation over time are related to growth in the Canadian economy. However, in addition to the federal contribution, each province or territory contributes its own resources. For example, in Ontario, Quebec, Manitoba, and Newfoundland, payroll taxes are used to supplement federal and provincial contributions. Given this financing mix, total spending within each province is ultimately determined by the provincial government. Federal contributions account for a shrinking proportion of total provincial health care spending and now account for less than 25 percent of total expenditures (Health and Welfare Canada 1991).

Results

During 1987, the United States spent 29 percent more per capita on personal health care and 29 percent more on hospitals than Canada (see Table 1). During the 1980s, the growth in per capita personal spending rose 9.8 percent per year in Canada, compared to 10.1 percent per year in the U.S. The difference in capita growth was larger within the hospital sector, increasing 8.8 percent in Canada and 9.9 percent in the U.S. The same results are evident when health spending is indexed by gross domestic product. Health care is growing faster than the general economy in both countries: between 1978 and 1987, the proportion of GDP devoted to health in Canada increased from 6.3 percent to 7.7 percent; an even

Table 1 Health Care Spending in the United States and Canada, 1978–1987

	Canada			United States		
	1978	1987	Average Annual Growth (percent)	1978	1987	Average Annual Growth (percent)
Personal Health Care per Capita	$574	$1,336	9.8	$724	$1,726	10.1
Hospital Spending per Capita	$280	$596	8.8	$329	$769	9.9
Personal Health Care as Percentage of Gross Domestic Product	6.3	7.7		7.7	9.6	
Hospital Spending as Percentage of Gross Domestic Product	3.1	3.4		3.5	4.3	

Note. Expressed in U.S. dollars using purchasing power parity: $1.12 Canadian = $1.00 U.S. in 1978, $1.23 Canadian = $1.00 U.S. in 1987.

Sources. Health and Welfare Canada 1991; Arnett et al. 1990; Gibson et al. 1984; unpublished data from the Health Care Financing Administration.

larger jump was observed in the U.S., as health expenditures rose from 7.7 percent to 9.6 percent of GDP.

Table 2 compares per capita growth in hospital spending within each Canadian jurisdiction and among the five states. I examine spending trends between 1978 and 1987, roughly reflecting the time period when the state payment controls were in place. Growth in per capita hospital spending varies widely within Canada and the U.S.: among the Canadian jurisdictions (the ten provinces and the Yukon and Northwest Territories), average annual growth in per capita hospital spending ranged from a low of 7.1 percent per year in Saskatchewan to a high of 10.6 percent in Alberta, while among the U.S. states, the hospital spending grew from between 8.3 percent in California to 10.1 percent in New York. The low rate of growth shown in California is consistent with previous evaluative studies documenting the effectiveness of the selective contracting program (Zwanziger and Melnick 1988).

Growth in California's per capita hospital spending was lower than the growth observed in nine of eleven Canadian jurisdictions. (Only Quebec

Table 2 Per Capita Hospital Spending of Selected American States and Canada, 1978–1987

Jurisdiction	Year		Average Annual Growth (percent)
	1978	1987	
New York	$350	$832	10.1
Massachusetts	$400	$880	9.2
Maryland	$270	$586	9.0
New Jersey	$260	$614	10.0
California	$338	$692	8.3
U.S. Weighted Average	$329	$769	9.9
Newfoundland	$263	$569	9.0
Prince Edward Island	$238	$490	8.4
Nova Scotia	$271	$632	9.9
New Brunswick	$258	$568	9.2
Quebec	$318	$643	8.1
Ontario	$271	$584	8.9
Manitoba	$273	$602	9.2
Saskatchewan	$259	$482	7.1
Alberta	$250	$618	10.6
British Columbia	$262	$547	8.5
Territories	$367	$899	10.5
Canada Weighted Average	$279	$596	8.8

Notes. Expressed in U.S. dollars using purchasing power parity: $1.12 Canadian = $1.00 U.S. in 1978, $1.23 Canadian = $1.00 U.S. in 1987.

U.S. totals represent revenues to nonfederal hospitals.

Sources. Health and Welfare Canada 1991; U.S. Bureau of the Census 1992: Table 710. Hospital revenues from unpublished data from the Health Care Financing Administration.

and Saskatchewan, whose expenses increased 8.1 percent and 7.1 percent, respectively, increased at a slower rate.) The growth in hospital costs in Maryland was the same as Newfoundland's and roughly equivalent to that of the Canadian median: five provinces increased at a slower rate, and four and the territories at a higher rate. In Massachusetts growth was slightly above the Canadian median. Growth in per capita hospital costs in New Jersey and New York exceeded the U.S. average, yet was lower than growth in Alberta and the territories.

The analysis presented in Table 2 examined per capita growth in hospital spending. However, some analysts have argued that international comparisons based on per capita health care spending are potentially misleading and that spending should, instead, be indexed by GNP (Barer et al. 1991). The rationale is, in part, based on previous empirical studies

Table 3 Hospital and Personal Health Care Spending as a Percentage of State and National Gross Domestic Product, Selected American States, 1980–1986

	Hospitals		Personal Health Care	
	1980	1986	1980	1986
New York	4.2	4.2	10.3	10.0
Massachusetts	5.3	4.9	11.3	10.9
Maryland	3.8	3.6	9.8	10.2
New Jersey	3.0	2.9	7.7	7.8
California	3.3	3.5	8.6	11.4
U.S. Average	3.5	4.0	8.6	9.8

Sources. Hospital revenues from unpublished data from the Health Care Financing Administration; state gross domestic product from U.S. Bureau of the Census 1992.

that find that the income elasticity of demand for health care exceeds one; that is, a 10 percent rise in GNP (income) would be associated with an even higher percentage growth in the health care sector. Thus, to account for different underlying rates of economic growth in each country, I compare the experience within the five American states to the Canadian provinces and territories, indexed by each jurisdiction's GDP.

In four of the five states examined, hospital spending as a percentage of GDP actually declined or remained constant between 1980 and 1986 (see Table 3). When measured as a percentage of state GDP, hospital spending declined in Massachusetts, Maryland, and New Jersey. Expenditures on hospitals remained a constant share of GDP in New York, and increased slightly in California. Though per capita growth in hospital spending was lower in California during the 1980s, growth in the California economy was slower than observed in the regulated states. The results presented in the rate-setting states differ sharply from the national experience. During the same time period, hospital expenditures increased from 3.5 percent to 4.0 percent of GDP nationally.

A similar pattern occurs in personal health care spending. Growth in such spending, expressed as a share of GDP, was lower than the national average in four of the five states. In New York and Massachusetts, spending on personal health care dropped as a share of GDP. However, rates rose slightly in New Jersey and Maryland, and jumped above the national average in California. Nationally, personal health care accounted for 8.6 percent of GDP in 1980 and 9.8 percent in 1986.

The experience among the Canadian provinces and territories yielded different results (see Table 4). Hospital spending increased as a percentage

Table 4 Hospital and Personal Health Care Spending as a Percentage of Provincial or Territorial Gross Domestic Product, Canada, 1980–1986

	Hospitals		Personal Health Care	
	1980	1986	1980	1986
Newfoundland	5.4	5.7	9.8	10.4
Prince Edward Island	4.8	5.1	9.9	11.0
Nova Scotia	5.0	5.2	9.7	10.3
New Brunswick	5.0	4.6	9.5	8.9
Quebec	3.9	4.0	7.3	7.9
Ontario	2.7	3.0	6.1	7.3
Manitoba	3.5	3.9	7.4	8.4
Saskatchewan	2.8	3.4	5.9	8.8
Alberta	1.7	3.1	3.8	6.3
British Columbia	2.8	3.2	6.5	7.9
Territories	2.4	3.4	4.5	5.5
Average	3.0	3.5	6.4	7.7

Source. Health and Welfare Canada 1991.

of GDP in ten of eleven jurisdictions. Increased spending was particularly high in Alberta and the territories. The only exception occurred in New Brunswick, where hospital spending fell from 5.0 percent to 4.6 percent of GDP. Overall, hospital spending increased from 3.0 to 3.5 percent of GDP during this time period. In addition to the upward trend in hospital expenditures, substantial variation in the level of hospital spending exists among the provinces. Hospital spending ranged from a low of 3.0 percent of GDP in Ontario to 5.7 percent in Newfoundland.

Personal health care spending within the provinces and territories followed a similar trend, accounting for a growing share of GDP in ten out of the eleven jurisdictions. We see a decrease in New Brunswick but sharp increases in Saskatchewan, where spending increased from 5.9 to 8.8 percent of GDP. Personal health spending also rose steeply in Alberta, from 3.8 percent to 6.3 percent of GDP. Overall, personal health spending increased from 6.4 percent to 7.7 percent of the Canadian GDP.

As a final analysis, I examined whether the pattern of health care spending relative to state GDP changed with the introduction of rate setting and selective contracting (see Table 5). New York State has employed hospital rate setting since 1969, though hospitals were reimbursed using the all-payer system between 1983 and 1985. The state decided not to seek a renewal of its federal waiver, and in 1986 it moved to Medicare's diagnosis-related group (DRG) system. This transition was, in part, moti-

Table 5 Percentage Growth in State Gross Domestic Product and Hospital Revenues, Selected American States, 1980–1986

	1980–1984		1984–1985		1985–1986	
	Gross Domestic Product	Hospital Revenues	Gross Domestic Product	Hospital Revenues	Gross Domestic Product	Hospital Revenues
New York	9.8	9.3	7.8	7.7	7.9	8.5
Massachusetts	10.5	10.4	9.5	5.0	8.8	4.6
Maryland	9.5	9.2	9.5	5.0	8.4	8.1
New Jersey	10.5	12.9	8.0	5.8	8.8	4.6
California	8.9	11.1	8.7	7.7	7.4	7.0
Remaining States	8.2	12.0	6.3	6.5	4.9	6.9

Source. Unpublished data from Health Care Financing Administration.

vated by a desire from the hospital industry to receive payment under Medicare's (relatively) more generous hospital payment system.

Hospital spending as a percentage of New York State GDP declined between 1980 and 1985 and, after moving into the Medicare system, increased relative to state income. These results are consistent with early estimates by the state hospital association, which indicate that the transition to Medicare would generate an influx of $400 million in new hospital revenue (Hospital Association of New York State 1985).

California adopted selective contracting during 1983, a period of relatively rapid growth in hospital spending. After adopting its competitive bidding scheme, hospital spending decreased as a share of state GDP. The slower growth in hospital spending accompanying the move to selective contracting is consistent with previous evaluative studies (see Zwanziger and Melnick 1988).

Maryland adopted its all-payer approach in 1977. Though I do not present baseline estimates, hospital revenues grew at a slower rate relative to state GDP from 1980 to 1986. Massachusetts and New Jersey adopted their all-payer rate-setting systems later than Maryland, in 1982 and 1980, respectively. During the initial years of the New Jersey experiment, hospital spending outpaced state GDP, although this trend was reversed between 1984 and 1986. Before it adopted its all-payer system in 1983, Massachusetts saw its hospital spending grow at approximately the same rate as its economy. After the adoption of the system, the growth in the state's hospital spending was substantially slower than its economic growth.

The experience of these five U.S. states differs from that of the remaining forty-five. From 1980 to 1984, immediately prior to the introduction of Medicare's DRG payment system, hospital spending increased nearly 4 percentage points faster than the general economy. After the adoption of Medicare's DRG payment system, the gap between the growth in hospital spending and national income in the remaining states narrowed.

Conclusions

Previous comparisons of hospital and personal health care spending in the U.S. and Canada have ignored the substantial diversity in experience within each country. The analysis I have presented indicates that the diversity in health spending among jurisdictions is as impressive as those reported among countries. Within the U.S., variations in the rate of hospital and personal health care spending appear related to several innovative state all-payer rate-setting programs and California's selective contracting system.

The analysis also reveals a lower rate of growth in health care spending in the "average" Canadian province relative to the "average" American state during the 1980s (General Accounting Office 1991b). Results commonly reported in the literature, however, are traced to spending trends in the forty-five U.S. states that did not enact significant expenditure controls. Cost growth in U.S. states that imposed central control over rates paid by health plans was equal to or lower than the growth observed in Canada. These results are similar to those found by the General Accounting Office (1991a) in the multipayer systems of France, Japan, and Germany. In each case, these countries have developed common rules applied to all payers that determine prices and overall spending. To a large degree, the all-payer approach is similar to the single-payer system; both develop rules guiding transactions among payers and providers. Both approaches reflect an underlying political decision to limit the growth in health care spending (Evans et al. 1991).

The success of California's selective contracting system in controlling the growth in hospital spending indicates that centralized, regulatory control may not represent our only road to salvation (see Table 5). However, though competitive bidding stemmed the rise in hospital spending, we see no impact on total health care spending.

Expenditure containment and growth ultimately reflect the outcomes of political bargaining among providers and payers. All-payer rate setting adopted by Maryland, Massachusetts, New Jersey, and New York and selective contracting in California represent attempts by these states to limit the growth in hospital and personal health care spending. At issue is whether the approaches selected to limit expenditure growth within a multiple-payer system are as effective as those in single-payer systems. The results presented above suggest that the growth in health spending within a multipayer system can be limited to the growth in state income. In each case, however, the state assumed a major role, either by coordinating hospital payment rates across payers or, in the case of California, by setting the stage for a competitive transformation of the hospital market.

My results indicate that a multipayer system can control health care spending, though they do not answer the more fundamental questions of what these controls sacrifice or whether higher levels and rates of growth in the remaining forty-five states are associated with better patient outcomes. Moreover, I do not compare access to medical care across states or between the U.S. and Canada. Other studies, however, have examined these features of all-payer rate-setting systems; Christine Spencer and I, for example, have reported on the impact of uncompensated care pools on maintaining or improving access to care among the uninsured. We found that pools increase access to hospital services among the uninsured and improve the financial condition of distressed hospitals (Thorpe and Spencer 1991). Uncompensated care pools do not, however, effectively substitute for health insurance.

In the final analysis, the results indicate that the growth in hospital spending in the U.S., at least, can be limited to the growth in income within its existing financing system. Fundamentally, such growth reflects political interactions among purchasers and suppliers in public and private markets. Thus, the "technology" of cost containment is perhaps less interesting or important than the "politics" of cost containment. Lower growth in spending does appear to require government, either at the state or national level, to assist in structuring the financing and payment system to achieve these results. Such changes tend to increase the bargaining strength of purchasers, generating a lower rate of growth. More directly, the existence of a single payer or common payment rules in an all-payer system *reflects* the augmented political power of purchasers relative to providers. With this augmented power, as experience within the U.S. shows, either a comprehensive regulatory approach or a competitive one could limit the growth in spending to the growth in state or national income. How a slower rate of growth might affect the health of the population remains, however, a critical area for study.

References

American Hospital Association. 1981, 1986. *Hospital Statistics*. 1981 and 1986 editions. New York: American Hospital Association.

Arnett, R. H., III, L. A. Blank, A. P. Brown, C. A. Cowan, C. S. Donham, M. S. Frieland, H. C. Lazenby, S. W. Letsch, K. R. Levit, B. T. Mapel, et al. 1990. National Health Care Expenditures, 1988. *Health Care Financing Review* 11 (4): 1–41.

Barer, Morris L., Pete Welch, and Laurie Antioch. 1991. Canadian/U.S. Health Care: Reflections on the HIAA's Analysis. *Health Affairs* 10:229–35.

Evans, Robert G., Morris L. Barer, and Clyde Hertzman. 1991. The 20-Year Experiment: Accounting for, Explaining, and Evaluating Health Care Cost Containment in Canada and the United States. *Annual Review of Public Health* 12:481–518.

Families USA. 1990. *Rising Health Care Costs in America*. Washington, DC: Families USA.

General Accounting Office. 1991a. *Health Care Spending Control: The Experience of France, Germany, and Japan*. Washington, DC: U.S. Government Printing Office.

———. 1991b. *Canadian Health Insurance: Lessons for the United States*. Washington, DC: U.S. Government Printing Office.

Gibson, R.M., K. R. Levit, H. C. Lazenby, and D. R. Waldo. 1984. National Health Care Expenditures, 1983. *Health Care Financing Review* 6 (2): 1–29.

Health and Welfare Canada. 1991. *National Health Expenditures in Canada, 1975–1987*. Ottawa: Health and Welfare Canada.

———. 1992. *National Health Expenditures in Canada*. Ottawa: Health and Welfare Canada.

Hospital Association of New York State. 1985. *Modelling Alternative Reimbursement Systems*. Albany, NY: Hospital Association of New York State.

Peltzman, Sam. 1976. Toward a More General Theory of Regulation. *Journal of Law and Economics* 19:211–40.

Thorpe, Kenneth E. 1992. Health Care Cost Containment: Results and Lessons from the Past 20 Years. In *Improving Health Policy and Management: Nine Critical Research Issues for the 1990s*, ed. S. Shortell and U. Reinhardt. Ann Arbor, MI: Health Administration Press.

Thorpe, Kenneth E., and Christine Spencer. 1991. How Do Uncompensated Care Pools Affect the Level and Type of Care? Results from New York State. *Journal of Health Politics, Policy and Law* 16:363–81.

U.S. Bureau of the Census. 1992. *Statistical Abstract of the United States, 1991*. Washington, DC: U.S. Bureau of the Census.

Zwanziger, Jack, and Glenn Melnick. 1988. The Effects of Hospital Competition and the Medicare PPS Program on Hospital Cost Behavior in California. *Journal of Health Economics* 7:301–20.

Commentary
Regulatory Regimes and State Health Policy

Robert B. Hackey

Kenneth Thorpe's analysis of trends in health care spending in Canada and the United States, which appears in this volume, raises several important questions about state health care regulation. Thorpe demonstrates that it is possible to contain costs in the context of a decentralized multipayer system of provider reimbursement, and he cites several U.S. states that were as effective in controlling costs over the past decade as Canadian provinces operating under a single-payer framework. Although Thorpe argues that "expenditure containment and growth ultimately reflect the outcomes of political bargaining among providers and payers," he does not specify the form these bargaining processes have taken or what their impact has been on states' ability to control hospital costs over the past decade. In the end, Thorpe's analysis leaves us with more questions than it answers. In particular, how can we account for significant differences in hospital expenditures between states with similar reimbursement methodologies? Under what circumstances are state governments able to control hospital costs effectively? And what lessons can state experiences with hospital regulation teach us about national health care reform?

The design of regulatory institutions, the policy preferences and economic interests of public and private decision makers, and the ability of public officials to modify providers' behavior all influence the effectiveness of state cost containment programs. The interaction between public officials and health providers reflects the larger relationship between state government and the private sector, since the development and implementation of hospital reimbursement policies occur in the context of a state's prevailing cultural and institutional setting. Because both political culture and the autonomy and capacity of political institutions vary from state to state, different regulatory outcomes (e.g., successfully controlling hospital costs) should emerge from different policy environments. In this context, the autonomy, capacity, and legitimacy of state regulation is often as important, if not more so, as the adoption of a particular reimbursement methodology in determining the success or failure of its cost containment initiatives (Hackey 1992).

The Institutional and Ideological Setting of State Hospital Regulation

Several features of a state's policy-making environment influence the development of hospital reimbursement policies. First, the policy-making capacity of political institutions responsible for the development and implementation of rate setting has an immediate impact on a state's ability to control hospital expenditures. A state's level of institutional capacity depends on stable (and adequate) budgetary and political support, the rate of personnel turnover, and the professionalism and expertise of regulatory policymakers. Second, if the governmental actors in the reimbursement process share a sense of mission, it improves a state's ability to control health care costs; if they do not agree over either the means or the ends of regulation, industry groups can play legislators, bureaucrats, and other participants off against each other in the hope of improving their bargaining position. Finally, when public officials can implement policies that run contrary to the preferences of powerful societal interests, state hospital cost containment efforts can be more effective. In states where policymakers lack either the autonomy or the authority to act against the preferences of provider groups, policy outcomes will resemble what happens with interest group liberalism (Lowi 1969) and regulatory "capture" (Stigler 1988; McConnell 1966), in which narrowly defined economic interests dominate the reimbursement process.

The legitimacy of state cost containment efforts has a powerful impact on the behavior of interest groups in the policy process. When state intervention in the hospital sector is seen as entirely legitimate, legal and legislative challenges to the regulatory system will be infrequent and less likely to succeed when they appear. Differences in the influence of public officials and providers also reflect variations in political culture from state to state, because the role, authority, and autonomy of political institutions are shaped by a state's prevailing political culture and traditions. In general, the more conservative states will be less receptive to government-sponsored solutions such as rate regulation that infringe on the decision-making powers of individuals and firms.

Regulatory Regimes and the Politics of Hospital Reimbursement

The relationship between state governments and the hospital industry falls into three distinct patterns, or regimes, which are biased either in favor of, or against, the development of effective regulatory policies to control hospital costs (Hackey 1992). Each regime represents a fundamentally different balance between the "relative bargaining strengths of purchasers and providers" (see Thorpe in this issue). At one extreme are the imposed regimes, which are defined by an extreme centralization of state regulatory powers, where public officials possess the authority to reshape the hospital reimbursement process to further the state's interests. In contrast, market regimes are notable for the relative underdevelopment of state regulatory authority and a hesitance on the part of policymakers to use the few powers granted to them. In states where regulation and traditional patterns of provider dominance remain in conflict, hospital reimbursement policy is governed by a negotiated regime.

Imposed Regimes

Under an imposed regulatory regime, the belief that the state has a legitimate role in regulating hospital reimbursement fosters an environment in which cost control initiatives can be successfully developed and implemented. Political support from the executive branch and the legislature also gives state officials more leverage with industry groups. Imposed regimes are highly institutionalized: low turnover among bureaucratic and legislative personnel responsible for health care reimbursement issues contributes to the development of specialized knowledge and a shared commitment to controlling health care costs.[1] For a state's hospital regulatory policies to be classified as an imposed regime, however, public officials must possess a well-defined set of policy preferences that they are able to implement consistently as public policy.

1. See, for example, Wilson's (1989: 95–110) discussion of the impact of a cohesive organizational mission on the performance of the U.S. Forest Service, the U.S. Army Corps of Engineers, and the Social Security Administration and Perrow's (1990) account of the effect of goal conflict and goal displacement on New York's response to the emerging AIDS epidemic during the 1980s.

Market Regimes

The relationship between providers, payers, and the state is fundamentally different under a market regime, where public officials possess little or no formal authority to regulate the hospital industry. Under these circumstances, regulatory agencies are unlikely to be catalysts of change, for the prevailing political culture favors private solutions to public problems, in the spirit of Grant McConnell's (1966) "orthodox tradition" as both a more efficient and less threatening solution than state intervention. Consensus on ideological and programmatic goals among participants and relevant publics in the health policy network is typically high, for the state imposes few requirements on either providers or payers; responsibility for negotiating reimbursement rates rests squarely with the private sector. A stunted bureaucracy also limits the state's ability to develop and implement innovative cost control policies, because both "managed competition" and rate-setting strategies typically require that government officials assume an activist role (Morone 1992).

Negotiated Regimes

The most common policy-making arrangements, however, fall somewhere between these two extremes, where the ability of public officials to change providers' behavior is limited by both institutional and ideological constraints. Under a negotiated regime, state efforts to control costs are often hampered by high personnel turnover, conflict over program goals, inadequate funding for state regulatory agencies, and ideological resistance to regulatory initiatives. Policy development and implementation has a strong corporatist flavor, as state officials must turn to industry groups for both political support and administrative assistance. Negotiated regimes thus reaffirm Huntington's (1968: 5) contention that the "primary problem of politics is the lag in the development of political institutions behind social and economic change."

The framework outlined above can shed some light on the questions posed by Thorpe's analysis, because the hospital reimbursement decisions that he discusses in California, Maryland, Massachusetts, New Jersey, and New York occurred in the context of either imposed or negotiated regimes. In each state, government officials adopted an activist role in the hospital reimbursement process, either by creating an all-payer rate-setting system or by designing an elaborate system of competitive bidding for health services (e.g., Medi-Cal). In the pages that follow, I explore the impact of differences in political culture and institutional arrangements on cost containment in two of those states, Massachusetts and New York, over the past decade.

New York

New York's experience with hospital rate setting can best be understood as an imposed regulatory regime. In no state was the "public utility" model of rate regulation more conspicuous than in the Empire State; by the early 1980s, the hospital industry had lost much of its capacity for autonomous decision making. While the state's initial forays into hospital rate regulation in the 1970s only set rates for Blue Cross and Medicaid, the scope of state regulatory authority gradually expanded to include all payers with the creation of the New York Prospective Hospital Reimbursement Methodology (NYPHRM) in 1982. When New York declined to renew its Medicare waiver after the expiration of NYPHRM I in 1985, subsequent versions of the state's prospective payment system operated as a "Medicare wraparound," setting rates for all non-Medicare payers.

Although the state's fiscal crisis during the 1970s provided the impetus for officials in the Department of Health (DOH) to engage in increasingly aggressive efforts to control the growth of hospital costs, the enormous expense of Medicaid insured that hospital cost control remained a policy priority. New York's fiscal obligation to Medicaid is staggering; throughout the 1980s, the Empire State led the nation in total Medicaid program expenses, per capita Medicaid spending, and the number of Medicaid recipients as a percentage of the state's population. The fiscal burden of Medicaid helped to forge a broad consensus among public and private payers over the importance of bringing hospital costs under control; with strong support from both the governor's office and the legislature over the past decade, officials in the Department of Health presided over a regulatory apparatus that presented hospitals with one of the most competitive, if not openly hostile, operating environments in the nation.

New York has a long tradition of regulatory activism in the health sector, dating back to the Metcalf-McClosky Act of 1964, which introduced one of the nation's most stringent certificate-of-need programs to curtail hospitals' capital expansion. Although providers have challenged both the Department of Health's regulatory decisions and its rate-setting powers, the department's regulatory authority has generally been upheld in court. The Hospital Association of New York State has vociferously opposed the state's reimbursement policies and has often found a receptive ear in the legislature, but endorsements from Blue Cross, business groups, and the governor's office generally supported the DOH's aggressive pursuit of cost control over the opposition of the hospital industry.[2] During the 1980s, the relationship between the state's hospital industry and the department reflect a level of animosity seldom seen in American politics. While hospitals fumed over the Department of Health's "micromanagement" of provider reimbursement and the lack of turnover among senior managers in the DOH, Commissioner Axelrod compared the state's hospitals to "seventeenth-century Germanic guilds" in speeches to the state's business community. Under these circumstances, as one hospital executive quipped, "it's tough to get people to be statesmanlike." By the end of the decade, the department had forced hospitals to shoulder the brunt of the cost for implementing new minimum operating standards, thwarted repeated efforts by providers to move the base year for calculating reimbursement rates, and successfully managed the transition from a per diem reimbursement methodology to a new case-based payment system using diagnosis-related groups (DRGs). Even after the unexpected retirement of Commissioner David Axelrod in 1991, the Department of Health remained firmly committed to controlling hospital costs.

The ability of policymakers over the past decade to resist industry pressures and persist in their efforts to keep hospital costs under control reflected the capacity of New York's policy-making institutions in the health sector. In particular, the institutionalization of expertise within both the DOH and the legislature's principal incubator for health policy development, the Council on Health Care Financing, provided state officials with a crucial advantage in reimbursement negotiations. While providers criticized low turnover in key policy positions within the Department of Health, the presence of a highly professionalized and experienced staff enabled the state to develop and implement innovative regulatory policies

2. In 1990, however, neither the governor nor the legislature was predisposed to wage a protracted battle over hospital costs because of the upcoming statewide election. Instead, the reenactment of the state's case payment system became an opportunity to appease powerful constituencies. The legislature rejected the DOH's proposal to pay providers on the basis of a "group price," where institutions' level of reimbursement is based on the average costs for a group of peer institutions rather than their own historical experience and pumped more than $300 million in additional revenues into the hospital reimbursement system over a three-year period. This decision, however, was unusual, and stands in marked contrast to the policies adopted by the legislature and implemented by the Department of Health in previous years.

Table 1 Personnel Stability under an Imposed Regulatory Regime, New York State Department of Health, Office of Health Systems Management, 1991

Name	Position	Appointed	Previous Departmental Experience
Raymond Sweeney	Director	1984	Executive deputy director (1981–83); associate director, DHCF (1979–81)
Brian Hendricks	Executive deputy director	1984	Governor's Select Commission (1983–84); deputy director, Health Planning Commission (1979–83)
Steve Anderman	Deputy director, DHCF	1982	Assistant director, DHCF (1979–82)
Mark Van Guysling	Assistant director, DHCF	1982	Assistant director, Bureau of Hospital Reimbursement, DHCF (1978–82)
William Gormley	Deputy director, DHFP	1989	Assistant director, DHCF (1979–88)
Nicholas Mangiordo	Deputy director, ALTCS	1989	Deputy director, DHFP (1979–89)
Michael Parker	Associate director, CON	1979	Director, Bureau of Facility and Service Review, DHFP (1976–78)

Note. DHCF: Division of Health Care Financing; DHFP: Division of Health Facility Planning; ALTCS: Alternative Long Term Care Strategies; CON: Certificate of Need Review Group, DHFP.

over the past decade (see Table 1). During the 1980s, New York led the nation in developing new DRG classifications for neonatal conditions and AIDS, significantly improved its DRG grouper in 1990, and began planning for improvements to be incorporated into the latest version of the state's case-based payment system (NYPHRM IV). In short, the technical sophistication and policy expertise of New York's health bureaucracy enabled it to respond to a changing environment by setting the state's policy agenda. In other states, however, state rate-setting programs were less dynamic and were unable to respond to new demands and pressures.

Massachusetts

Massachusetts's experience with rate regulation illustrates the perils of regulatory policy-making in an unstable political environment. Less than a decade after the introduction of all-payer rate setting, hospital rate regulation self-destructed and was effectively discredited as a cost control strategy in the eyes of payers, providers, and former legislative supporters. In 1991, the Weld administration's proposal to deregulate the reimbursement system passed comfortably in both the House and the Senate, effectively ending the state's foray into hospital regulation. Few mourned its passage. The demise of rate setting in Massachusetts presents a puzzle: Why did Massachusetts and New York have such different experiences with all-payer rate setting, despite the similarities between their reimbursement methodologies? Furthermore, what led Massachusetts to turn its back on regulation scarcely a decade after it came to national prominence?

Although the state's authority to regulate hospital reimbursement expanded considerably over time, support for regulation in Massachusetts depended on a fragile coalition of payers, providers, and business groups brought together to support the state's first all-payer system (Chapter 372) in 1982 (see Bergthold 1988). After the passage of Chapter 372, the Massachusetts Rate Setting Commission (MRSC) took a less active role in policy development as the locus of decision-making authority shifted to the legislature. In sharp contrast to New York, the institution with the most experience regulating health providers was relegated to a marginal role, since subsequent reenactments of the all-payer system in 1985 (Chapter 574) and 1988 (Chapter 23) actually specified the terms of the contracts between providers and payers. In the legislative arena, however, hospital reimbursement soon fell victim to the vagaries of the political process as payers, providers, and business groups pursued their own narrow economic interests.

The origins of all-payer rate setting in Massachusetts also constrained the state's ability to implement policies opposed by powerful societal groups. The state was a reluctant participant in the process which produced Chapter 372; legislators simply ratified an agreement hammered out under the prodding of the state business community, led by the Massachusetts Business Roundtable (MBRT) (Bergthold 1988). Chapter 372 reflected the concerns of the state's business community that hospital costs were spiraling out of control. The all-payer system provided hospitals with a strong incentive to cut operating costs, control admissions, and shift patient care to less expensive, outpatient settings when it linked reimbursement to patient volume and imposed new "productivity" incentives on hospitals. Business supported both Chapter 372 and its successor, Chapter 574, as a welcome step toward cost reduction. When the all-payer system came up for renewal in 1988, however, the political environment had changed. Hospitals demanded a relaxation of the strict productivity requirements and sought additional funding to offset rising labor costs for nurses and other allied health personnel in exchange for their support of the Dukakis administration's health care reform agenda. In the end, the passage of the universal health care bill (Chapter 23) was a watershed for rate regulation in Massachusetts: its generous treatment of providers was a bane to business groups and a boon to providers. The coalition that had framed Chapter 372 collapsed after the passage of Chapter 23. After losing badly in the legislative debates in 1988, business effectively withdrew from health policy debates to pursue other issues, such as worker's compensation and tax reform.

Blue Cross, for its part, felt increasingly constrained because the regulatory framework embodied in Chapter 23 prevented the company from flexing its muscle in a more competitive bidding process. By 1988, the state's cumbersome proto-DRG system appeared anachronistic and inflexible to providers and payers alike. High personnel turnover and budget cutbacks, however, prevented the MRSC from either improving the system or developing a worthy successor; with few resources, the MRSC was overwhelmed with the day-to-day administration of the payment system. Staff cutbacks, a statewide hiring freeze, and the attractiveness of opportunities in the private sector drained the MRSC of several of its most talented managers; leadership of the MRSC's Bureau of Hospitals changed hands four times between 1985 and 1990, while other key positions remained unfilled. The arrival of the Weld administration in 1990 sealed the fate of rate setting, for the governor and his staff sought to eliminate, not enhance, the MRSC's regulatory authority as part of a general campaign to "downsize" state government.

Massachusetts's experience in controlling costs during the 1980s reflects the turmoil and instability of a changing political environment. The state was more effective in controlling the growth of hospital expenditures in the early years of the all-payer system, when the various parties shared a consensus on both goals and means. As this consensus began to fray in the mid-1980s, the legislature made significant concessions to the hospital industry in order to win reauthorization of the reimbursement system, undermining the system's ability to control costs. From 1982 to 1986, hospital expenditures in Massachusetts increased, on average, at slightly more than a 7 percent annual rate, reflecting the stringency of

Table 2 Hospital Expenditures under Selected State Rate-setting Programs, 1982–1989

State	1982 (dollars)	1986 (dollars)	1987 (dollars)	1989 (dollars)	Percentage Change 1982–86	Percentage Change 1987–89	Average Change 1982–86	Average Change 1987–89
Maryland	1,769,362	2,266,202	2,455,947	3,022,679	28.08	23.08	7.02	11.54
Massachusetts	3,582,627	4,598,913	4,944,140	6,160,608	28.37	24.60	7.09	12.30
New Jersey	2,926,344	4,137,488	4,458,193	5,813,699	41.39	30.40	10.35	15.20
New York	9,436,920	13,179,965	14,182,866	17,362,865	39.66	22.42	9.92	11.21
Rhode Island	431,032	593,767	651,505	788,259	37.75	20.99	9.44	10.50

Notes. Expenditures are for short-term general and other special hospitals.
Data obtained from the American Hospital Association's annual survey of U.S. hospitals.

the new cost control mechanisms introduced by Chapter 372. After 1986, however, the Bay State was much less successful in controlling costs, as annual increases in hospital costs nearly doubled, averaging more than 12 percent from 1987 to 1989. Although Medicaid placed a heavy burden on both Massachusetts and New York, the stringency of NYPHRM's all-payer reimbursement methodology successfully limited the growth in program outlays. In New York, Medicaid expenses increased 147 percent from 1975 to 1988, compared to a whopping 332 percent increase during the same period in Massachusetts (HCFA 1988). While hospital expenditures increased in all of the states described in Table 2, the rate of growth in Massachusetts and New Jersey far exceeded that in New York, where strong political support and an experienced policy-making team continued to campaign for cost control at the end of the decade.

Conclusion

In the end, state efforts to control hospital costs have much to teach policymakers about national health care reform. More than three decades after rising health care costs first became an issue of public concern, policymakers and the public continue to search for a "quick fix" to the nation's health care dilemma. Too often, our search for solutions begins, and ends, with various methods for reorganizing the health care system (such as HMOs), reforming provider payment (DRGs), or rationalizing the production of health services (HSAs, PSROs, and PROs). Thorpe's analysis, however, suggests that no single reimbursement methodology, in and of itself, holds the key to controlling health care costs. Instead, the problem is a political one, linked to the peculiar institutional and ideological context of American health policy.

Successful cost control, therefore, depends not on whether providers are reimbursed by a single payer or multiple payers, paid prospectively or retrospectively, or whether reimbursement is computed on a per diem, per case, or global budget basis. As Foster (1982) notes, the rate of reimbursement can be set at a high or low level under any payment methodology. Cost control is inextricably linked to the capacity and autonomy of regulatory institutions, for without adequate authority and expertise, government will be hard pressed to design and implement an effective health care financing system. The experiences of Massachusetts and New York over the past decade also lend credence to Sapolsky et al.'s (1987: 135) observation that "it is less difficult to bring together a talented group for designing a new program than it is to hold one together for the arduous task of program implementation and refinement." Decentralizing cost control responsibilities is desirable, because it would permit continued experimentation with various methods of organizing and financing health care services, despite the states' inability to significantly improve access to health services (see Stone 1992). Any proposal for national health care reform which leaves policy implementation in the hands of the states, however, is likely to require institution building, for not all states possess the institutional leverage to negotiate effectively with providers and payers. If a decentralized strategy is to succeed, the federal government must be willing to bolster the states' regulatory capabilities; without technical expertise and a clear mandate to control costs, neither state nor federal efforts are likely to reduce health care expenditures significantly in the years to come.

References

American Hospital Association. 1982–89. Annual surveys of U.S. hospitals. New York: American Hospital Association.

Bergthold, Linda A. 1988. Purchasing Power: Business and Health Policy Change in Massachusetts. *Journal of Health Politics, Policy and Law* 13:425–51.

Foster, Richard W. 1982. Cost-based Reimbursement and Prospective Payment: Reassessing the Incentives. *Journal of Health Politics, Policy and Law* 7:407–20.

Hackey, Robert B. 1992. Trapped between State and Market: Regulating Hospital Reimbursement in the Northeastern States. *Medical Care Review* 49 (3): 355–88.

HCFA (Health Care Financing Administration). 1988. *Medicare and Medicaid Data Book*. Washington, DC: U.S. Government Printing Office.

Huntington, Samuel. 1968. *Political Order in Changing Societies*. New Haven: Yale University Press.

Lowi, Theodore. 1969. *The End of Liberalism*. New York: Norton.

McConnell, Grant. 1966. *Private Power and American Democracy*. New York: Knopf.

Morone, James A. 1992. Hidden Complications: Why Health Care Needs Regulation. *American Prospect* 10 (Summer): 40–48.

Perrow, Charles. 1990. *The AIDS Disaster*. New Haven: Yale University Press.

Sapolsky, Harvey, James Aisenberg, and James A. Morone. 1987. The Call to Rome and Other Obstacles to State-Level Innovation. *Public Administration Review* 47 (March/April): 135–42.

Stigler, George. 1988. The Theory of Economic Regulation. In *Chicago Studies in Political Economy*, ed. G. Stigler. Chicago: University of Chicago Press.

Wilson, James Q. 1989. *Bureaucracy: What Government Agencies Do and Why They Do It*. New York: Basic.

I am grateful to Jim Morone of Brown University and Michael Sparer of Columbia University's School of Public Health for their helpful comments and suggestions. This research was generously supported by a grant from the Dean's Fund at St. Anselm College.

The Unknown States

Michael S. Sparer

Rarely heard in the debate over health care reform is a discussion of health care politics at the state level. This lack of analysis is surprising. Not only do state treasuries fund a large share of the nation's health care bill, but also state officials play a key policy role. The Medicaid program, for example, delegates to state governments broad authority to determine who in their state receives coverage, what medical services are covered, and how much medical providers are paid for delivering care. State officials also supervise the nation's private insurance system, regulate the quality of care rendered by most medical providers, and work to reduce the glaring gaps in the nation's health care delivery system.

Given the imporatnce of state-level politics and the scant attention it typically receives, it is refreshing to read Kenneth Thorpe's essay. As Thorpe reminds us, there is extraordinary variation in the health care policies of the fifty states, and there is much to be learned by studying the politics that produces such policies. But Thorpe's quantitative analysis only hints at the complicated politics of reimbursement policy, and in this commentary I flesh out in more detail the stories of cost containment in New York and California (two of the states Thorpe examines). I then corroborate Thorpe's observation that the politics of cost containment is more interesting and important than the technology of cost containment and suggest that reformers cannot develop workable cost containment (or other health reform) policies without taking into account the realities of state-level politics.

The Politics of Cost Containment:
Some Preliminary Observations

Thorpe argues that New York and California have done a relatively good job of cost containment. New York, says Thorpe, adopted a successful all-payer hospital reimbursement system (in 1983), enforces rigorous certificate-of-need requirements, and does a good job of controlling Medicaid expenditures. California, adds Thorpe, implemented the innovative "selective contracting system," which demonstrates that "centralized, regulatory control may not represent our only road to salvation." Thorpe concludes from these examples that the key to cost containment is not to change financing systems (from multipayer to single-payer) but is instead to strengthen government's ability to dominate the political battles over reimbursement policy.

On one level, Thorpe is surely right: If government chooses cost containment as a high-priority goal, and if government dominates the political battles over reimbursement policy, then cost containment will follow. But government's ability to dominate reimbursement policy depends primarily on the policy-making environment within which state officials operate. And such environments vary, not only by state but also by the particular policy under consideration.

Consider, for example, nursing home reimbursement policy. State officials seem poised to dominate this policy arena: after all, Medicaid is the primary third-party payer of nursing home bills. Why then does a nursing home in New York receive over $120 per day per Medicaid patient (which represents the highest rate in the continental United States), while a similarly situated facility in California receives only $65 per day?[1] Why then did New York in 1989 spend $1.3 billion more on skilled nursing care than did California ($2.34 billion to $1.08 billion), even though it had 17,000 fewer nursing home patients than did California (U.S. HCFA 1990)? What explains this policy puzzle?

The explanation, I suggest, is rooted in the contrasting political environments in the two states. In New York, Medicaid bureaucrats operate

1. In New York City, the average rate is even higher: $142 per day. The New York figures were obtained from a New York State Department of Health report (1991). The California figures were obtained during a telephone interview with Joseph Klun, Rate Development Branch, California Department of Health Services, 7 June 1991, and from materials received from Eugene Knoweful, of the Rate Development Branch, in February 1992. The disparity in rates is mildly deceptive, since the New York rates include the cost of certain "ancillary services" (such as physical therapy) that are not included in the California rate. Nonetheless, the percentage of the difference explained by this variable is, by all accounts, quite small.

within a fragmented, decentralized, and interest-group-dominated polity, in which nursing home owners, union officials, and patient advocates all exert significant influence. As a result, patients in New York receive (relatively) good care, employees receive (relatively) high wages, and providers receive unusually high reimbursement. In California, in contrast, Medicaid officials enjoy significant bureaucratic autonomy and can ensure that policy is driven by the goal of cost containment. As a result, state officials developed a flat rate reimbursement system (under which facilities receive the same low rate regardless of their actual costs), imposed minimal regulatory oversight over nursing home behavior (enabling facilities to cut costs by cutting patient care), and permitted facilities with low costs to make a profit (Sparer 1992).

These disparate policy-making environments not only influence state policy decisions; they also influence federal efforts to impose national reforms. Congress, for example, recently enacted a series of nursing home quality-of-care reforms, which were to take effect on 1 October 1990. The reforms required nursing homes throughout the country to meet minimal standards on several counts, from staff-patient ratios, to patient rights, to staff training. California officials, anxious to avoid higher nursing home costs and unwilling to impose a strict regulatory regime on providers, embarked upon an all-out effort to evade the new mandate. Governor Wilson even appealed directly to President Bush. And while the final chapter on the reform legislation is as yet unwritten, California's effort to avoid implementation is ongoing.

The comparison of nursing home politics in New York and California suggests several lessons. First, American federalism encourages a health care system with extraordinary variation, even between similarly situated states. We need to consider more carefully whether such variation is good or bad (or sometimes good and sometimes bad). Second, federal legislation which seeks to overcome the constraints and biases that dominate state-based politics is difficult to implement. Third, implementation is particularly difficult if states not only must change their practices but also must use state dollars to pay for such changes. And fourth, state officials will (and should) always play key roles in our health care system. But we need to think more carefully about what that role should be. For example, if the federal government financed a national health insurance system and state officials regulated the quality of health care, California officials would surely be less opposed to federal efforts to establish minimum levels of care.

In any event, I return to these themes toward the end of this commentary. First, however, I explore in some detail the efforts by New York and California to contain hospital costs, a subject much discussed in Thorpe's paper.

The Politics of Hospital Reimbursement:
The Case of New York

Has New York done as good a job at hospital cost containment as Thorpe suggests? Yes, although its most successful cost containment effort came in 1976, long before the state implemented an all-payer reimbursement system. What explains the state's success? Once again, the policy-making environment is the key (or, put another way: context, context, context).

The story begins in 1969, when New York enacted legislation that ended (for Medicaid and Blue Cross) the practice of reimbursing hospitals retroactively for their actual costs and substituted instead a requirement that rates be developed prospectively by state bureaucrats. The rate-setting legislation was prompted by a proposal, promoted by Blue Cross, to impose a thirty-three-month freeze on hospital rates. The state's hospitals obviously opposed the freeze, and they had the law on their side: federal law required that hospitals be reimbursed (by Medicaid) for their "reasonable costs," and such costs would not stay frozen for nearly three years. After much negotiation, the parties compromised: the freeze was reduced to nine months,[2] the rate-setting legislation was enacted, and the federal government permitted New York's "demonstration project" to proceed.

New York's new reimbursement system did not, however, produce the significant savings that were expected. Instead, the early 1970s saw a continual rise in hospital costs. Why the higher costs? Three explanations seem persuasive. First, the health department regulations implementing the legislation were unexpectedly generous to the hospital industry. For example, the state exempted from the new system "capital costs, costs of schools of nursing, costs of interns and residents, and costs of ancillary services." 10 NYCRR 86.14(b). These exemptions were particularly helpful to the large (and politically powerful) teaching hospitals (Law 1974: 105). Second, politically powerful health care unions persuaded state officials to build generous wage increases into the Medicaid and Blue Cross rates, even though the increases far exceeded the level of inflation. And third, the tendency of New Yorkers to have unusually long inpatient stays was accentuated by the per diem reimbursement system, since a hos-

2. Even the shortened freeze was subsequently struck down by the courts.

pital's costs typically decrease after the first few days of hospitalization, often to well below the Medicaid and Blue Cross rates (Berry 1976).

The era of rising costs came to an abrupt end, however, with the 1976 hospital cost containment legislation. This legislation, prompted by the 1975 fiscal crisis, signaled a suspension of politics as usual. Indeed, providers later claimed they were sandbagged, as state officials acted quickly and secretly to develop a plan to respond to the crisis. The legislation used a three-pronged strategy. First, it closed several loopholes in the rate-setting methodology, in an effort to reduce the per diem rates paid to hospitals (for example, ancillary costs were henceforth to be treated similarly to routine costs). Second, it required increased utilization review, to ensure that persons receiving hospital care actually needed hospital care. And third, it encouraged agency efforts to enforce strictly certificate-of-need laws and to institute a program to close "unnecessary" hospitals; as a result, twelve New York City hospitals, with approximately 4,500 beds, were closed between 1975 and 1979 (Thorpe 1988: 366).

The cost containment legislation was so successful that hospitals throughout the state were soon facing their own fiscal crisis (Thorpe 1988: 366). Hospitals responded by shifting costs to the (unregulated) commercial health insurers and by canceling affiliations with Blue Cross. The effort to shift costs increased the tension between insurers, hospitals, and Blue Cross. Ironically, however, it also created an alliance among the three groups: all were united in the effort to challenge the state's hospital reimbursement scheme. By mid-1977, the alliance included also the health care unions (which had done very poorly in their 1976 negotiations), New York City officials (who were spending more and more city dollars in an effort to keep public hospitals afloat), and health care advocates (who noted the precarious fiscal condition of hospitals that served the poor).

With the state's fiscal crisis easing, and the antistate coalition pressing hard, the legislature in 1978 ended its short-lived experiment with draconian cost containment. First, it liberalized some of the more restrictive elements of the 1976 cost containment package. Second, it delegated the task of revising and overseeing the hospital reimbursement system to a new pluralistic agency, called the Council on Health Care Financing, which was composed of members of the legislature, the hospitals, Blue Cross, the commercial insurers, the unions, and the advocates. Third, it provided short-term relief to the commercial insurers by regulating (for the first time) the rates charged to such insurers.

The politics of hospital policy-making had clearly changed. The single-minded quest to control costs, which dominated during the fiscal crisis, was replaced by pluralistic bargaining, aimed at reviving the hospital industry and stabilizing the insurance industry. In this context, the council soon developed a consensus on two goals: first, a single payment methodology for all payers (which would minimize cost shifting); and second, a surcharge on hospital revenue, with the funds collected to be used to subsidize hospitals for a portion of their uncompensated care and to offer financial support for hospitals in fiscal distress.

There was, to be sure, lengthy debate over the mechanics of the new system, particularly with respect to the formula by which the bad debt and charity pool would be distributed. Eventually, however, the council reached agreement on the specifics of a proposal, and in 1983 the New York Prospective Hospital Reimbursement Methodology (NYPHRM) went into effect. Within months, the financial condition of the state's hospitals had improved significantly (New York State Council on Health Care Financing 1986: 20). Indeed, while Thorpe now suggests that all-payer systems produce reduced costs, the all-payer system in New York represented a dramatic (and probably warranted) retreat from a truly effective cost containment experiment.

The Politics of Hospital Reimbursement: The Case of California

The selective contracting program is often touted as evidence that free-market competition can reduce health care costs. But selective contracting works so well not because California's big hospitals compete vigorously for Medi-Cal business but because powerful and autonomous state officials dictate to these hospitals the price they can charge for Medi-Cal clients. The California experience thus supports Thorpe's thesis that centralized regulatory control leads to cost containment: it is not, as he suggests, an exception to the rule. Indeed, Medi-Cal officials spent the fifteen years prior to selective contracting trying unsuccessfully to snare the centralized authority they now enjoy.

The story begins in the late 1960s and early 1970s with the first efforts to constrain state expenditures on indigent hospital care. State officials took a three-pronged approach: first, transfer costs to county governments; second, institute strict utilization review procedures; and third, seek federal permission (much like New York) to move away from Medicare-styled reasonable-cost reimbursement, substituting in its stead a state-established cap on expenditures.

The state-county dispute was rooted in the state's decision, in 1966, to develop the so-called county option program, under which counties paid a small percentage of the overall Medi-Cal bill, but the state guaranteed that county medical expenditures (for Medi-Cal recipients and others) did not exceed (in real dollars) what the counties spent in 1964. This agreement was an obvious target for cost-cutting state officials (like Ronald Reagan). By the mid-1970s, the county option program was gone, the county contribution to the Medi-Cal bill had skyrocketed, and counties were spending over 35 percent of their property tax collections on indigent health care. The result was the California tax revolt of 1978, otherwise known as Proposition 13, a state takeover of county Medi-Cal costs, and a growing fiscal crisis for the state (Solish 1989: 107). The "new federalism" approach to cost-containment (shift the costs to the counties) had clearly failed.

The state's second cost containment effort was a strict prior authorization and utilization review program. In 1970, for example, the state required prior authorization for all nonemergency hospitalizations, and even emergency admissions were subject to immediate oversight and review. Such oversight was relatively effective: in 1981, for example, 28 percent of all requests to extend hospital stays were denied. Moreover, in 1978, treatment authorization denials saved Medi-Cal over $16 million (Aging Health Policy Center 1983: 85). Despite these savings, however, utilization review alone did not and could not significantly constrain rising costs.

Finally, in the mid-1970s, Medi-Cal officials proposed a frontal attack on rising costs: a fixed annual cap on hospital reimbursement increases. Such a system would provide state officials with the same control over hospital rates that they had successfully wielded over nursing home rates. But the new system was never implemented. Instead, the federal courts ruled on two separate occasions that the fixed cap system violated federal Medicaid law, even though federal Medicaid officials sided with the state. California Hospital Association v. Obledo, 602 F.2d 1357 (9th Cir. 1979); California Hospital Association v. Schweiker, 559 F. Supp. 110 (C.D. Cal. 1982), aff'd 705 F.2d 466 (9th Cir. 1982).

Frustrated by the failed efforts at rate regulation but encouraged by President Reagan's support for innovative state-based initiatives, the California legislature in 1982 enacted the selective contracting program. The program was heralded as a path-breaking effort to introduce competition into the hospital industry: State officials would estimate the number of hospital beds needed for Medi-Cal patients; hospitals would bid for Medi-

Cal contracts; hospitals without contracts would provide only emergency room care to Medi-Cal patients (for which they would receive cost-based reimbursement); and the competition for business would encourage efficiency and savings.

Selective contracting as implemented, however, was hardly a case study in competition. Instead, and to the contrary, selective contracting provided a backdoor route for powerful state officials to set (and thereby lower) reimbursement rates. The most powerful such official was William Guy, the so-called czar of the hospital contracting system. Guy's mission was to negotiate the first round of hospital contracts; after that, the California Medical Assistance Commission (CMAC) would take over.

Guy was in a powerful bargaining position: most of California's large hospitals needed Medi-Cal contracts (particularly given their relatively low occupancy rates). Using this leverage, Guy decided to implement a policy of "no net increases" in overall hospital expenditures, an even tougher fiscal cap than had previously been rejected by the federal courts. Such a policy was enormously distressing to hospitals used to double-digit cost-of-living increases. But Guy was unwilling to retreat. And in November of 1982, he rejected bids proffered by San Francisco's three largest hospitals, hospitals that serviced 40 percent of San Francisco's Medi-Cal population. News of the rejection traveled quickly. In the words of one commentator,

> Exclusion of these hospitals sent a message to hospitals in the rest of the state that the state did not so highly value participation (and access for recipients) that it would accept bids that were not competitively priced. The state clearly had chosen to exercise much of the market power it had, and the hospitals now understood that fact. In the days following the San Francisco outcome, the state was flooded with phone calls from hospitals in other areas reducing their bids. The San Francisco area bidding process was reopened, and—this time—the three excluded hospitals submitted acceptable rates. (Abt Associates 1987: 46)

In July, 1983, CMAC assumed the task of administrating the selective contracting program; it adopted and implemented the hard-nosed negotiating model developed by Bill Guy. As a result, by the mid-1980s, the program was generating approximately $350 million in savings per year and was doing so without adversely affecting recipient access to care or the quality of care provided (Johns et al. 1985: 41).

The States and National Health Reform:
The Ongoing Tension

State officials are strong supporters of federally financed national health insurance: the thought of shifting rising health care costs to the federal treasury is irresistible. By and large, however, state officials are anxious to retain their authority to set policy, regulate quality, and administer programs. The stage is thus set for an important debate over the role states should play in a reformed health care system. But participants in this debate need to understand the degree to which key players at the state level (politicians, bureaucrats, providers, insurers, business leaders, union officials, and consumer advocates) have developed institutional arrangements that vary by state and that fundamentally affect policy. These institutional arrangements pose challenges for any reform agenda.

Consider, for example, the argument that state officials should be given *increased* authority to establish health care policy (perhaps with federal financing of such policies, to rescue the average state budget). This view draws strength from three strands of American thought: first, that the delegation of decision-making authority to the states is "democratic"; second, that public policy should, where possible, fit local needs and conditions; and third, that local autonomy encourages innovative ideas, enables such ideas to be "tested," and allows state officials to evaluate and implement ideas that "work." [3] Nonetheless, the comparison of reimbursement policy in New York and California suggests, if only preliminarily, two ongoing problems with this model. First, the problem of inappropriate interstate variation is not limited to the usual suspects: reimbursement policy, like eligibility and benefit policy, is irrationally inconsistent. It is absurd that a nursing home in New York receives twice the reimbursement of its counterpart in California. Moreover, even if (as Thorpe argues) five states have effectively contained hospital costs, what about the forty-five that have not? Second, state actors are not as free as the "laboratory" model suggests to experiment boldly with new policies. Indeed, it is extremely difficult for even the very best state policymakers to escape their state-based political environments. This is particularly true in states like New York, where state officials are but one player in a pluralistic environment.

The New York–California comparison should give equal pause, however, to those who believe that federal legislation can (or should) undo with the stroke of a pen policy-making environments that have existed

3. I am grateful to Deborah Stone for guiding me to this typology.

for years. Federal legislation that seeks to overcome the constraints and biases of state-based politics is difficult to implement, particularly if states not only must change their practices but also must use state dollars to pay for such changes.

The task (and the challenge) is to rework the division of labor between states and the federal government in a way that acknowledges and accounts for the realities of state politics. The goal is to minimize inappropriate interstate variation and to maximize useful interstate variation. (For example, the home care system in New York City should look very different from its counterpart in rural Idaho. Local needs do differ.) In this task, the Canadian system provides a helpful model, with its effort to encourage provincial flexibility within several overarching federal principles. But a workable American model is achievable only if we study more carefully the black box of state-based politics. Without such an inquiry, reform efforts will be uninformed, poorly planned, and inevitably disappointing.

References

Abt Associates. 1987. *Medicaid Program Evaluation: Inpatient Hospital Reimbursement*. Cambridge, MA: Abt Associates.

Aging Health Policy Center. 1983. *State Discretionary Policies and Services in the Medicaid, Social Services, and Supplemental Security Income Programs*. University of California at San Francisco.

Berry, Ralph E. 1976. Prospective Rate Reimbursement and Cost Containment: Formula Reimbursement in New York. *Inquiry* 13(3): 288–301.

Johns, L., R. A. Derzon, and M. Anderson. 1985. *Selective Contracting for Health Services in California: Final Report*. Washington, DC: Lewin and Associates and the National Governors Association.

Law, Sylvia A. 1974. *Blue Cross: What Went Wrong?* New Haven, CT: Yale University Press.

New York State Council on Health Care Financing. 1986. *Annual Report of the New York State Council on Health Care Financing*. Albany: New York State Council on Health Care Financing.

New York State Department of Health. 1991. *Bureau of RHCF Reimbursement: Average 1991 Rates by DOH Region*. Albany: New York State Department of Health.

Solish, Martha. 1989. Los Angeles County Public Hospitals. In *Competition and Compassion: Conflicting Roles for Public Hospitals*, ed. S. H. Altman, C. Brecher, M. G. Henderson, and K. E. Thorpe. Ann Arbor, MI: Health Administration Press.

Sparer, Michael S. 1992. Health Politics and American Federalism: A Comparison of the Medicaid Programs in New York and California. Ph.D. dissertation, Department of Politics, Brandeis University.

Thorpe, Kenneth E. 1988. Health Care. In *The Two New Yorks*, ed. Gerald Benjamin and Charles Brecher. New York: Russell Sage Foundation.

U.S. HCFA (U.S. Health Care Financing Administration). 1990. *Medicaid State Tables for Fiscal Year 1989*. Washington, DC: U.S. HCFA, Division of Medicaid Statistics.

Part 6

Lessons from Abroad

Who Gets What? Levels of Care in Canada, Britain, Germany, and the United States

Colleen M. Grogan

Abstract Americans view universal coverage as a reality only if a minimum benefit package is explicitly defined, and discussions about expanding access take place under the slogan of minimum benefits. The policy environment is different in Canada, Britain, and Germany. There, health care costs are controlled and benefits provided under universal coverage plans. Yet the medical services provided in these countries result not from difficult decisions about rationing care at a "minimum" benefit level but from difficult political decisions about the structure of the health care system. Institutional factors rather than explicit policy influence the implicit health priorities in these countries. The United States, in contrast, develops policies that explicitly designate a minimum level of benefits.

In the last decade the health policy debate in the U.S. has focused largely on controlling health care costs. The problem of access to health care is addressed only when the issue is couched within the larger concerns of cost escalation. Discourse about access, when it occurs, has centered on how to make health care accessible and at the same time control costs. This debate leads to the question—Access to what? What *is* an acceptable level of health care?

It is not surprising, therefore, that when several American states have considered or passed a state health care plan for the uninsured, it has been presented under the heading of "basic" or "minimum" health care benefits. For the first time, at least in the public arena of U.S. health care policy, the notion of explicitly setting limits on the provision of health care services (often euphemistically called "rationing" care) is being discussed. While this trend is not surprising, given the cost-conscious policy environment of the past decade, it is important to note that such explicit discussion of limiting medical service is unique to America.

In general, there are two main strategies that governments can pursue to limit the utilization of medical services and thereby control costs. First, they can limit care by category—by designating either specific groups, such as the elderly, or specific diseases or medical procedures, such as heart transplants, that will not be paid for by the government. This is an explicit form of limitation, because the government creates a set of policies specifying who or what is not covered. The United States is gradually adopting this strategy.

The second strategy is not explicit: it limits the supply of medical services through policies for reimbursement (payments to medical facilities and providers) and the acquisition of technology. In general, countries providing universal health care coverage tend to pursue this second strategy to control the cost of care.

My purpose in this paper is to explore why Americans tend to view universal coverage as a reality only if a minimum benefit package is explicitly defined. In the first section of this paper, I will briefly document the U.S. policy environment, where expanding access is discussed under the slogan of minimum benefits. I go on to analyze how health care costs are controlled and benefits provided under universal coverage plans in three countries—Canada, Britain, and Germany. From my analysis, I argue that medical services provided in these countries result not from difficult decisions about rationing care at a "minimum" benefit level but rather from difficult political decisions about the structure of the health care system. Institutional factors rather than an explicit health priority policy influence the implicit health priorities in these countries. I conclude by offering some reasons why the United States focuses on policies that explicitly designate a minimum level of benefits.

Access Policy in the American States

Due to chronic inaction at the federal level, many states have been forced to grapple with the issue of care for people who are covered by neither private health insurance nor Medicaid. At the same time, there has been an effort under the "New Federalism" of the 1980s for the federal government to shift a greater burden of the costs of social services such as Medicaid to the states. Moreover, the cost of the state-administered Medicaid program has continued to increase substantially over the past two decades. Missouri, for example, has since 1983 spent 80 cents of every additional dollar levied in the state for social services on the Medicaid program (*Nation's Health* 1991). All this is happening at a time when most states are projecting moderate to serious revenue shortfalls.

Despite these depressed economic forecasts and serious budget deficits, many state legislatures have continued to address the issue of expanding access to health care. The headlines of two adjacent articles about American state health policy in the April 1991 edition of *The Nation's Health* illustrate this tension between expanding access and controlling costs: "Mandates on Medicaid Trouble Governors" and "Emphasis on Improving Access." At least six states have passed or seriously considered legislation to expand access to all of their residents, and many states have at least focused on improving access for population groups such as children or workers employed by small businesses. However, the cost/access dilemma persists, and states tend to consider the expansion of access to health care only under the rubric of "basic" health care benefits.

For example, all the states that have considered a state health care plan have done so in conjunction with some minimum benefit design. Oregon is considering explicitly rationing care to make medical services accessible to a greater number of persons (Garland and Hasnain 1990; IHPP 1991a). The New York State Department of Health (1990) also proposed a minimum package in its Universal New York Health Care proposal (UNY*Care): "UNY*Care will specify a basic package of benefits which will serve as a standard for all benefit packages. . . . While this coverage will specify a minimum, the minimum will be sufficiently high to encourage acceptance by all parties as the basic standard of care" (p. 11). When the state of Washington passed a health plan, it created a new agency to administer the plan and gave this agency the explicit responsibility of determining the minimum benefit package for the plan. Massachusetts created a similar agency, the Department of Medical Security, and charged it with this responsibility as well. Minnesota's Health Care Access Commission, appointed by the governor to address the issue of Minnesota's uninsured, advocates "a basic set of health care benefits" in its recommendations for a state health plan (Quam 1991: 2). A report (Geoghegan and Allenby 1990), prepared for the California governor and legislature by the secretaries of the California State agencies of health and welfare and business, transportation, and housing, stated that "the design of a benefit package is crucial to overall viability and affordability of legislated health care coverage. The schedule of benefits should be restricted to those services that are medically necessary" (p. 10). A California task force, in fact, developed a list of essential basic services which was included in the appendix of the report.

Even states that have focused their attention on expanding access to specific population groups have done so under this framework of minimum benefits. The Intergovernmental Health Policy Project (IHPP 1991b)

Table 1 Provisions of Basic Benefit Laws in Fifteen American States.

Basic Benefits	AR	FL	GA[a]	IL	KS[b]	KY	MD	MO	MT	NM	ND[c]	RI	VA	WA	WV
Inpatient Hospital	x[d]					x[e]	x[f]		x	x[g]		x[h]	x[i]	x	x[j]
Emergency Medical															x
Outpatient Hospital							x		x						x
In/Outpatient Physician Care in Hospital						x									x
Physician Services															
Primary Care Visits	x						x		x	x		x	x		x
Prenatal Care	x						x		x	x		x	x		x
Well Baby Care							x		x	x		x	x		
Obstetric/Maternity Care	x	x[k]					x		x	x		x	x		x
Newborn Metabolic/ Sickle Cell Screening												x			
Adopted Children	x			x											
Child Health Supervision		x[k]						x[f]							
Children's Preventive Services	x														
Newborn Children	x			x				x[f]	x	x		x			
Mammograms				x				x[f]		x		x		x	
Pap Tests												x			
Mental Health		x[k]					x	x[f]	x			x			x
Substance Abuse		x[k]										x			x

Home Nursing Care	x[k]	x	x
Other Primary/ Preventive Care	x	x	x
Ambulatory Surgical Center Services	x[k]	x	
Surgical Procedures and Devices Incidental to Mastectomy	x[k]		
Maximum Annual and/or Lifetime Benefit	x	x	x

Source. IHPP 1991b: 3.

Note. States are designated by their zip code abbreviations; the names read, from left to right: Arkansas, Florida, Georgia, Illinois, Kansas, Kentucky, Maryland, Missouri, Montana, New Mexico, North Dakota, Rhode Island, Virginia, Washington, West Virginia.

a. The law authorizes the state insurance commissioner to establish a model basic health insurance plan that provides coverage for primary health care services designed to prevent the need for more expensive health care services.

b. The law does not specify individual benefits that must be part of the basic package. Instead, small-employer benefit plans are required to provide so-called Part I coverage, defined as coverage up to a statutory maximum for necessary care and treatment of sickness or injury in excess of $5,000 for an individual or $7,500 for a family.

c. The law does not specify any minimum benefits but requires that the exempted mandated benefits be made available at the option of the individual or employer, for which an additional premium for each coverage can be charged.

d. At least fifteen days.

e. At least fourteen days.

f. Up to ten days.

g. The law does not mandate the inclusion of any specific benefits or coverage, but limited mandate health insurance policies must offer this benefit.

h. Up to twenty-five days.

i. Up to twenty days.

j. At least thirty days.

k. The basic policy is not required to contain this benefit, but the law requires that insurers make it available to the policy-holder for an appropriate additional premium.

recently reported that since the beginning of 1990, the legislatures in fifteen states have enacted laws authorizing insurers to market basic benefit plans to small business employers (usually fewer than twenty-five employees). As of May 1991, basic benefit health plan bills were under active consideration in at least ten more states. Table 1 shows the benefits that must be included in the basic benefit plans in the fifteen states that have enacted laws. All these laws assume that explicitly defined basic benefit plans are key to the problem of affordability for small firms. This presumption—that an adequate minimum benefit package must be explicitly defined *before* health care protection can be expanded to more population groups—has become an acceptable and popular position in the U.S. health policy arena.

Benefits in Countries with Universal Access

Comparative studies of foreign health care systems have become commonplace as Americans search for pieces of the cost/access puzzle (see Morone 1990). Popular conclusions derived from some comparative studies warn that universal coverage is not without costs—in terms of both reduced quality (Aaron and Schwartz 1984) and increased expenditure (Enthoven and Kronick 1989). Britain is most commonly used as the example of a country which rations health care to control the costs of universal access. (Recently, claims of rationing in Canada have also been presented—see Aaron and Schwartz 1984 and Todd 1989). These discussions tend to imply that countries that have designed universal access policies have systematically limited the provision of particular services.

Yet these countries did not define a minimum benefit package when their national health plans were enacted. To the contrary, "comprehensive benefits" was and still is their motto. While these countries have made explicit decisions about long-term care and dental and prescription drug coverage, they have not made explicit policy decisions on which specific medical services will or will not be provided (e.g., transplants or prenatal care). It is not an explicit benefit structure that has enabled these countries to control their health care costs but the structure of the health care system itself.

In political rhetoric, *comprehensive benefits* does not mean *unlimited care*. There is implied at least devotion to the principle of a "minimum" level of care and this minimum level is slightly different in each country. In this section I discuss how health care costs are controlled and what bene-

Table 2 Services Provided through Medical Benefit Packages
in Canada, Britain, and Germany

Services	Canada	Britain	Germany
Inpatient Care	x	x	x (copay)
Ambulatory Care	x	x	x
Health Education and Promotion	x	x	x
Long-Term Care for Chronically Disabled Elderly	x	x	Means-tested
Dental Care	Some provinces	x	x (copay)
Prescription Drugs	Some provinces	x (copay)	x (copay)
Chiropractic Care	Some provinces	x	x
Optometric Care	Some provinces	x	x
Private Health Insurance	x	x	x

Sources. U.S. DHEW 1980; Henke 1989; Potter and Porter 1989.

fits are provided under universal coverage plans in Canada, Britain, and
Germany. Table 2 illustrates the breadth of service coverage in these countries. All three cover inpatient services, ambulatory care, and community-
based services (health promotion, education, and prevention). However,
key differences in benefit coverage occur with long-term care; dental, chiropractic, and optometric care; and prescription drug coverage. Britain is
the most generous in terms of benefits *covered*: it provides all the services
shown in Table 2, regardless of age, income, or geographic location. In
Canada, coverage differs by geographic location (among the provinces).
In Germany, most services are covered, but they are much more likely
to include cost-sharing provisions (though the amount that the consumer
copays for these services is minimal by U.S. standards).

Expenditure and utilization data (shown in Tables 3 and 4) provide
some indication as to how countries have decided to spend their health
care budget. For example, Germany's relatively high utilization and funding of inpatient, ambulatory, and pharmaceutical care, combined with its
relatively low funding of services such as community-based care, suggest a strong emphasis on curative services. Britain's lower use rates and
proportionately higher allocations to community-based services suggest a
greater emphasis on preventive services. Canada, on the other hand, tends
to emphasize traditional, physician-related services; this is indicated by its
lack of coverage for pharmaceutical, chiropractic, optometric, and dental
services. There are no public policies in these countries which explicitly

Table 3 Proportion of Public Expenditures on Health in Britain, Canada, Germany and the United States, by Type of Care, 1987

	Canada	Britain	Germany	U.S.[a]
Inpatient Care (percentage)	59	57	43	47
Ambulatory Care (percentage)	22	11	27	31
Pharmaceutical (percentage)	4	10	20	7
Other[b]	15	22	10	15
Percentage of Gross Domestic Product	8.6	6.1	8.2	11.2
Average Physician Income[c]	$88,566	$39,571	$110,615[d]	$132,300

Source. OECD 1989.

a. Proportion of total health expenditures from government and private sources.

b. *Other* includes community-based care, therapeutic appliances, collective services (such as armed forces medical care), public health programs, biomedical research and development, as well as administrative outlays.

c. In U.S. dollars.

d. Data for 1986.

Table 4 Utilization of Health Care in Britain, Canada, Germany, and the United States, by Type of Care, 1987

	Canada	Britain	Germany	U.S.
Inpatient				
Admission Rates				
(percentage of population)	14.5	15.8	21.1	14.7
Average Length of Stay	13.2	15.0	17.1	9.6[a]
Ambulatory				
Visits per Capita[b]	6.4	4.5	11.5	5.3
Pharmaceutical				
Average Number of Medicines				
per Capita		7.3	12.2	

Source. OECD 1989.

a. Data for 1983.

b. Data for 1986.

state particular health service priorities: the organization of the health care system itself serves to emphasize certain types of care over others.[1]

1. It is likely that unique cultural beliefs in each country also affect health service priorities; however, because cultural differences are very difficult to measure, I will focus only on institutional factors in this paper.

For example, the budget allocation process implicitly shapes health priorities in these countries. The amount allotted to hospitals, physicians, and technology, for instance, determines the priority of preventive care over secondary or tertiary services within the system.

Hospital Reimbursement

While Canada and Britain have comparable rates of inpatient admission and length of stay, Germany's inpatient rate is substantially higher (see Table 4). Schulenburg (1983) suggests three plausible reasons for these high inpatient use rates in West Germany. First, Germany makes a rigid distinction between office-based and hospital-based physicians. A patient is required to have an admission prescription written by an office-based physician to receive hospital care. Because of this differentiation between office-based and hospital-based physicians, the flow of information between the two is often incomplete, and many inpatients undergo repeats of diagnostic examinations they have already received from office-based physicians before they were hospitalized. Second, the per diem hospital reimbursement method (see Table 5) encourages, or least does not discourage, long inpatient lengths of stay. Third, German hospitals (excluding teaching hospitals) are prohibited from offering outpatient care—

Table 5 Structural Characteristics of Universal Access Plans in Canada, Britain, and Germany

Characteristics	Canada	Britain	Germany
Hospital Reimbursement	Capitation	Capitation	Per diem
Physician Reimbursement	Fee for service	Capitation/ salary	Fee for service/ expenditure cap
Freedom to Choose a General Practitioner	Yes	Limited	Yes
Freedom to Choose a Specialist	Yes	No	Yes

Note. Capitation: provider receives a fixed fee per person; *fee for service*: provider receives a fixed fee for each service; *per diem*: provider receives an amount equal to total costs divided by the total number of days of care provided to inpatients over the same period; *expenditure cap*: a group of providers is assigned a fixed expenditure level, which its total reimbursements should not exceed.

Admissions

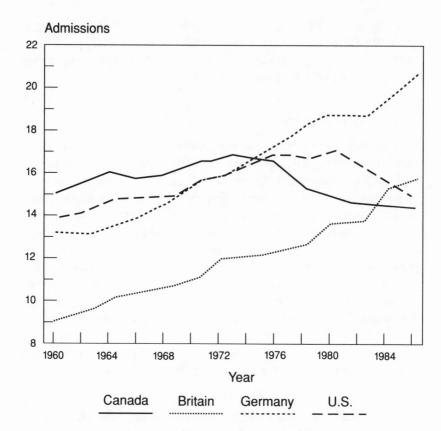

Figure 1 Inpatient Admissions for Canada, Britain, Germany, and the United States, as a Percentage of Population, 1960–1986
Source: OECD 1989.

a restriction that makes it difficult to substitute inpatient services with outpatient care. We can see from Schulenburg's explanation that the emphasis on inpatient care in Germany is an institutional effect rather than an explicit German policy. In other words, Germany's emphasis on inpatient care results from reimbursement and manpower policy decisions, not from an explicit decision that long inpatient treatments are medically appropriate.

In contrast to Germany, Canada and Britain exercise greater control over inpatient expenditures and use rates (Table 5). Britain is the prime example of a country that controls health care costs by limiting the supply of medical services. Because its Department of Health and Human Services has central authority over hospital budgeting allocations, the supply

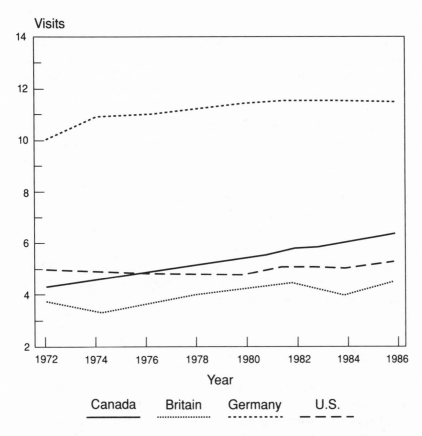

Figure 2 Outpatient Visits per Capita for Canada, Britain, Germany, and the United States, 1972–1986
Source: OECD 1989.

of inpatient services is more easily controlled in Britain than in many countries. Notice in Figure 1 that Britain's inpatient admission rate was, until recently, substantially lower than in either Canada, Germany, or the United States.

Analyzing Canadian use rates over time reveals that inpatient use rates have decreased since 1976, while patient contacts (as measured by visits per capita) have continued to increase (see Figure 2). It is likely that Canada's capitation method for reimbursing hospitals has influenced these trends, allowing the country to reduce its emphasis on inpatient care. Several government studies conducted in the 1970s (shortly after the enactment of Canada's national health legislation) concluded that acute care services were overutilized and should be replaced by more appropriate and less costly alternative services (Letouze 1975). For example, the Manitoba white paper on health policy stated, "By containing the 'acute care bed ratio' to an optimum level, and by supplementing the 'acute care bed' with less expensive alternatives, standards could be maintained and large savings produced" (p. 13).[2] Perhaps as a result of such policy statements, several Canadian hospitals either closed or reduced the number of acute care beds. However, while Canada's shifting of resources to ambulatory care may reflect a political decision about the appropriate allocation of resources, the shift does not represent an explicit allocation policy specifying the appropriate *amount* of ambulatory versus inpatient care. Such a policy is more characteristic of health insurance policies in the U.S. For example, an insurance policy explicitly emphasizing ambulatory care might allow generous reimbursement for ambulatory care, but restrict the number of reimbursable inpatient days. As illustrated in Table 1, basic benefit plans offered to small business employers (in states that have passed legislation exempting mandated benefits) include provisions of this nature.

Physician Reimbursement

While several studies have documented the effect of various reimbursement policies on physician behavior and consumer demand, it is important to realize that reimbursement policies implicitly direct the health priorities in a country. They serve not only to determine the income level of health professionals but to influence the proportion of resources allocated to each health service sector.

Although most countries adopt a mixture of reimbursement methods that differ between hospital-based and community-based physicians, those that predominantly use a fee-for-service method, such as Germany and Canada, have relatively high professional earnings (Culyer 1989). Average physician income figures, shown in Table 3, support this conjecture. Interestingly, and not coincidentally, the four industrialized countries that do not use fee-for-service as a principal means of payment (Britain, Denmark, Italy, and Sweden) have the lowest ratios of average doctor income to gross domestic product per capita (Culyer 1989). If the amount paid to health providers affects the cost of medical services, clearly, one way for

2. See Letouze 1975 for similar comments in provincial government publications from Ontario, Quebec, and Nova Scotia.

countries to control costs is to restrict the amount paid to health providers rather than restrict the particular services they can provide.

The relatively high rates for ambulatory care in Germany and low rates in Britain undoubtedly reflect a number of demand factors—many of which may be cultural, such as patient expectations, and therefore not easily explained. However, given that payment methods affect physician behavior and use rates, such differences are not surprising. We can also expect the number of services provided per capita by general practitioners (GPs) to be lower in countries where the capitation system predominates, such as Britain. Theoretically, the capitation method provides an incentive for physicians to limit the services provided so as not to exceed their allocated budget. Fee-for-service methods as used in Germany and Canada, on the other hand, encourage the provision of services because the physician's income is tied to the number of services she or he provides.

The number of annual per capita contacts with a specialist is comparatively higher in Germany (5.0) and Canada (2.5) than in Britain (1.2) (Culyer 1989). Again, such a finding is not due to a benefit policy in Britain that limits the number of specialty visits per year; rather, it emerges from various manpower policy provisions. For example, while neither Canada nor Germany restricts access to specialists, a specialist in Britain can only be seen on the recommendation of a GP (see Table 5). Such a restriction is quite different from an explicit policy about benefits, because once the patient is referred there is no question about service coverage.

Technological Acquisition

Rather than explicitly state which technological services should or should not be provided, Canada, Britain, and Germany control the degree to which patients gain access to technological services through three main institutional mechanisms: (1) the referral system and the location of technological services, (2) the rate of technological acquisition, and (3) reimbursement policies.

The location of technologies such as laboratory and diagnostic imaging procedures (excluding a limited range of basic tests) is restricted to hospitals and a defined set of approved private facilities in Canada, Britain, and Germany. Canada restricts physicians through the reimbursement system from acquiring certain technologies. In general, physicians are reimbursed for professional services and "technical" expenses (or capital plant). Technical reimbursement covers the costs of equipment, supplies, and support personnel. However, reimbursement for technical costs is not automatic. For example, if a physician installs a CT scanner, the costs associated with operating the equipment would not be reimbursed (Evans 1985). In Britain, access to technologies is also tightly controlled, not only through the general practitioner who acts as the gatekeeper to the system, but also by designating specific technological functions to specific hospitals. The NHS provides two types of hospitals: secondary care hospitals where acute services or services for severe physical and psychiatric illnesses are provided, and tertiary care hospitals (or regional centers of expertise) providing specialty care requiring expensive technology or infrequently required procedures (Potter and Porter 1989). In general, National Health Service patients only obtain access to high-technology services through specific referral channels—GP to hospital consultant in secondary hospital, to hospital consultant in tertiary care center.

In countries with universal access, technological policies tend to restrict access to high-technology services through the referral system while maintaining comprehensive coverage of services. This is very different from the U.S. approach of providing open access to technological services but instituting specific restrictions on which type of services and how much service will be covered under the numerous different insurance plans.

Table 6 shows that countries vary substantially in their reliance on certain technological medical procedures. McPherson (1989) found that surgical utilization rates, standardized by age and sex, varied up to sevenfold among these countries and suggests that use rates vary because of differences in the method of payment, supply of resources, availability of manpower, and reimbursement and referral patterns. Differences in demand for these surgical services also partly explain these variations; so do differences in cultural expectations and physician practice style. Note that the differences in use rates are not accounted for by explicit policies restricting access to certain technological services.

Technological medical procedures can be thought of as having three main dimensions: the probability of correcting the health problem, the degree to which they maintain health or save lives, and their relative cost. When a technology is high in two dimensions but low in one, countries with universal access tend to choose among three scenarios, depending on the configuration of dimensions. In the first scenario, a technology is reliable, maintains health, but is not expensive (ampicillin for bacterial infections, for example). Most countries will adopt it without any significant debate. In the second scenario, a technology is lifesaving and expensive but varies in its probability for success. It tends to be assigned a low priority or a selective priority under a system of universal coverage

Table 6 Admission Rates for Selected Procedures, 1980

Procedures	Number of Admissions per 1,000 Population		
	Canada	Britain	U.S.
Tonsillectomy	89	26	205
Coronary Bypass	26	6	61
Cholecystectomy	219	78	203
Inguinal Hernia Repair	224	154	238
Exploratory Laparotomy	105	116	41
Prostatectomy	229	144	308
Hysterectomy	479	250	557
Operation on Lens	139	98	294
Appendectomy	143	131	130

Source. McPherson, 1989 obtained from OECD 1989.

Note. Data are unavailable for Germany.

and centralized decision making. An example would be heart transplants. Selective priority means that the procedure may be performed on a select number of patients who have a relatively high probability for success but is withheld from patients for whom the chances of success are quite low. Because physicians enjoy a relatively high degree of clinical autonomy in these countries, they are usually granted the power to determine these success rates. Coronary bypass admission rates per thousand population, as shown in Table 6 (twenty-six for Canada, six for Britain, and sixty-one in the U.S.), illustrate this relationship—in the U.S., where technological use and acquisition are not controlled, the use rates for coronary bypass are substantially higher. In the third scenario, a technology is reliable and expensive but not lifesaving or life-extending (for example, cosmetic face-lifts). It is, therefore, more likely to be considered a luxury benefit (Halper 1985).

While this relationship between the characteristics of a technology and the likelihood of its adoption (or use) is purely speculative, it does provide a plausible explanation for the observed differences in procedure use rates between countries with universal coverage and the U.S. For example, cosmetic surgery is not covered in either Canada, Britain, or Germany. Heart transplants are given a much lower priority in these countries (as evidenced by use) than in the U.S. And preventive services, which are considered reliable and life-extending but are not expensive (for example, pre- and post-natal care) are usually provided free of charge in all three

Table 7 Treatment of End-Stage Renal Disease Failure in Canada, Britain, Germany, and the United States, 1986

Treatments	Canada	Britain	Germany	U.S.
Number of Patients Treated per Million Population	336.4	242.0	333.0	522.0
Patients on Dialysis[a] per million Population		64.0		283.1
Percentage of Patients on Home Dialysis[a]		60.4		17.8
Percentage of Patients with Functioning Transplants	48.3	49.7	17.2	23.9
Number of Patients with New Grafts	33.9	28.6	26.6	37.3

Source. OECD 1989.

a. 1984 data, obtained from Potter and Porter 1989.

countries. There are some anomalies, such as the coverage of spas by some sickness funds in Germany, which would be considered a luxury good in Canada, Britain, and the U.S. However, the coverage of spas is illustrative more of cultural differences than a refutation of this relationship. From a German's perspective, spas might fall under the rubric of a reliable, life-extending, and relatively inexpensive form of treatment.

Difficult allocative decisions arise for countries when a technology, such as dialysis treatments for end-stage renal disease (ESRD), ranks high in all three dimensions—it is reliable and life-extending or lifesaving, but costly. Halper (1985) contends that these technologies appear to governments financing them to be too valuable to be ignored and yet too costly to embrace fully. The result is that use of these technologies among countries with universal coverage and centralized technological acquisition decision making usually lies somewhere between two poles. Table 7 shows that while Britain, for example, has a lower rate of hemodialysis (though a higher proportion of less expensive home dialysis), in its treatment of ESRD it has a higher rate of transplantation and a comparable level of patients with new grafts. It is important to note that Britain does not have an explicit policy regarding the provision of hemodialysis; rather, such allocation provisions (between dialysis, transplantation, or new graft treatment) are decided implicitly by physician practice styles, which, in turn, are affected by political budget allocation decisions.

Conclusion

In this paper I have documented the policy environment of the United States and noted that explicit discussion about limiting medical services is unique to America. Other countries provide "comprehensive" coverage of medical services with universal access while controlling costs through various institutional policies. These policies affect the way in which the health system is structured, and it is this structure that determines the extent of medical services rather than any explicit discussion.

The term *comprehensive* takes on a different meaning in each country. Comprehensive benefits do not mean unlimited care. The right to health care in Canada, Britain, and Germany does not mean the right to all medical treatments. While most services provided in these countries are covered, the extent to which services are offered varies substantially across countries. Equity in health care in reality means a commitment to providing some common, adequate level of care. As yet, however, no country has explicitly determined what this level is.

Why do Americans tend to view universal coverage as a reality only if a minimum benefit package is explicitly defined? The basic health plan has become increasingly popular to state legislators because it requires neither major government intervention or expanded bureaucracy nor additional taxes or new public outlays (IHPP 1991b). In essence, Americans appear to believe that putting explicit limits on care is inevitable *because* the opportunity to restructure the system is no longer a choice. Therefore, the real question becomes not why Americans now believe in setting limits to medical care utilization (most policymakers are, in fact, uncomfortable with the notion of rationing care), but, rather, why a major restructuring of the health care system (either at the state or federal level) is usually not considered an option. There are three possible interrelated answers to this question.

First, the economic situation in the American states has clearly set the stage for such reasoning. It is quite true that the fiscal condition of the federal and state governments, as well as current health expenditure levels, necessitate controlling health care costs. Because health care policy reforms have not successfully controlled costs in the past, there is a general sense of government incompetency in providing an efficient delivery of health care services. Therefore, policy options which rely on minimal government intervention, such as authorizing insurers to provide basic benefit policies, are viewed more favorably.

The second possible reason has to do with timing. In some respects, the experience of Germany, Canada, or Britain may not be relevant, because they enacted their health care plans at a time when health care costs were not a major concern. The U.S. is operating in another era, when expensive technologies are abundant, but the public purse is small. Restructuring the system for technological acquisition might be possible for future technologies but would be difficult to implement with technologies already in large supply.

The problem of timing is related to the third reason for the U.S.'s reluctance to restructure—the U.S. has put off the politically difficult decision of universal access to the point where such a commitment becomes more and more difficult to make. This perhaps most prominent reason for why restructuring the system is not considered an option is rooted in American political culture. Morone (1990) writes in his analysis of American political culture and its effect on U.S. health care policy, "Because Americans distrust both politics and politicians, they tend to seek solutions which do not rely on either." Americans, he says, search for nonpolitical solutions: solutions which appeal to the desire for scientific accuracy—automatic, self-enforcing solutions which present the illusion that, if applied correctly, they will yield the correct result without politics; in the search for these solutions, they prefer hidden or implicit policy choices. Morone cites the example of the prospective payment system, in which open political debate over hospital budgets or fees is substituted by a set of "scientifically" derived formulae—the diagnosis-related groups (DRGs), which classify hospital patients into diagnostic categories for which fees are negotiated in advance. While important political judgments are the backbone of DRG policy, Morone points out, they are hidden within the methodology. The recent upsurge of articles dealing with methods for setting medical care priorities, using measures such as quality-adjusted life years (QALYs), has set the stage for states to replace political questions about rationing with a "scientific" formula.

This method of avoiding overt political conflict is unique to America. The methods of controlling costs in Britain, Canada, and Germany are derived from a series of political conflicts. Evans (1990), in fact, argues that this conflict is the key to the Canadian success in controlling costs. Politicians do not avoid political controversies over nonavailable services; on the contrary, the allocation of health care resources is at the center of the health care debate in these countries. As Morone (1990) points out, these countries' politicians are held accountable for difficult political decisions—hospital budget allocations, physician reimbursement, and decisions about which technologies should be acquired.

Given America's unique political culture, its procrastination over the issue of universal access, and the current financial situation of American government, it is not surprising that little if any attention has been paid to the notion of reorganizing the health care system. The federal and state governments have expanded access in the past and attempted to control costs within the existing institutional framework. The practice of explicitly designing benefit structures is perhaps more in line with American health policy than one might initially presume. The current search for a minimum benefit package is based on the notion that the U.S. can find a scientific formula, like QALYs, as the solution to philosophically fraught questions of who gets what, when, and where.

References

Aaron, H. J., and W. B. Schwartz. 1984. *The Painful Prescription: Rationing Hospital Care*. Washington, DC: Brookings Institution.

Culyer, A. J. 1989. Cost Containment in Europe. *Health Care Financing Review* Annual Supplement (December): 21–32.

Enthoven, A., and R. Kronick. 1989. A Consumer-Choice Health Plan for the 1990s: Universal Health Insurance in a System Designed to Promote Quality and Economy. *New England Journal of Medicine* 320:94–101.

Evans, R. 1985. Illusions of Necessity: Evading Responsibility for Choice in Health Care. *Journal of Health Politics, Policy and Law* 10 (3): 439–67.

————. 1990. Tension, Compression, and Shear: Directions, Stresses, and Outcomes of Health Care Cost Control. *Journal of Health Politics, Policy and Law* 15 (1): 101–28.

Garland, M. J., and R. Hasnain. 1990. Health Care in Common: Setting Priorities in Oregon. *Hastings Center Report* 16 (5): 16–18.

Geoghegan, J. K., and C. L. Allenby. 1990. *A Report to the Governor and Legislature*. Sacramento, CA: California State Transportation and Housing Agency and Health and Welfare Agency.

Halper, T. 1985. Life and Death in a Welfare State: End-Stage Renal Disease in the United Kingdom. *Milbank Memorial Fund Quarterly* 63 (1): 52–93.

Henke, K. 1989. Respondent to Johnson's article. *Health Care Financing Review* Annual Supplement (December): 93–6.

IHPP (Intergovernmental Health Policy Project). 1991a. Oregon Releases Revised Priorities List. *State Health Notes* 111 (March).

————. 1991b. 'Bare Bones' Insurance Plans: Filling the Small Business Gap. *State Health Notes* 113 (May).

Letouze, D. 1975. Hospital Bed Closures: A Review of the Canadian Experience and a Report on the Ontario Situation. *Hospital Administration in Canada* 17 (11/12): 28–32.

McPherson, K. 1989. International Differences in Medical Care Practices. *Health Care Financing Review* Annual Supplement (December): 9–20.

Morone, J. A. 1990. American Political Culture and the Search for Lessons from Abroad. *Journal of Health Politics, Policy and Law* 15 (1): 129–43.

The Nation's Health. 1991. April.

New York State Department of Health. 1990. *Universal New York Health Care (UNY*Care) A Proposal: Revision I.* Albany, NY: New York State Department.

OECD (Organization for Economic Cooperation and Development). 1989. International Compendium. In *Health Care Financing Review* Annual Supplement (December): 111–94.

Potter, C., and J. Porter. 1989. American Perceptions of the British National Health Service: Five Myths. *Journal of Health Politics, Policy and Law* 14 (2): 341–65.

Quam, L. 1991. Health Insurance for All. *Minnesota Journal* 8 (6): 2.

Schulenburg, J. M. G. 1983. Report from Germany: Current Conditions and Controversies in the Health Care System. *Journal of Health Politics, Policy and Law* 8 (2): 320–51.

Todd, J. S. 1989. It Is Time for Universal Access, Not Universal Insurance. *New England Journal of Medicine* 321:46–7.

U.S. DHEW (U.S. Department of Health, Education and Welfare). 1980. *Responses of Canadian Physicians to the Introduction of Universal Medical Care Insurance: The First Five Years in Quebec.* DHEW 80-3229. Hyattsville, MD: U.S. DHEW, National Center for Health Services Research.

This research was supported, in part, by the Health of the Public Program, a program of the Pew Charitable Trust and the Rockefeller Foundation.

Canada: The Real Issues

Robert G. Evans

Abstract Canadians are, by and large, satisfied with their health care system. It is for them a symbol of their community and distinguishes them from the United States. Unlike the health system of that country, it is universal, comprehensive, and accessible, and it costs less as a percentage of GNP to run. The difference between the two systems is rooted in differences in funding. By providing coverage of medically necessary care under a single nonprofit payer (the provincial governments, with guidance and some funds from the federal government), the Canadian system avoids the large overheads and profit incentives that make a fragmented private insurance industry so expensive and inequitable. Whereas health insurance in Canada is socialized, care is not: patients are free to choose among providers, physicians are primarily in private practice, and hospitals are independent, nonprofit institutions overseen by boards of trustees. Canada and the United States view the challenges confronting the Canadian system differently. To Canadians, the real issue is how to improve the management of a popular, effective, and heretofore affordable system, so as to preserve it in a more hostile economic environment. The specific areas of concern are common to all health care systems in the developed world but bear little resemblance to the misleading images of Canada fabricated in the United States for internal political purposes. For Canadians, the proof of their system is that it works, while millions in the United States go without.

Canada's system of universal public insurance for health care is by far the nation's most successful and popular public program. Far more than just an administrative mechanism for paying medical bills, it is widely regarded as an important symbol of community, a concrete representation of mutual support and concern. In a nation subject to strong divisive forces rooted in both geography and history, the health insurance system is an important unifying idea as well as an institution. It expresses the fundamental equality of Canadian citizens in the face of disease and death and a commitment that the rest of the community, through the public system, will help each individual with these problems as far as it can. "There is no social program that we have that more defines Canadianism or that is more important to the people of our country" (Peterson 1989; see also Evans 1988a).

Perhaps as important to the establishment of national identity, the Canadian health insurance program also clearly distinguishes Canada from the United States, where the health care funding process is quite different. The fact that Canada has developed such a different system suggests to Canadians that, despite most outward appearances, we are in fact a separate people, with different political and cultural values. Even better, our form of organization *works* and, compared to most other systems, works very well, while the American alternative is generally regarded in Canada as a disaster.

Still, even successful systems face challenges and conflicts. In this paper, I want to turn to what Canadians see as the real issues for Canadian health policy. In the United States, a richly financed lobby throws its weight against publicly financed health care for all citizens (known as the "Canadian model"). Defending the American status quo by attacking the alternatives, these threatened interests fabricate and market an image of the Canadian system—endless queues, merciless rationing, primitive technology, physicians (and patients) fleeing for the border—which ranges from grossly distorted to blatantly false. Such claims may be effective interest group politics in the United States—but they have little to do with health care policy debates in Canada.

Canada in Perspective

The North American experience with health insurance represents a vast social experiment, carried on over several decades, in which two countries with very similar societies have adopted very different ways of funding health care. These funding approaches have been superimposed on remarkably similar health care delivery systems. The forms of organization of hospitals and of professional practice are almost identical, and the two countries share similar training and accreditation systems for personnel.

Thus the major differences in health system performance which have emerged over the last twenty years can be attributed to the influences of the different funding systems. Prior to the 1970s, the two systems were showing very similar performance. Since the universal public plans went into effect in Canada, the two systems have increasingly diverged, and the gap is now about 3 percentage points of GNP.

The shift in performance in the Canadian system is concentrated in spending for the services of physicians and hospitals (about 50 percent of the total), which are covered by the distinctively Canadian form of health care insurance. Although each of the provinces provides some form of assistance with dental care and prescription drugs (when provided out of hospitals), it is usually for only part of the population, or for part of the costs.

Canada does not skimp on health care: excluding the United States as an obvious outlier, Canada actually spends more per capita than any other nation, although its differences from most of the major European nations are not great.[1] Nevertheless, the Canadian experience shows that it is possible to place a limit on the economic expansion of a health care system in a North American environment, without significant modification of the process of health care delivery, by unifying the payment process through a public system. Moreover, it is possible to do so through a set of programs that are overwhelmingly popular politically.

Canadian Health Care Services

The Canadian public insurance program is often portrayed, particularly in the United States, as "socialized medicine." This is inaccurate. Canada has "socialized insurance." Public agencies in each of the ten provinces of Canada pay for all of the costs of "medically necessary" hospital and medical care received by their residents. These payments are made from general government revenues, raised through taxation.

The services, however, are provided primarily by private physicians, who are in independent fee-for-service practice, and by nonprofit hospitals that are "owned" by, or at least under the direction of, boards of trustees. Every Canadian resident is covered by a provincial plan, and both patient and provider have free choice. Normally, however, a patient will contact a general practitioner—roughly half of Canadian physicians are general or family practitioners. The general practitioners either provide diagnostic and treatment services themselves or refer to a specialist.

---

1. If health care in Canada is "underfunded," as is routinely claimed by Canadian physician associations seeking higher fees and now by the American "anti-Canada" lobby, then a fortiori, so is every other country in the world. Everyone is out of step but Uncle Sam. Yet few in the United States or out of it regard its health care system as a model.

The Ins and Outs of Funding

At no point will the patient be required to pay a fee or make any other financial contribution. The physicians involved, including those who own private diagnostic facilities, will be reimbursed according to fee schedules negotiated at periodic intervals—usually annually—between each provincial ministry of health and the corresponding provincial medical association. The schedule in each province is binding on all physicians working in that province, and physicians do not bill their patients additional amounts above these rates.[2]

Hospitals, on the other hand, do not receive reimbursement for particular items of service. Each hospital negotiates an annual global budget with the provincial reimbursement agency, from which it pays all staff salaries and costs of equipment and supplies. These global budgets are to cover operating costs only; they do not include an allowance for capital costs, either depreciation or interest charges. There are separate provincial capital budgets from which contributions are made to hospitals for new construction or major equipment purchases.

The Canadian funding system is, strictly speaking, not a national system but a system run cooperatively by the federal and provincial governments. The federal government has, with limited exceptions, no constitutional authority over matters of health. Thus, the public insurance plans are actually operated by each of the provincial governments, which have full administrative and fiscal authority and responsibility. But the federal government makes substantial financial contributions to the provinces in respect of such plans (historically about 40 percent of total costs, but falling), on condition that the provincial plans conform to certain broad federally defined standards. It is thus possible to speak of, and describe, a "Canadian" system, even though each of the ten provincial plans has some distinctive features.

The federal standards to which each provincial plan must conform in order to qualify for federal contributions are

1. Universality
2. Comprehensiveness

---

2. These fee schedules, and the associated rules for reimbursement, differ somewhat from one province to another, but a resident of one province who receives services in another province remains fully covered. The government of the province of residence reimburses the costs of the care at the rates of the province of care. Care outside the country is reimbursed at the cost of equivalent care in the home province.

3. Accessibility
4. Portability
5. Nonprofit administration

Universality was initially defined, when first the hospital and then the medical insurance programs were being phased in province by province, as "almost" all provincial residents (95 percent, rising over time to 99 percent). But the standards now require 100 percent coverage of provincial populations. This is of particular importance in the provinces (now down to two) that still require their residents to pay premiums as part of the public health insurance system.

The provincial government is legally entitled to raise funds for the program any way it chooses, including through premiums. But no one can be denied services, or even charged for them, for failure to pay premiums. Payment is legally required, and unpaid premiums are subject to collection, but payment is not a condition of coverage. Moreover, premiums have never been risk-related.

In early years, however, when most provinces still charged premiums, there was some concern that very low-risk individuals might carry private insurance and stay out of the public plan. Since this would defeat the purpose of risk spreading over the whole population, private insurance for services covered under the public plan was made illegal. Private insurance persists for services not included under Canadian Medicare— dentistry, prescription drugs out of hospitals, and costs outside Canada above those reimbursable by the public plans—but (except for dentistry) these are relatively small amounts.

Nor is there any "private" system of health care, operating side by side with the public plan. All physicians and hospitals, like all patients, work within the public *payment* system, but the *delivery* system is still, from most points of view, "private."

In some provinces it is still technically possible for a physician to withdraw from the public plan and see patients on a purely private basis, with neither being reimbursed by the public plan. But their patients would have neither public nor private insurance; such care would thus appeal only to a very select group. Furthermore, the physicians must be "all in" or "all out" of the public plan. They cannot play both sides of the street, as is common in European systems with a private system. In consequence, no private market has developed, even where it is permissible. This suggests a more general principle, that "private" markets in medicine can persist only where they can be supported directly or indirectly by a public system.[3]

Comprehensiveness requires that provincial plans cover "all medically necessary" services. Such services as semiprivate or private hospital accommodation, when not necessitated by the patient's medical condition, or elective cosmetic surgery, are not included under the public plans. Similarly, the services of nonphysicians—optometrists, naturopaths, chiropractors, and other practitioners—are implicitly excluded from the federal definition of "medical necessity," and need not be covered. A province may cover other professional services of whatever type and on whatever terms it chooses; but the federal government imposes no conditions and makes no contribution toward such care.

The increasing interest in the effectiveness, or lack of it, of much contemporary medical care is likely to infuse more content into the principle of "medical necessity." Many of the services provided by medical practitioners and associated stays in hospital appear to be in part or whole unnecessary. Strictly speaking, then, they should not be covered by the public plan. In practice however, the test of necessity of a service has been (with very limited exceptions) that a properly licensed physician was willing to provide it and a patient to accept it.

The concept of "medical necessity" might receive further consideration in the future, if provincial governments decided simply to "deinsure" services of no demonstrable health benefit. Physicians might still offer such services as carotid endarterectomy or cardiac bypass grafts for one- or two-vessel disease, but patients would be required to pay the full costs themselves.

Accessibility has been a particularly contentious area, encompassing two major disputes between physicians and governments—extra-billing and hospital capacity. Do direct charges to patients impede access to needed care and violate the principle of accessibility? And do attempts to moderate the expansion of beds and technology constitute a form of "rationing," which effectively does the same, even if care is "free"? To date, the answers given by Canadian opinion and practice to these questions are "Yes" and "Not necessarily." The former question appears, for

3. It is conceivable that all the specialists of a particular type in one region might withdraw from the public plan, forcing patients to choose between paying privately or going without entirely. This has from time to time been threatened, by small subspecialty groups, but provincial governments have made it clear that they would use their legislative authority to force the members of such a "conspiracy" back into the plan.

the moment, settled, but the latter is wide open and takes up a major share of Canadian political debate. On the first point, practice originally varied from province to province, depending on the political strength of the medical associations at the time the medical insurance plans were introduced.[4] In Québec, at one end of the spectrum, physicians who billed patients for amounts above the negotiated schedule were not reimbursed at all by the public plan, nor were their patients. At the other, in Alberta, physicians were free to collect their official fees from the public agency and then extra-bill their patients in any amount they wished. Other provinces permitted some form of extra billing but on more or less restrictive terms.

The Canada Health Act of 1984, however, provided that any provincial government which either charged patients for covered services or permitted anyone else to charge for them would lose an amount from its federal grant equal to the estimated total amount of such direct charges. Since that time, all provinces have negotiated or imposed an end to extra-billing and removed any other direct charges for covered services.[5] The act responded to growing concerns and some evidence (hotly disputed by physicians) that extra-billing was beginning to spread and was becoming an increasing impediment to access to care for those in greatest need.

The second issue is conceptually more difficult. Canada has historically maintained a relatively large supply of hospital and other institutional beds and a correspondingly high rate of use. Nationwide, there are about 6.75 public general hospital beds per 1,000 population, two-thirds in short-

4. Physicians consistently favor, and lobby energetically for, the right to extra-bill above the fee schedule and to impose other forms of direct charges. This appears to be the position, not only of their professional associations, but also of a majority of individual physicians and is not at all peculiar to Canada. If it were true, as some rather simple-minded economic conceptions of patient behavior continue to assume, that such charges would lead to a reduction in overall rates of utilization of the services charged for, then they would tend to lower the incomes of the physicians who advocate them. The universal enthusiasm of physicians—at least in fee-for-service environments—for charges to patients is prima facie evidence that such charges are *not* effective in limiting overall utilization.

5. There is a significant exception to this penalty, however, with respect to long-term care. Patients in extended-care hospitals are considered as receiving room and board services, which substitute for services they would otherwise be paying for (a substitution which does not usually occur in the case of acute care). Since almost all such patients are elderly and on some form of public pension intended to provide minimum support, the allowable charges to patients in extended care are set at a level to recoup most of the public pension, leaving a basic "comfort allowance." The charges bear no relation to the actual cost of providing care, which is met from public budgets. This exception emphasizes the point that "prices" are seen and used as income distribution mechanisms, not as resource allocators. It is thus quite consistent with the penalties for extra-billing, which is also seen as a matter of income distribution, between physicians and patients, rather than a way of allocating access to services. (To the extent that such charges *do* allocate access, by "deterring" use, they are generally seen as an inappropriate mechanism.)

term units and one-third in long-term units or extended care hospitals. Days of care provided are about 2,000 per 1,000 population, with just over 60 percent in short-term units—a smaller proportion of days because occupancy rates in short-term units average about 80 percent, compared with over 95 percent in long-term facilities.

Students of health care utilization have generally concluded that the Canadian pattern represents overuse, relative to medical need, and public policy in all provinces has been, on balance, directed towards reducing hospital use.[6] Similarly, the introduction and dispersion of expensive new technical facilities and procedures has been restrained through the public control of both capital and operating budgets in hospitals, and the negotiation process that determines what shall be included in the fee schedule.

Yet the supply of physicians has increased steadily, and this increase interacts with the rapid extension of technology to create a constant pressure for more and newer "tools of the trade." Physicians' incomes, in a fee-for-service environment, depend on their billing opportunities, and these in turn, for many specialties, depend on their access to (publicly provided) capital and associated (publicly paid) nurses and technical staff. Thus the pressure mounts for expansion, and failures to expand in line with the ambitions of the medical profession are labeled "cutbacks."

It is generally agreed that "access" means, not the provision of all services imaginable for everyone, but rather services according to need. The political struggle is then over the processes by which need is to be defined. To the medical profession, need is whatever a physician says it is. If they require more, and more costly, services, then so be it. Someone— the government, the patient, the rest of the community—should raise the necessary funds. Governments, on the other hand, are increasingly arguing that the test of necessity is effectiveness, the demonstrable effect of intervention on health outcomes, not merely a physician's opinion. Furthermore, they are becoming aware of the large and growing body of research evidence which indicates that there is often little or no connection between the physician's opinion and the demonstrated effectiveness of the services provided.

Since this conflict between professional autonomy (and economic self-interest) and payers' concern for value for money (and economic self-

6. Certainly the Canadian rates greatly exceed the corresponding American averages, which are themselves well above the experience of populations served by American health maintenance organizations. Yet Canadian physicians continue to claim that they need more beds, and occupancy rates are near the limits of de facto capacity.

interest) is a central issue in virtually every developed country in the world, the application of the principle of access in the Canadian system is likely to remain contentious for a very long time to come.

Portability of benefits is an important principle in terms of its symbolism for national unity, but has not been particularly contentious, being largely a technical problem. Political issues have arisen only in the one or two cases in which a metropolitan region spans a provincial border, or a significant region of one province receives its tertiary care from a large city in another. If the fee schedules are markedly different, either providers or payers may object to the financial transfers involved.

More potentially troublesome is the issue of payment across the border with the United States. As noted in the discussion of accessibility, provincial governments limit the proliferation of hospital capacity and particularly of expensive diagnostic equipment, by funding them through hospital capital and operating budgets, not through fees per item of service. A hospital which wishes to acquire an MRI machine, for example, or a lithotripter, must not only receive planning approval from its provincial ministry of health, it must also convince the ministry to provide the capital funds. Private physicians can in principle purchase and use such equipment, but if there is no corresponding procedural item in the fee schedule, they cannot be reimbursed (by government or patient) for its use.

The result is that physicians claim a shortage of capacity, while in the United States beds and facilities are in surplus. (The price, however, does not fall in the U.S.!) And it is certainly true that the per capita availability and use of major diagnostic equipment is much greater in the United States, although whether this represents a shortage in Canada, relative to the needs of the population, or a surplus in the United States, or both, is another matter.

One could imagine, then, an increased flow of patients across the border in response to the increasing gap between Canadian and American patterns of care. This would place provincial governments in the difficult position of either paying for such additional care, and thus losing control of their total outlays, or permitting the development of a de facto private system of care alongside the public, for those who can afford to pay the American price.

In practice, however, this does not seem to be developing as a significant problem, with the exception of one or two border cities, and one or two particularly contentious procedures. The reality of care use is that patients do not in general "demand" particular procedures; they seek the recommendations of their physicians. The latter can, and do, sometimes refer patients to the United States and then energetically publicize the incident as part of a continuing struggle with provincial governments over the availability of health resources. But this sort of political theatre does not correspond to any large underlying movement of patients or dollars.[7]

Nonprofit administration, the final principle, has drawn very little commentary in Canada, because in most parts of the country the private health insurance industry was relatively underdeveloped at the time the public plans were introduced. In each of the provinces there were nonprofit insurers, sponsored originally by the hospital and physician associations, similar to the Blue Cross plans in the United States, and the hospital and medical insurance business of these plans was simply taken over by the public agencies. In some cases the provincial plans continued to work through the previous carriers as intermediaries, but this arrangement was found to be both unnecessarily costly and inefficient.

The emphasis on nonprofit administration arises out of the observation in the report of the federal Royal Commission on Health Services (1964), the massive investigation which predated the extension of public coverage from hospital care to physicians' services, that the private insurance plans that were then just developing paid out relatively low proportions of their premiums in benefits. What a private insurer regards as a "loss ratio," and something to be minimized, the rest of the community sees as that proportion of what is paid to the insurer that actually goes to pay for medical care, as opposed to being taken up in overhead costs. A "good" plan, from the community's perspective, is one which *maximizes* the loss ratio and minimizes the cost of insurance.

The commissioners concluded that private, for-profit insurers operated under incentives which tended to increase this form of overhead cost, adding to the expense of health care without adding to the resources available to provide it. This inherent tendency is strongly reinforced in a competitive environment with multiple insurers. Regarding the costs of the insurance mechanism as unproductive overhead, the commissioners recommended instead centralized, nonprofit administration. And, as if to confirm their reasoning, the costs of the insurance mechanism have steadily escalated

7. Such theater can, however, have powerful political effects, because one or two such incidents can be very emotionally gripping. The results can be significant in terms of effects on allocations of health care resources among particular programs.

in the United States, while remaining stable or falling (as a proportion of GNP) in Canada.

The administrative costs borne by U.S. hospitals and physicians' offices have gone up rapidly as they attempt to cope with an increasingly complex payment and regulatory environment. Thus, a significant proportion of the recorded expenditures for hospital and medical care are in fact costs generated by the payment mechanism, though not as explicitly reported costs of prepayment and administration. An increasing share of the sums Americans *think* they are spending on hospital and medical care, is going in fact to pay for administrators, accountants, lawyers, public relations specialists, and other forms of personnel, whose services are not usually considered as contributing to the health of patients (Himmelstein and Woolhandler 1986).

Increasing numbers of U.S. *physicians*, as well as payers and patients, are beginning to believe that they might be better off under a Canadian system. The key component of expenditure which has caught their attention is the relative cost of the insurance process. Health expenditures in the United States keep going up, but providers feel—rightly—that their share is not going up as fast, yet they are bearing the full brunt of the various measures intended—so far unsuccessfully—to limit cost escalation.

Of course providers have always preferred nonprofit administration. The Blue Cross/Blue Shield plans were originally established by hospitals and medical associations in the United States. What providers did not want, however, was a *single* nonprofit payer, negotiating on behalf of the public generally, rather than under provider control. And officially, they still do not (Todd 1989). The Canadian form of nonprofit administration, by contrast, comes in combination with "socialized insurance"—sole-source payment by an agency with both incentives and authority to try to keep down the costs of care, i.e., provider incomes, as well as the costs of insurance.

But if a fragmented payment system, like that of the United States, inevitably leads to escalation of expenditures, insurance costs, regulations, interference, and a deteriorating practice environment, then the Canadian form of payment might not be so bad.

In Canada the question is beginning to be raised whether administrative expenses might not be *too* low; one observer has coined the term "administrative anorexia" for the attitude of the provincial governments and their agencies towards spending on management. A recent analysis of the Canadian system advances the thesis that, while not underfunded, it is very seriously undermanaged (Rachlis and Kushner 1989). They raise the same issues as the debates over accessibility—which services are worth paying for, for whom, and what information and processes of analysis are needed in order to decide.

It must be emphasized, however, that these are quite different from the problems facing a private insurer. The private insurer is forced by the laws of the competitive marketplace to devote a great deal of effort to determining who *not* to insure—that is, the worst risks. The private insurance market does not, cannot, cover those in most need of care.[8]

Under a universal public system, this problem of identifying individual risk status disappears and, along with it, the whole complex apparatus of rate making and policy design. The private marketplace generates a multiplicity of different types of coverage in order to minimize the extent to which those in low-risk categories pay to support those at high risk. But the public insurance system expresses the community's decision to do precisely that, to use the resources of the healthy and wealthy to support the poor and ill. So the principal services of the traditional private insurance sector are worthless, because their "product" is not what the community wishes to buy.

In its place, however, is the problem of determining the needs and priorities of those to be cared for and the effectiveness of the services offered. Provincial governments are clearly responsible for purchasing care on behalf of their populations. Achieving "value for money" in this process may well require a buildup of managerial capacity and the creation of new administrative structures, within the overall framework of nonprofit administration.

Canada's Policy Agenda

The functioning of the Canadian health care system is constantly in the forefront of public debate with ministers of health and premiers of provinces, who are held accountable in the provincial legislatures and in the press for any problems or misadventures which occur.

At present, the health care policy agenda in Canada is being driven

8. Unless of course they happen to be quite well off. But in general they will not be, because both illness and risk of illness are closely correlated with poverty, not wealth. The 37 or more million Americans who are uninsured, and the other 20 or 40 million who have insufficient insurance to cover the costs of any serious illness, are not an unfortunate aberration or oversight in a private insurance system, but rather a natural and inevitable outcome of the operation of competitive market forces. This point has been made very clearly both by American advocates of a public system, e.g., Fein (1986), and by advocates of a radically reformed competitive private system, e.g., Enthoven (1989).

by a set of interlocked problems, none of which are particularly new, or peculiar to Canada.

These problem areas can be summarized in several categories or clusters. These categories are not conceptually consistent with each other, indeed some turn out to be partial subsets of others. They are, however, the labels that tend to be employed in the public debate, and under which most of the research results are assembled.

1. Cost control
2. Coping with an aging population
3. Coping with the extension of technology
4. Manpower policy—surpluses of physicians and shortages of nurses
5. Improving the effectiveness and efficiency of health care delivery
6. Extending our concern from the delivery of medical care to the enhancement of health

Cost Control

This problem has faced every society in the industrialized world. If the modernization and growth of a country's general economy can outstrip that of its health care system, it need not be overly concerned with health care cost control. This has not, however, been the situation in North America or Western Europe, where all countries have had to wrestle, over the last decade or more, with the problem of moderating the growth of health spending in order to protect resources for other social and private priorities. And any country modernizing its health care system must consider how it will deal with the inherent tendency of such systems to expand without limit, in the absence of strongly enforced external constraint (Evans 1990, 1991).

Within the last five to ten years, however, all developed societies, except the United States, appear to have found some response, if not necessarily a permanent solution, to this problem (Schieber and Poullier 1989). Sweden has actually significantly *reduced* its share of national income spent on health care. The process of control, in every country, has been accompanied by considerable difficulties and political conflict, and it is always possible that the health care system will break out of the controls which each society has placed on it, but, for the moment, a degree of stability prevails.

The processes whereby the provincial governments in Canada have imposed this degree of control for nearly twenty years, with the exception of the "recession breakout" of 1982, are three in number. First, as noted above, the nature of the Canadian payment system permits it to function very economically in terms of administrative costs, and these have not been rising over time.

Second, the medical fee schedules negotiated between the provincial medical associations and governments have grown much more slowly than fees in the uncontrolled American environment. Over time, fees in Canada have risen at a rate more or less in line with general price inflation; when physicians can set their own fees freely, fees rise substantially faster. At the same time, the elimination of extra-billing has prevented physicians from exploiting this alternative form of fee inflation.

In response, physicians in Canada do appear to have increased their volumes of billings per physician somewhat faster than in the United States, in order to keep their incomes rising, but they have not been able to offset fully the slower increase in fees (Barer 1988). Fee schedules have helped this process, by limiting the reimbursement of diagnostic services outside hospitals—most physicians cannot simply set up their own laboratories, for example—and also by preventing implicit "fee splitting" between laboratories and referring physicians (Reinhardt 1987).

On the other hand, these controls over the tendency of physicians to engage in "procedural multiplication," particularly when fee inflation is contained, are by no means complete, and Canadian provincial governments are increasingly exploring ways of imposing more explicit "caps" on total outlays for physicians' services. Two provinces—Québec and British Columbia—have already done so, and it is likely that more will follow (Lomas et al. 1989; Evans 1988b).

Furthermore, it appears quite clear that the volume of physicians' services billed for in a province rises more or less in proportion to the increasing numbers of fee-for-service physicians. Thus control of cost escalation is directly connected to manpower policy, and in Canada these have been seriously inconsistent.

Finally, a very important part of the control of health care costs has been the system of global budgeting for hospitals, which enables this component of the health budget to be subjected to absolute "cash limits." The result has been a steady decline in acute care utilization, which nevertheless remains high relative to United States experience, and a much less rapid proliferation of new and very expensive, high-technology interventions. Canadian provinces do acquire the most recent technology, but such equipment tends to be confined to the teaching hospital centers and does not proliferate throughout the regional hospital system or into free-standing facilities. Thus the availability per capita of such equipment tends to be lower than in countries such as the United States, Germany, or Japan.

The Aging of the Population

This is perhaps the most frequently cited source of serious problems, now and particularly in the future, for the Canadian and most other health care systems. Yet it is the area in which the rhetoric is in fact most misleading. The usual argument is that elderly people require more, and more costly, health care services, on average, than do younger people. At the same time, the proportion of elderly and, particularly, very elderly people in the population is growing, as birthrates have fallen and life expectancies have risen. Both these observations are true. But the common conclusion, that the costs of caring for the elderly will therefore necessarily exceed the willingness or ability of industrialized economies to pay for them, does not follow.

The aging of the population in Canada and in the rest of the industrialized world, is a very important phenomenon over a time span of decades. But its effects on health care use are slow. In Canada, the aging of the population would add about 1 percent per capita per year to health costs, *if* the utilization patterns of each age group remained unchanged, and only the population age structure changed (Woods, Gordon Management Consultants 1984). This is well within the normal, or at least historical, economic growth rates of industrialized economies and could easily be accommodated, with a constant share of such growth being devoted to health care.

However, per capita rates of utilization and costs of health care services for the elderly are rising rapidly for each age group (Barer et al. 1987; Evans, Barer, et al. 1989; Barer, Pulcins, and Evans 1989). Elderly people *are* accounting for a rapidly increasing share of our health care effort and resources. But the reason is not primarily that there are so many more of them. The real change is in how much is done to and for the elderly— they are being subjected to many more, and more intensive, interventions, often of unproven effectiveness.

The question is what benefits are being derived from the services that are being applied in increasing numbers to the care of the elderly. That brings us to the questions of technology, of effectiveness and appropriateness of care, and indirectly to issues of manpower or personnel. The demographic transition, at least as it applies to the past decade and the next, is in fact a smokescreen that obscures more fundamental questions of the basis on which utilization decisions are made and the costs and benefits of the results.

The Extension of Technology

The extension of technology is simply part of this more general set of issues. Technology per se is neither good nor bad; new knowledge and capabilities in principle merely expand our range of choices. The rhetoric surrounding technology often suggests that we are somehow compelled to apply whatever is discovered, at whatever expense. But the technology does *not* define its own range of application. Some new technologies have the capability to *reduce* significantly health costs—if conservatively applied and limited to areas of demonstrated effectiveness. The real problem of a trade-off between technological "advance" and cost control arises when new and expensive techniques (or for that matter old and not-so-expensive techniques) are employed and paid for in circumstances in which there is no evidence that they will do any good.

Thus the problem posed by new technology is primarily evaluative and organizational, rather than economic. First, how do we determine whether the technique does more good than harm, and for which patients? This requires careful analysis of the biological effect of the associated interventions; it also requires developing techniques for eliciting the preferences and values of potential patients. And second, once such information is available, how do we ensure that utilization decisions by providers and patients actually reflect this information?

A number of students of the benefits and costs of new technology have concluded that there is ample capacity in the health care systems of industrialized societies to support all the new technology that one might want—if one could get rid of the minimally effective, useless, or harmful interventions now being provided and paid for. The problem is to find an organizational framework, and decision processes, which will lead to this result—the fifth problem category, detailed below ("Improving the Effectiveness and Efficiency of Health Care Delivery").

Coming back to the Canadian experience with cost control, it has been noted that the intensity of service, or the inflation-adjusted expenditure per person, has risen relatively slowly in Canadian hospitals. The control of hospital costs through global budgets has been associated with a slower rate of increase in the number of procedures performed, and/or their expense, than in the United States.

This raises the question of the appropriateness and effectiveness of the care being provided. Are Canadians being denied potentially effective treatments that would increase the length and/or improve the quality of their lives? Or are they being protected against the over-enthusiastic application of interventions that would be useless at best, quite possibly harmful, and certainly expensive? One can find advocates of both points of view.

The second point of view has the assumptions which underlie the use of global budgets, namely that (1) physicians and hospital administrators, when they do not have enough resources to do all that they would like to do, react by eliminating the least useful or most harmful services first; (2) although they will always claim the contrary, they really do have enough resources to do all that is worth doing and probably more besides; and finally (3), if (2) should cease to be true, other sources of information will bring this fact into the open, so that budgets can be adjusted as needed.

On the other hand, detailed information on the effects both of the care that is being provided in Canadian hospitals and of the care that is *not* being provided is remarkably scarce (as it is in most other countries). We should study this area much more closely—the same point emerges when one looks closely at the changing patterns of care of the elderly. But the growing evidence of the very substantial use of inappropriate and actually harmful high-technology procedures in the more richly endowed United States emphasizes that the relative limitation placed on the diffusion of technology by the Canadian funding system may very well be a benefit of that system.

Manpower Surpluses (Physicians) and Shortages (Nurses)

The least successful area in health care policy in Canada has been the formulation and execution of manpower policy. As noted above, the supply of physicians has been rising steadily relative to the population and is projected to do so for the foreseeable future, on the basis of the training capacity now in place. There are now nearly 60,000 "active civilian" physicians in Canada, or about one for every 450 people, and the ratio of physicians per capita is rising about 2 percent per year. This growth places continuing pressure not only on the budgets for physicians' services, but also on the available hospital bed space and associated facilities (Barer, Gafni, and Lomas 1989). The "physicians per bed" ratio is rising steadily, so that each physician *perceives* a growing shortage of capacity, available to him or her.

This problem was easily foreseeable, and was in fact foreseen, in the early 1970s. The collapse of the birth rate in the mid-1960s has been followed by a continuing decline ever since. The population forecasts of the early 1960s were grossly in error, but were the basis for a significant increase in medical school capacity in the late 1960s and early 1970s. These increases were not scaled back when it became apparent that there had been a permanent and large change in population trends, although as early as 1975 changes were made to reduce drastically the rate of physician immigration.

Medical school representatives cloud the political issue with numerous false claims (Lomas et al. 1985): more physicians, they claim, are needed for an aging population. True; but aging is currently adding only about one-third of 1 percent per year to use, not 2 percent (Woods, Gordon Management Consultants 1984). In fact, the increasing physician supply is resulting in the increase in servicing rates among the elderly, as more and more physicians struggle to keep busy and maintain their incomes. They also claim that increasing numbers of female physicians and changing lifestyles, will lead to more physicians being needed to provide the same services. This would result in a fall in gross fee billings per physician, after allowing for changes in the level of fees, and this is not happening.

Thus Canada's present medical school capacity was put in place to serve a population which was forecast to be, by 1991, nearly 10 million people larger than that which is actually here.

Some reductions in training places are occurring, but slowly and painfully, because the benefits of reduction, in terms of savings, accrue over a number of years, while the political costs are immediate.

Nursing manpower presents the opposite picture, of growing shortages. Nursing shortages and surpluses alternate from year to year, or even month to month, depending upon the provincial government electoral and budget cycle. When funds for hospitals are plentiful, there is usually a "shortage" of nurses to fill the new jobs created. When fiscal times are tougher, the "shortage" disappears, along with the jobs. All that is happening is that the process of supply adjustment is less flexible than hospital budgets. But over the long run, larger forces are at work.

There are nearly a quarter of a million nurses registered in Canada, or about one per 100 persons, but only about one-half are employed full time in nursing. There are another 80,000 nursing assistants, but only about half were employed in hospitals in 1986, and their numbers are falling. Nursing manpower has been barely keeping up with population growth, though the adjustment for aging has much more impact on need for nurses than for physicians.

The collapse of births in the mid-1960s has just reached the twenty- to twenty-five-year-old age cohort, from which nursing has traditionally recruited. A greater proportion of the population now works, but not enough to offset the decline; and career opportunities for females are increasing all the time. The demographic change has, in fact, resulted in a long-run shortage situation for nursing, which has become apparent only very recently. (Though it, too, could easily have been forecast from the 1960s birth data.)

The lack of cooperation, and sometimes even communication, between the educational and health care systems, located in different ministries and institutions, has been a major source of the serious inadequacies in health manpower policy. In this field, errors can have consequences for a whole generation.

Improving the Effectiveness and Efficiency of Health Care Delivery

Throughout the discussion above, we have noted that a number of apparently separate problems—population aging, the extension of technology, manpower—actually reduce to special cases of the more general issue: What sorts of health care services do we wish to have produced, and for whom?[9] These questions, as noted, ultimately turn on a combination of technical and value information: What will particular services actually *do*, in the way of good or harm? and, What do actual or prospective patients want?[10]

To date the Canadian health care system has addressed these questions only indirectly. "All medically necessary" services are free, implying that effectiveness, somehow defined, is the overriding criterion. But, as noted earlier, this has been determined implicitly as whatever a physician is willing to offer and a patient to accept. We have discovered, as has every other industrialized nation, that (1) the indirect definition of "need" is indefinitely expansible within the relevant range, particularly for elderly

9. The struggle over income shares (how much we will have to pay the producers) is largely—though not entirely—a separate question, though providers try hard to confuse the two. For example, it is claimed that aggressive bargaining over fees by provincial governments will threaten the quality of care of patients. More generally, the economic and professional objectives of providers are virtually always framed in terms of ill-specified but very important effects on "quality of care."

10. The latter is not in itself wholly decisive. Since in every industrialized nation, most or all of health care is collectively funded and could not in fact be funded any other way, it also matters what the rest of us are willing to pay for. But that will presumably be heavily influenced by the answers to the first two questions.

people, and (2) overall utilization rises with the availability of facilities and personnel and presses against any resource constraints, but (3) the aggregate levels and patterns of utilization that result are highly variable and bear no identifiable relation to any external definition of the "needs" of the population served.

The Canadian response has been to try to impose capacity constraints on the availability of facilities, sources of payment, and (much less successfully) personnel. The assumption, as noted above, is that when subjected to these constraints, the providers of health care will themselves choose to provide the services which respond to the greatest needs. Thus, the payers for services can avoid the very difficult and politically very dangerous task of establishing explicit priorities and protocols, and the fiercely defended autonomy of the physician need not be challenged.

This approach is slowly changing, however, in the face of accumulating evidence that patterns of care use in Canada bear no more systematic relation to indicators of need than they do in any other jurisdiction, and increasing pressure for more resources from the providers of health care themselves—the consequences of the physician supply increase and the extension of technology. As the relatively arbitrary limitations on facilities and resources are challenged more and more intensely by providers, provincial governments are becoming increasingly interested in the extensive research evidence of ineffective and inefficient care delivery as a basis for counterattack.

From the Delivery of Medical Care
to the Enhancement of Health

The Canada Health Act of 1984 defines the objective of Canadian health care policy as "to protect, promote, and restore the physical and mental well-being of residents of Canada, and to facilitate reasonable access to health services without financial or other barriers" and refers to "outstanding progress" through the system of insured health services. But it also declares that further improvements will depend on a combination of improved individual lifestyles and "collective action against the social, environmental, and occupational causes of disease."

Equalizing access to health care, or at least removing the financial barriers, and significantly increasing the overall quantity of resources available have not equalized health status across the population. There remain significant inequalities in life expectancy and health status across different socioeconomic groups. Furthermore, there are sources of mortality and morbidity which are beyond the reach of health care services as conventionally defined. A public *health* policy, as different from a *health care* policy, would have to go much deeper into the determinants of health and illness, and carry out a much wider range of interventions than simply the expansion (or contraction) of particular health care services.

This is clearly recognized within the federal Department of National Health and Welfare. Most provincial ministries of health have a similar understanding, although they are so heavily involved in the day-to-day and year-to-year operations of the health care system that they do not always have the luxury of pursuing the broader issues. In general, however, these broader issues of inequalities in determinants of health have been honored with much rhetoric and careful thought, but very little money.

The problem is that the relentless pressure for expansion from the health care system, independently of any contribution it may be demonstrated to make to the health of the population, absorbs the lion's share of both current resources and any additional that may become available. Thus, cost containment in health care becomes a precondition for any new initiative in other areas of health. By a cruel irony, an overextended health care system may become a threat to health.

Conclusion

In summary, the Canadian approach to health care funding has been very successful in equalizing access to health care services, though less so in equalizing access to health. This appears to be a common experience in the industrialized countries, reflecting the fact that population health is not determined simply by the availability or use of health care. The health status of the Canadian population, insofar as that is known (which is not very far), compares well on the usual indicators of life expectancy and infant mortality with the rest of the industrialized world, and continues to improve (though not as fast as Japan!).[11]

The public insurance system has not only assisted access to health care, it has also played a very important role in "nation building" and community solidarity, as it emphasizes a fundamental equality among citizens. Greater wealth or position buy many things, but they do not buy more or better health care. Moreover the economic burden of this system is shared, through the general tax system, according to ability to pay. Since

---

11. Life expectancy for Canadians at birth is about eighty years for females and seventy-three for males. Infant mortality is about 7.3 deaths per 1,000 births.

there are no direct payments, people who must bear the burden of illness and injury do not have to carry an additional economic burden as well.

Going beyond assuring access and improving the lives of individual citizens, the Canadian system has managed to contain the costs of health care for an extended period of time. Equilibrium is a crucial test of the sustainability of a funding system. Furthermore, it has done so in a way that has reconciled the interests of citizens as payers and citizens as patients and is consequently overwhelmingly popular politically. Even most physicians working in the Canadian system prefer it to the known alternatives—they would just like more money (and more hospital facilities and more equipment and the right to extra-bill patients, etc.). But one should not always infer the views of the ordinary physician from the rhetoric of professional associations.

On the basis of this experience, which is not so different from that of a number of European countries, we can conclude unequivocally that centralized, public funding systems "work," although they will require an increasing degree of explicit collective intervention in the determination of the content of medical practice. Whether this will be "public" or "private," or, more realistically, a balance between the two, depends upon whether the medical profession can bring itself to develop *and enforce* scientifically based standards upon its members, or whether the public sector will have to take on this role by default.

On the other hand, we can conclude, equally unequivocally, from the United States experience that a private or pluralistic funding system does not work; it produces neither effective health care, nor equity, nor public satisfaction, and cannot even meet the most fundamental test of stable and sustainable cost. It is conceivable that some pluralistic system might be developed in the future that would be capable of harnessing competitive forces to improve health care system performance. But at present such systems exist only in the imaginations of those with an overriding ideological commitment to the private marketplace—they cannot be shown to have been seriously tried, much less to have succeeded, in the real world.[12] What has been tried, in the United States, has failed.

12. The work of Enthoven should be excluded from this generalization. His proposals represent the most thoughtful and carefully worked out example of a competitive system that takes account of the sources of failure in ordinary conceptions of "market" systems of health care funding and attempts to develop realistic ways of dealing with them. But his scheme is very subtle and sophisticated, and its feasibility of implementation in a highly adversarial (and often ignorant) environment is very far from clear. In any case, even he offers a totally untried alternative, which may appeal where the status quo is generally recognized as intolerable, and where such admittedly imperfect but battle-tested systems as the Canadian one are ruled out on ideological grounds.

References

Barer, M. L. 1988. Regulating Physician Supply: The Evolution of British Columbia's Bill 41. *Journal of Health Politics, Policy and Law* 13 (1): 1–25.

Barer, M. L., R. G. Evans, C. Hertzman, and J. Lomas. 1987. Aging and Health Care Utilization: New Evidence on Old Fallacies. *Social Science and Medicine* 24 (10): 851–62.

Barer, M. L., A. Gafni, and J. Lomas. 1989. Accommodating Rapid Growth in Physician Supply: Lessons from Israel, Warnings for Canada. *International Journal of Health Services* 19 (1): 95–115.

Barer, M. L., I. R. Pulcins, R. G. Evans, C. Hertzman, J. Lomas, and G. M. Anderson. 1989. Trends in Use of Medical Services by the Elderly in British Columbia. *Canadian Medical Association Journal* 141 (1): 39–45.

Blendon, R. J. 1989. Three Systems: A Comparative Survey. *Health Management Quarterly* 11 (1): 2–10.

Culyer, A. J. 1982. The NHS and the Market: Images and Realities. In *The Public-Private Mix for Health: The Relevance and Effects of Change*, ed. G. McLachlan and A. Maynard. London: Nuffield Provincial Hospitals Trust.

Enthoven, A. 1989. What Can Europeans Learn from Americans about Financing and Organization of Medical Care? *Health Care Financing Review*, Annual Supplement: 49–63.

Enthoven, A., and R. Kronick. 1988. A Consumer Choice Health Care Plan for the 1990s (Parts I and II). *New England Journal of Medicine* 320 (1 and 2): 29–37, 94–101.

Evans, R. G. 1983. The Welfare Economics of Public Health Insurance: Theory and Canadian Practice. In *Social Insurance*, ed. L. Soderstrom. Amsterdam: North-Holland.

———. 1984. *Strained Mercy: The Economics of Canadian Health Care*. Toronto: Butterworths.

———. 1988a. We'll Take Care of It for You: Health Care in the Canadian Community. *Daedalus: Journal of the American Academy of Arts and Sciences* 117 (4): 155–89.

———. 1988b. *Squaring the Circle: Reconciling Fee-for-Service with Global Expenditure Control*. Health Policy Research Unit Discussion Paper 88-8D, University of British Columbia, Vancouver.

———. 1990. Tension, Compression, and Shear: Directions, Stresses, and Outcomes of Health Care Cost Control. *Journal of Health Politics, Policy and Law* 15 (1): 101–28.

———. 1991. Life and Death, Money and Power: The Politics of Health Care Finance. In *Health Politics and Policy*, 2d ed., ed. Theodor J. Litman and Leonard S. Robins. Albany, NY: Delmar.

Evans, R. G., M. L. Barer, C. Hertzman, G. M. Anderson, I. R. Pulcins, and J. Lomas. 1989. The Long Good-Bye: The Great Transformation of the British Columbia Hospital System. *Health Services Research* 24 (4): 435–59.

Evans, R. G., J. Lomas, M. L. Barer, R. J. Labelle, C. Fooks, G. L. Stoddart, G. M.

Anderson, D. Feeny, A. Gafni, G. W. Torrance, and W. G. Tholl. 1989. Controlling Health Expenditure: The Canadian Reality. *New England Journal of Medicine* 321 (9): 571–77.

Fein, R. 1986. *Medical Care, Medical Costs: The Search for a Health Insurance Policy.* Cambridge, MA: Harvard University Press.

Himmelstein, D. U., and S. Woolhandler. 1986. Cost without Benefit: Administrative Waste in U.S. Health Care. *New England Journal of Medicine* 314: 441–5.

Lalonde, M. 1974. *A New Perspective on the Health of Canadians.* Ottawa: Health and Welfare Canada.

Lomas, J., M. L. Barer, and G. L. Stoddart. 1985. *Physician Manpower Planning: Lessons from the Macdonald Report.* Ontario Economic Council Discussion Paper Series, Toronto.

Lomas, J., C. Fooks, T. Rice, and R. J. Labelle. 1989. Paying Physicians in Canada: Minding Our Ps and Qs. *Health Affairs* 8 (1): 80–102.

National Leadership Commission on Health Care. 1989. *For the Health of a Nation: A Shared Responsibility.* Ann Arbor, MI: Health Administration Press.

Peterson, D. 1989. Opening Address. International Conference on Quality Assurance and Effectiveness in Health Care. Toronto, 8–10 November.

Rachlis, M., and C. Kushner. 1989. *Second Opinion: What's Wrong with Canada's Health Care System and How to Fix It.* Toronto: Collins.

Reinhardt, U. E. 1987. Resource Allocation in Health Care: The Allocation of Lifestyles to Providers. *Milbank Quarterly* 65 (2): 153–76.

Schieber, G., and J.-P. Poullier. 1989. International Health Care Expenditure Trends: 1987. *Health Affairs* 8 (3): 169–77.

Todd, J. S. 1989. It Is Time for Universal Access, Not Universal Insurance. *New England Journal of Medicine* 321 (1): 46–7.

Woods, Gordon Management Consultants. 1984. *An Investigation of the Impact of Demographic Change on the Health Care System of Canada—Final Report.* Prepared for the Task Force on the Allocation of Health Care Resources, Joan Watson, Chairman. Toronto: Woods, Gordon.

This is a substantially revised version of a paper presented at the international symposium, "What Can Be Learned from the Experiences of the Health Care Systems in Developed Nations?" held in Taipei, Taiwan on 18–20 December, 1989. A different, revised version is appearing in the *Yale Law and Policy Review*; some parts will also be included in *Health Financing and the Role of Health Insurance in Developing Countries: Lessons from the More Affluent Countries*, edited by D. W. Dunlop and J. Martins and published by the Economic Development Institute of the World Bank.

Response

Lessons from the Frozen North

Theodore R. Marmor

Let me begin by noting that I am in broad agreement both with what Robert Evans has written in the essay included in this volume about the funding and delivery arrangements of Canadian national health insurance and with his efforts to clarify how Canadian experience illustrates wider generalizations. That last concern seems especially important for his topic—the drawing of lessons from Canada and the health insurance experiences of the developed nations of the Organization for Economic Cooperation and Development (OECD).

There are two kinds of lessons obviously worth drawing. First are medical care generalizations that hold for a number of countries, nations that themselves vary widely in cultural disposition, political arrangements, and economic character. Generalizations of this kind—for instance, the claim that countries almost invariably do not enact national health insurance systems with the approval of their major physician organizations, or the conclusion that democratic regimes do not impose unfamiliar methods of payment upon most doctors at the start of a national health insurance program[1]—highlight what will likely be constraints on health policy-making in a variety of countries.

The second sort of policy lesson is country-specific. When one has good reason to think there are specially powerful similarities between two nations, particular institutional practices and their effects are worth

1. See, on these generalizations and comparative health policy studies more generally, Marmor et al. 1978: 59–80; Marmor 1983: chap. 2. For a more recent and revised statement of my views, see Klein and Marmor 1986.

studying in great detail. (Such a study took place in the case of Australia learning from Canada, with Australian architects of their national health insurance program studying carefully the provisions of the Canadian system as it evolved through the early 1970s. The grounds for such detailed study included their common status as Commonwealth nations, similar cultural traditions and similarly profound alterations of their English backgrounds by non-English immigration since World War II, comparable levels of wealth and economic dependence on extractive industries, and so on. These were very similar nations, and the collaboration developed from that base.)

With that said, what about Evans's characterization of Canadian experience in connection to both sorts of questions? He rightly asserts that Canada's public health insurance has substantially provided equal access to health care for all of its citizens. And it has done so without Canada's medical costs spiraling upwards in a relentless fashion. Canada is, however, the second or third most expensive medical care system in the world. Though it has stabilized the share of gross national product (GNP) going to health care during the 1980s (at roughly 8.5 to 9 percent), it is by no means a model of asceticism (except by comparison with the United States). Whether the Canadian system has promoted the efficient use of resources is more complicated to answer. But it has not induced the substitution of nonphysicians for primary care; indeed, both the increased supply of physicians and the rules of the payment system have made that harder in Canada than elsewhere.[2]

My more specific responses to Evans's discussion of Canadian lessons are these:

First, from Canada's example, the best alternative for covering special groups—like the elderly, disabled, partially employed, etc.—is to include them within one national system. Evans is particularly strong on this point, asserting, rightly in my view, that Canadian national health insurance (NHI) has played a very important role in the nation's sense of "community," treating its citizens, for health care purposes, as fundamentally equal (p. 40). No one fears economic ruin from health care expenses in Canada, because it is for all practical purposes free on use (and its costs spread among the entire community), and no one faces the stigma of "charity care," whether private or public.

Second, the Canadian lessons about how to control costs are, in one sense, straightforward and, in another, not so clear. The obvious lesson

2. The best historical guides to Canadian experience include Taylor 1978; Andreopoulos 1975; and Evans and Stoddart 1986.

drawn is that Canada, along with other OECD nations, controls costs ⎞
through centralized, public funding. That is not, of course, strictly true, ⎠
since Canada's federal system creates ten different units of financial administration. But what is important is that, within each jurisdiction for
payment purposes (the provinces and territories), there is one accountable funding unit, not plural ones as in the United States. To the extent
that other nations have this concentration of payment responsibility, as
for example in Britain, they lend support to this broad claim of what
lesson should be drawn about "how to control health expenditures at a
macro level."

There is, however, a complexity here that Evans does not take up in his
paper. Single-payer systems have, at least by comparison with the United
States, produced relatively more restrained health care expenditures in the
last fifteen years. But what about them is at work? Why should this be
the case? Without knowing that, there is too much of a black-box quality
about the explanation—the results so to speak, but not the reasons.

This is, of course, a complicated subject in political economy, and I
can only sketch out what I take to be the outline of an answer here.[3]
What I would emphasize is the distribution of the winners and losers from
increases in health care expenditures. Everywhere, there are pressures
to spend more on medical care. It is presumed, though with increasing expert skepticism, that more medical care will mean better health.
So the question is, how are expenditures for what is presumed social
improvement constrained? In pluralistic systems of finance, payers are
more interested in their own costs, not the costs of health care. Any cost
shifted represents a 100 percent gain to that payer; hence the competition in such systems to have someone else pay whenever possible. In the
United States, that means attention to cost sharing by patients (shifting
costs backward), government requiring private insurance to pay Medicare
benefits for certain retired workers (shifting costs sideways), and the reverse, as when companies reduce or eliminate their health benefits and
turn employees into charity cases for local hospitals and doctors. Under
such systems, total costs are reckoned at the end of the year—discovered,
not chosen; the results are expensive, as the American experience amply
illustrates.

What are the implications of this analysis for understanding the Canadian experience with centralized "single-payer" funding? It appears there

3. This is the subject of the chapter entitled "The Politics of Medical Inflation," in Marmor 1983. The point is elaborated in my recent testimony to the Senate Finance Committee
(Marmor 1992a).

are two forces at work: competitors for the public dollars that might be available for medical care and politically powerful constraints on shifting costs back to patients. To have competition for the tax dollars collected, medical care must be administered by a general level of government with other responsibilities. It might be argued, for example, that the Swedish form of public funding is less constraining than either the English or the Canadian, precisely because its county government has medical care as its dominant responsibility and hence has few other organized, bureaucratic competitors for the income tax dollars that the county councils have raised almost exclusively for medical care. Put another way, as the proportion of the jurisdiction's public expenditure going to health care approaches 100 percent, the restraint on costs weakens. The grounds for this claim are that the political costs of mobilizing taxpayer restraint on merit goods like medical care are higher than the costs of mobilizing restraint from other government departments who will suffer in their budgets if medical care expenditures rise more quickly than tax revenues.[4]

The theory addresses as well the most obvious source of cost control relaxation in single-payer financing: increasing consumer cost sharing as a revenue-raising device. The Canadian example is quite telling on this point. The commitment to equal access has been strong enough to withstand the rather persistent efforts to introduce patient charges—or at least permit extra-billing—and that means the health professions face what amounts to a unified "consumers' cooperative" in bargaining over what the health budget will be in any particular year. Provincial governments have been quite interested—from time to time—in off-loading this pressure onto patient charges. The Canada Health Act of 1984, as Evans points out, reasserts the presumption against such practices and backs it up with financial penalties to provinces that allow extra-billing. Without the law's force, it is safe to say that Canadian physician expenditures would no doubt have grown more rapidly than they have through increased patient payments.[5]

4. This raises the question of functional substitutes for the constraining effects of cabinet competitors for public funds. In the German case, there is a clear presentation of costs and benefits to the bargainers representing sickness funds and professional associations. The cost of care is identified clearly and yearly increases—and the immediate payment implications—produce the organizational incentives to weigh costs and gains that are comparable to the form discussed above. I want to make clear that the single payer of the Swedish model is not indifferent to cost; it just takes longer to organize the paying stakeholders. Recent Swedish restraint on their quite high health care expenditures is testimony to the capacity to act that exists when the will is mobilized. See Poullier and Schieber 1989 on recent OECD cost developments in health care.

5. There is an interesting Canadian feature here that helps to distinguish genuine cost control from cost shifting. The Canadian financial sanctions for extra-billing by physicians are simple:

Put together, this is a case for monopsony bargaining over the price and volume of health care in a political jurisdiction. It rests on the notion that every marginal dollar of expenditure for health care is income for identifiable and organized health care providers. As a result, the payer side must have correspondingly concentrated interest in those marginal dollars to balance the stakeholders, who regard each unit of expenditure as income, not as cost. The balancing of these interests does not mean health care expenditures will assume a particular level and stay there. But it does appear to provide the necessary condition for establishing some equilibrium in expenditure levels. (Whether some system will emerge that can, as Evans explicitly wonders, "harness" competitive forces to improve health care performance is at best speculative.)[6] What has emerged so far has not had this effect, and Canada provides another illustration of the general type of arrangement that throughout the industrial world has, in fact, restrained costs.

I have so far addressed cost control questions at the macro level. At a micro level, cost control raises issues of medical care supply and payment details. Evans argues explicitly that Canada's sharp increases in physician supply have strengthened the pressures for increased utilization and expenditures over recent decades. Other work, by Christel Woodward and Greg L. Stoddart (1989), estimates that the Canadian physician supply increased by over 70 percent since the mid-1970s, with the supply of physicians exceeding the growth in population by 2.3 percent per year. What is fascinating is that this rate of growth in physician numbers practically matches the increased per capita utilization of health care services over the same period. Evans's warning, which I fully share, is that a belief in the restraining effect on expenditure of excess numbers of competing physicians is a very serious, expensive mistake.

What about hospital bed supply? Here, the Canadian experience is best thought of in connection with more recent American developments. The trend in length of stay is downward in both the United States and Canada, with Canada's level still considerably higher. But it is clear that there are

---

every dollar a province allows in extra-billing reduces the federal block grant by a dollar. If any of the provinces believed physician contentions that patient cost sharing would reduce needless and wasteful medical care at a rate where there was more than a dollar's reduction in care given for every dollar of penalty, they presumably would have permitted cost sharing to continue. None has. Robert Evans made this nice point in a personal communication.

6. This is particularly relevant in the United States in light of the 1992 presidential election campaign. Clinton has committed himself to a plan that expands access, constraining costs using both budgetary limits and managed competition. For an example of the celebration of managed competition as a promising tool for cost control, see *New York Times* 1992.

very substantial variations, and therein lies a clear lesson for others wondering about how much to augment the supply of hospitals in advance of expanding financial access to care. The relevant lesson seems something like this: the "undersupply" of hospital beds may well be the single most important prod to primary and preventive care that lies within a nation's range of policy-relevant tools. How long one must stay in hospital varies not just with the relevant medical condition but with the availability of alternatives to hospital use. This is relevant not only to the beginning of life—births—but to the treatment of the frail old. What Canada shows beyond doubt is that an ample supply of hospital beds, combined with increases in the old old, produces a substantial increase in the use of hospital beds for what is nursing home care. (Beyond that, there is a simply wasteful use of amply supplied hospital beds: e.g., patients coming in one or two days before surgery to "get ready.")

Evans does not take up the redistribution of health care supply across communities. Perhaps it is safe to say that the huge distances and spread-out population of Canada do not present obvious parallels to the circumstances of more urban nations.

Evans does, however, comment substantially on methods of payment for health care. He strongly endorses the global (as opposed to line-item) budgeting of hospitals as against the per diem method of insurance funding that had been the pre-NHI norm in the West. There are no panaceas here and each funding mechanism has the vices of its virtues. But among the virtues of global budgeting is ease in knowing what is committed to health care—particularly its most expensive component. Global budgeting in Canadian practice involves a trade-off between the increased predictability (and controllability) of hospital spending and greater autonomy in hospital decision-making about how to spend the global budget. There are ample means in the Canadian system to restrain capital expenditures (separately budgeted) and additional means through decisions on operating costs that will be included in the global amount. But Canadian analysts, as Evans argues, seem now to agree that Canadian use of hospital beds (as opposed to the use of technology within hospitals) has been unnecessarily ample. This is but one example of where Evans argues that Canadian performance on health might be improved by less rather than more expenditure.

In sum, Evans has sharply portrayed a medical care system that works, that delivers decent care to an entire population at outlays that, while always pressuring decision makers, are relatively stable and quite amazingly popular. If ever there was an example of a public institution that was both expensive and admired, it is Canadian national health insurance. None of these features, he points out, depend on peculiarly Canadian features—whether of politics, society, or economics. The particular institutional details do, of course, show their origins, but other nations could extract the essential features of the Canadian system and adapt them to their institutional architecture. Whether they would have similar effects depends on whether the new user differs in some significant way from those nations whose practices conform to the Canadian pattern as well.

Evans is by no means oblivious to tensions and troubles within the system he sketches. But there are two areas where I think considerable amplification would be helpful to those unfamiliar with Canadian practices.

One is the degree of conflict that successful instances of public cost control experience on a regular basis. To the degree cost control "works," it is disappointing to the aspirations of health professionals. They, in turn, can reach out to publics for support in making sure that the restraints in cost do not "lower" the quality of care. The fights over this—and issues like "abuse" by patients or doctors—make the regular determination of hospital budgets and, especially, doctors' fees very contentious matters. It is of the greatest importance to anticipate such contentiousness and, within the limits set by the budgetary restraint goals themselves, to design formats, select negotiators, and employ modes of public explanation that do not worsen the pain which such struggles cause. This is not the place to say much more about the subject, but it is worthwhile, I believe, to give it pride of place in planning.

A second issue, which Evans fails to raise at all, is the legal liability environment and its impact on patterns of utilization. This was not an issue of any great moment when I began to study Canadian health arrangements in the early 1970s. The price per physician of malpractice insurance was, by American standards, incredibly modest. But, as Woodward and Stoddart (1989) recently argued in connection with alleged "abuses" through unnecessary testing and procedural elaboration, defensive medicine may well have something to do with the relentless increases in per capita utilization that Canada has experienced over the past two decades. Some of it, undoubtedly, arises from physician-induced demand, itself a product of increased physician numbers, tough bargaining on fee schedules, and the income aspirations of doctors who can feel with some justification that more elaborate care is what their patients "want" (as against need). But some of the utilization pattern is consistent as well with substantial increases in legal liability. That, too, requires attention, particularly in fee-for-service systems, where doing more both increases income and brings whatever protection there is from extensive servicing as a defense against inadequate professional care in a malpractice suit.

Taken together, Canada supplies a model of an admittedly imperfect, but successfully functioning health care system. Since very little of its performance seems to rest on magically Canadian properties, it is precisely the sort of programmatic experience that can be usefully studied, with good value, for comparative purposes.[7]

References

Andreopoulos, Spyros, ed. 1975. *National Health Insurance: Can the U.S. Learn from Canada?* New York: John Wiley.

Evans, Robert G. 1992. Canada: The Real Issues. *Journal of Health Politics, Policy and Law* 17 (4): 739–62.

Evans, Robert G., and G. Stoddart, eds. 1986. *Medicare at Maturity: Achievements, Lessons and Challenges.* Calgary: University of Calgary Press.

Klein, Rudolph, and Theodore R. Marmor. 1986. Cost v. Care: America's Health Care Dilemma Wrongly Considered. *Health Matrix* 4 (1): 19–24.

Marmor, Theodore R. 1983. *Political Analysis and American Medical Care: Essays.* New York: Cambridge University Press.

———. 1992a. The Problems of American Medical Care Reform: The Case for Universal Coverage and Single Payor Financing. Hearing on comprehensive health care reform before the Committee on Finance of the United States Senate, 17 June.

———. 1992b. Commentary on Canadian Health Insurance: Lessons for the United States. *International Journal of Health Services* 23 (1): 45–62.

Marmor, Theodore R., Amy Bridges, and Wayne L. Hoffman. 1978. Comparative Politics and Health Policies: Notes on Benefits, Costs, Limits. In *Comparing Public Policies: New Concepts and Methods*, ed. Douglas E. Ashford. Beverly Hills, CA: Sage.

New York Times. 1992. The Bush-Clinton Health Reform (editorial), 10 October, p. 20.

Poullier, Jean-Pierre, and George J. Schieber. 1989. International Health Care Expenditure Trends: 1987. *Health Affairs* 8 (3): 169–77.

Taylor, Malcolm. 1978. *Health Insurance and Canadian Public Policy: The Seven Decisions That Created the Canadian Health Insurance System.* Montreal: McGill-Queen's University Press.

Woodward, Christel, and Greg L. Stoddart. 1989. Is the Canadian Health Care System Suffering from Abuse? CHEPA Working Paper Series 19 (Commentary). McMaster University Center for Health Economics and Policy Analysis.

7. For two recent examples see Marmor 1992a, 1992b.

Universal Health Insurance That Really Works: Foreign Lessons for the United States

William A. Glaser

Abstract The United States has serious and worsening problems in the delivery and financing of health care. The debate about reform has inspired many schemes that are persuasive in their presentation, but they are unrealistic: some cannot be enacted by Congress, others would not improve existing arrangements, most are imaginary inventions with uncertain outcomes. The most politically prudent and the most effective course is to emulate the methods used successfully and available for full analysis in other developed countries. America created its successful social security system in this fashion, and statutory health insurance should be added now. All or most groups would be required to join. Financing would come from social security payroll taxes, supplemented by government subsidies. Basic acute care services would be equally available to all. The existing insurance companies would remain as fiscal intermediaries. Doctors and hospitals would continue to work much as they do now. They would prosper from more utilization, few bad debts, and less administrative trouble. The payment and work of doctors would be governed by collective negotiations between the insurance carriers and the medical associations. The payment and work of hospitals would be governed by a mixture of government regulations and negotiations with the carriers. Costs would be controlled by coordinated decision making by the payers, the providers, and government. The system would not turn over services and financing to government.

American health care has become so chaotic that the country cannot fail to adopt a national health plan soon—or so everyone says. Costs skyrocket, insurance coverage diminishes, confusion spreads, and complaints multiply.

Let us debate the issues, everyone says, and a consensus will emerge. Many schemes are offered in journals and in conferences, in the hope they will save the country and will make the reputations of their inventors. Each is complex, each is supposed to be unique, and nearly all are imaginary, so that one cannot judge their feasibility in actual practice. The following paper will describe a fundamental reform that is not imaginary but that can be observed and evaluated in real life, in the principal developed countries of Western Europe. America's successful social security system was copied from Western Europe after careful study, and health care financing can be added to America's social security in the same way.

Employment Group Insurance

When a country enacts social security and a health financing system, it usually strengthens and expands its previously voluntary and private arrangements: The mutual aid funds and insurance carriers remain as financial administrators; many or all persons are now required to join; premiums become taxes, to guarantee adequate financing; hospitals and doctors remain autonomous. All European countries have enacted such arrangements. (A few have replaced "national health insurance" with government-managed and tax-financed "national health services.") Complete details appear in Glaser 1991; the history is summarized in Köhler et al. 1982.

Alone among developed countries, the United States went in a partially different direction. It enacted the social security pension, disability, work accident, and unemployment programs of Europe, but political deadlocks blocked statutory health insurance. Trade unions after World War II pressed employers to buy group health insurance as a fringe benefit of employment. Eventually it was assumed that these private arrangements would cover the entire American labor force and its dependents (Munts 1967). Government would intervene only to cover the persons without jobs, in the form of Medicare and Medicaid. A uniquely American arrangement was supposed to achieve the same results as those of national health insurance and of national health services.

Group coverage through the workplace has always left many Americans without third-party protection. Persons covered experience cuts in benefits, when employers try to reduce their labor costs. Instead of pressing for the national health insurance common in Europe, American reformers have tried to make employment-based insurance universal and more generous. Since the mid-1970s, every bill for statutory health insurance introduced into Congress has required all employers to arrange group insurance for all their employees, either by contracting with a carrier or by paying equivalent premiums to a public fund (an arrangement known as "play or pay"). The principal example during the 1980s was the Kennedy-Waxman Bill (Feder 1981). The national commission to design health care financing for America recommended mandating employment-based insurance, either by individual group contracts with carriers or by "play or pay" (Pepper Commission 1990), and a variant (HealthAmerica) was sent to the floor of the Senate by the Committee on Labor and Human Resources in 1992. Hawaii and Massachusetts enacted such obligatory employment group laws within their jurisdictions (Lewin 1992; Goldberger 1990), and other states have considered them (for example, Beauchamp and Rouse 1990). Reforms proposed by many individuals rely on mandating employment group insurance (for example, Enthoven and Kronick 1989).

Political Obstacles

None of these schemes can accomplish the goal of full coverage of the population. The first problem is that none can be enacted by the United States Congress. The principal source of the uninsured is employment in small business. Most of these owners do not want to provide any fringe benefits for their workers. They are ideologically committed to self-help: they believe everyone should pay for his own health care and insurance. Many of these employees are part-time or occasional workers, not included in any pension or health plans that small firms might have.

Small business is very influential in the United States House of Representatives and in all lower houses of state legislatures. No mandate of truly universal employment group health insurance with standard benefits can be enacted by Congress or by any state legislature. In order to reduce the number of negative votes, the authors of bills (such as Kennedy-Waxman) exempt all very small business (for example, with six or fewer employees), phase in moderate-size small business (for example, with six to twenty-five employees) over a long period and require them to offer a lower level of benefits.

The political compromises result in such a low requirement of benefits that government must subsidize the covered employees of small business, as well as paying in full for the workers in completely exempt firms. This contradicts the theory of employment group coverage and falls victim to American government's need to reduce deficits. For example, the Massachusetts Health Security Act permitted small business to opt out of insurance coverage of its workers by paying the state government a tax of $1,680 per worker per year—the origins of the enfeebling play-or-pay method—and the state government was expected to pay for full benefits for the worker and his entire family. Even this was too much for small business, who pressed the new governor and the legislature to repeal the act before implementation. Even if it had been carried out in its original form in Massachusetts, the workers and dependents in the small business sector would have received limited benefits (Blendon et al. 1992). The much-touted Prepaid Health Care Act of Hawaii is incomplete too: employers need not include in their groups dependents, part-time workers, and seasonal workers.

Defects in Design

If it could be enacted, universal employment group insurance would preserve on a larger scale all the defects in the current American health insurance system, going far beyond the present omission of the uninsured alone. (Some of these technical weaknesses are evident in U.S. House of Representatives 1990 and in Congressional Budget Office 1991.) Following are several basic defects in America's current employment group insurance that would persist.

The system will still lack any methods of financial redistribution. Each employed group will continue to be experience-rated (if an insurance company is the carrier) or will pay only its own costs (if the employer self-insures). There will be no equalization mechanism, so that the more affluent groups, industries, and geographical regions contribute to the costs of the less affluent.

Preferred-risk selection of groups by insurance companies will continue. The insurance industry will still have large marketing costs to find and sign up the healthier and more affluent groups.

Benefits would vary among employer groups, according to their affluence and philosophy. In a supposedly universal system, workers would be unequal in their benefits and cost-sharing. Within each firm, owners and managers might continue to give themselves more generous benefits than they give their workers—discrepancies that Congress tried to reduce in 1986 but then re-authorized, because of lobbying by small business. Hospitals and doctors would continue to experience the great complexity and administrative burden of dealing with patients with different coverages and reimbursement procedures. Under most proposals, the state governments would continue to be the regulatory authorities, and wide variations would persist across the country in benefits, financial oversight, and subscriber protection.

Within the same firm, workers can experience changes in coverage and cutbacks from year to year. If he changes jobs, the worker's benefits and administrative procedures change. All this leaves the worker and his family with great uncertainties and unexpected denials.

During the first decades of employment group insurance, American employers paid for all benefits of workers and dependents. Americans became accustomed to think that health care was "free." Contributory plans became common only during the 1980s, but trade unions have fought all but the lowest premiums. Bills for mandatory employment group insurance usually permit employers to recover from the workers no more than one-quarter of the premiums. This will give employers an incentive to shop among insurance carriers for the thinnest benefits. During economic recessions, businessmen's associations have an incentive to press for cutbacks in the law. Because of their low contributory premiums, the American people will continue to lack a full understanding of health care costs.

The personnel departments of business firms will continue their arduous work of negotiating benefit packages with unions and shopping among insurance carriers or third-party administrators for the best deals. Business firms wish to reduce their involvement in the frustrating health financing sector, not increase it.

Medicare and Medicaid—with all their regulations, disputes, and bureaucracies—will continue without change.

All-payer management is prescribed by few of the national employment group bills. Under most proposals, reimbursement rates will continue to differ among payers, hospitals will still shift costs from the less generous to the more generous payers, and recriminations will continue.

The health sector will remain an unorganized mosaic of groups and carriers. Each will try to minimize its own costs, whether by limiting benefits or by "managed care" arrangements with hospitals and doctors. But the entire system is unmanaged, and costs will continue to grow. The many different managed care arrangements will continue to increase the administrative costs of hospitals.

"The Canadian Model"

Once the American and Canadian health financing markets were closely connected and much alike. But Canadian industry was never prosperous enough and Canadian trade unions never strong enough to develop an extensive set of employer-paid fringe benefits throughout the country. Outside of a few industrial sites, the scattered Canadian population did not develop the mutual aid funds that became the foundation of European statutory social insurance. Canadian hospitals were owned and managed by nonprofit associations and municipalities, doctors were self-employed, governments had limited power, and the country wanted to avoid the British path to a national health service.

Instead, several western Canadian provincial governments subsidized the hospital inpatient bills of their citizens from their general budgets. The method spread, the national government agreed to share the costs during the 1950s, and soon all hospital operating and capital costs were paid for from provincial government budgets. All physician bills came to be reimbursed from provincial government budgets after the same evolution (Taylor 1978; Evans and Stoddart 1986).

Frustrated by the uncontrolled growth of American health costs, several influential members of Congress during the late 1980s asked why the United States could not learn from Canadian cost containment. With less spending, Canada delivered advanced care to its entire population, and people seemed satisfied. A rush of American researchers and policy analysts then wrote descriptions of Canada, and several proposals for reform of the United States recommended "the Canadian model" (especially Himmelstein and Woolhandler 1989).

Political Obstacles

Whatever its merits in Canada, the Canadian health financing system will never be enacted in the United States. The Kennedy-Corman Bill of the late 1970s proposed financing from general revenue and exclusive administration of payment by state governments, but it never reached the floors of Congress (Waldman 1976: 121–37). Enactment now continues to be unlikely for several reasons.

Since health financing is part of Canadian government budgets, the leaders of the hospital and physician sectors must conform to the priorities of the Parliament, the Treasury, and the Ministry of Health. The medical profession in all countries avoids such subordination to laymen and to politicians. Health financing often becomes a political controversy in the Canadian mass media and in election campaigns. Fearing this situation, the American Medical Association responded to the mounting interest in the "Canadian model" by attacking it in many issues of the *American Medical News* and in a national advertising campaign.

Financing is generous during periods of growth and tight when government must control its deficits. When their programs began, Canadian hospitals and doctors thought they would always be guaranteed full operating costs and increasing incomes, but limits were imposed during the late 1970s and 1980s. At first, Canadian hospitals negotiated prospective budgets with provincial governments, but now the latter impose what they can afford to pay (Glaser 1981, 1987: 179–88). At first, the provincial medical associations negotiated their fees with provincial governments, but some governments (particularly Quebec and Ontario) then invoked their budgetary constraints and legal sovereignty to dictate the final results. (After a decade of disputes, Quebec, Ontario, and Manitoba in 1991 reluctantly agreed to resolve deadlocks by arbitration.) Conversant with Canadian history, aware of the same evolution in American Medicaid, and fearing stringent across-the-board cost containment in the future, American hospital and medical associations would fight creation of any such single-payer governmental arrangements in the United States.

In each Canadian province, the Ministry of Health pays the hospitals, the ministry or a public corporation pays the doctors, and the insurance companies play no role. The carriers must specialize in supplementary benefits, such as dentistry, pharmaceutical drugs, private hospital rooms, and so on. The American insurance industry can easily block enactment of such an arrangement in the United States.

Learning from Appropriate Foreign Experiences

Americans devoted to a slightly reformed status quo declare it superior to government-run national health services (as in Great Britain and Sweden) and superior to their image of a capital-starved Canada (Enthoven and Kronick 1989: 94; Sullivan 1990). Their argument seems compelling. But it misleads the policy debate, since the apologists ignore the most politically feasible and the most successful alternative, that is, the statutory health insurance arrangements that much of Europe has been using for a century.

Shortly after Germany enacted the first social security laws for pensions and health insurance, scholars and public officials throughout Europe and North America made site visits and wrote reports about the German precedent and the arrangements that each country subsequently enacted. The United States government sponsored several of these lessons-from-abroad reports and drafted typical European social security proposals (Commissioner of Labor 1911; Willoughby 1898; Rubinow 1916). During the 1920s, state officials and professors of economics conversant with the European programs enacted social insurance in Wisconsin and proposed it in New York. They accompanied the Roosevelt administration to Washington and designed the social security law of the national government. The author of the latest lessons-from-abroad book (Armstrong 1932) was the principal drafter of Old Age and Survivors Insurance (OASI). In order to avoid a fight with the medical association that would lose votes in Congress and antagonize the Supreme Court, the Roosevelt administration temporarily set aside the health insurance component of social security.

After World War II, statutory health insurance for the entire population was proposed by presidents and by others in 1950, the early 1960s, and the early 1970s. Because of the growing belief that employment group insurance might cover the entire population without legislation, a limited version of statutory health insurance was enacted for the retired alone in 1965. After 1974, the idea of statutory health insurance was forgotten and was replaced by schemes to force laggard employers to cover all their workers. However, it is not possible to achieve the goals of national health insurance in this fashion, as explained above. The policy debate over health financing reform should rediscover its original road.

Statutory Health Insurance for the United States

Following is a brief summary of a statutory health insurance system for the United States, based on the experiences of other countries. Unlike nearly all other entries in the current American policy debate, the following proposal is not my personal imaginary nostrum, but it is derived from the actual operations and successes of other developed countries. This paper—like every article—can only state highlights and must focus on its topic. For complete details about the organization, financing, benefits, problems, and effects of European statutory health insurance see Glaser 1991, the many sources cited therein, and my other publications.

The proposal synthesizes the experience of many countries and is not based on only one. The American policy debate lately has noticed foreign events, but it focuses on one country at a time. The vogue of "the Canadian model" in 1989 was superseded by discussion of a "German model" in 1991. However, cross-national lesson drawing is doomed if one thinks it refers only to reproducing one other country's total system in the United States (for reasons explained in Glaser 1978: 233–47). The lesson-drawing task consists of discovering the consensus of how nearly all developed countries solve the problems they share with the United States, adapting it for the American situation, and identifying the supports and barriers to implementation. This article and the entire research project reported in Glaser 1991 are based on the experience of the successful systems in Germany, France, the Netherlands, Belgium, Switzerland, and Japan, and on the early experiences of countries that finally substituted national health services (Great Britain, Italy, and Spain).

Statute

As in other countries, Congress would pass a law specifying:

- Certain groups in the population must be covered by national health insurance.
- They have free choice of insurance carrier.
- They and their employers must pay payroll taxes.
- Minimum benefits are guaranteed the subscribers.
- Subscribers have free choice of licensed doctors, hospitals, and other providers.
- Conditions are listed for participation by doctors, hospitals, and other providers. Usually all licensed practitioners are eligible. Procedures for exclusion are specified.
- Conditions are listed for participation by insurance carriers. Usually all mutual aid funds, mutual insurance companies, and stock companies are eligible.
- How claims, provider reimbursement, and other administrative and financial matters are managed.

The law would be part of the Social Security Code, replacing the present Titles XVIII and XIX for Medicare and Medicaid.

Ideally, Congress should enact framework laws and delegate details to the executive branch and to negotiations between payers and providers. That was the custom of Congress before the 1970s, when suspicion of the executive branch and exposés about fraud led Congress to its current practice of fine-tuning everything. In no other country does parliament prescribe so many details. The American practice leads to constant demands by interest groups, legislative entrepreneurship by individual congressmen and senators, and constant overload of the legislature.

Ideally, Congress should enact a law, let it settle down, and avoid annual tinkering. Current practice invites interest groups to demand frequent self-serving revisions, prevents administration from stabilizing, and sows uncertainties and disputes.

Coverage

Usually statutory health insurance evolves over many decades. A country starts with miners and other factory workers and at intervals adds all other blue-collar workers, white-collar workers, the self-employed, farmers, leading managers, the pensioners, and the unemployed. By now, every country has almost complete coverage.

The United States, too, has added occupations successively to the original 1935 coverage of the Old Age and Survivors Insurance (OASI), so that now everyone is covered. Therefore, perhaps the United States will include all occupations under statutory health insurance from the start.

Pensioners

Everyone would remain in his chosen health insurance carrier after retirement. Benefits would not differ by age. Once a few countries (such as Holland) kept special financial accounts for the pensioners who did not bring in normal payroll taxes, but this distinction has been abolished. Whether the elderly person is still working or is retired makes no difference.

The age of sixty-five would no longer be associated with a change in coverage and financing in the United States. Its special significance is an artifact of America's unique decision to create special statutory health insurance for the retired alone. The Americans at that time mistakenly expected that everyone would remain under private employment group coverage until all retired at sixty-five. Lifelong coverage would eliminate the present gap for most Americans who retire before sixty-five, drop out of their workplace groups, create dilemmas for their employers, and must wait several years for Medicare.

The elderly and disabled pensioners incur high costs but do not bring in high payroll taxes. Part of the shortfall is raised by the sickness fund from payroll taxes levied on those who are economically active, whose tax payments are higher than their medical costs. The rest of the shortfall is covered by public subsidies.

Under national health insurance, Medicare would be abolished. The nation would be spared Medicare's large administrative bureaucracy, its stream of incomprehensible regulations, and its endless disputes. The Department of Health and Human Services would maintain a less intrusive and less overloaded agency to oversee the performance of the insurance carriers, to formulate guidelines about procedures and costs, and to oversee the machinery deciding provider reimbursement. Compared to the Health Care Financing Administration, the new agency would be more responsive to subscribers and to providers.

Poor and Unemployed

As in the case of the pensioners, those temporarily without jobs would remain in their original sickness funds. The working poor would be covered at all times, thereby solving America's crisis of the working uninsured. Once many countries had public welfare programs to deliver or pay for the medical care of the poor—that is, arrangements like Medicaid—but now all countries include these persons under normal statutory health insurance with the standard benefits. Rich and poor would differ in income and in living standards, but they would have the same basic health coverage and the poor would receive mainstream services.

As in the case of the pensioners, the financing system would cross-subsidize the medical costs of the poor. The economically active would bring in payroll taxes exceeding their costs. Government would add subsidies. Medicaid would be abolished, and state governments would be relieved of a millstone.

Payroll Taxes

As in all social security programs, funds are raised primarily from taxes proportionate to earnings. The United States already uses them for Medicare Part A, and they would merely increase for a comprehensive program. The rates could be equal for employee and employer (as in American Medicare and Germany), or they could be higher for employers (as in most countries). In most countries a single nationwide rate is enacted annually by parliament as part of the tax and budget legislation, but Germany allows each health insurance carrier to set its own. Since the carriers break even without profits or losses, the rates can rise or fall each year, after calculations by actuaries and legislation in parliament. In contrast, American social security practice employs prolonged freezes and occasional automatic minute increases if a formula reveals an excessive decline in the reserves.

Financing must be redistributive, to cover the high costs of the elderly, disabled, and poor. Medical costs have increased so much that France and Belgium have eliminated the earnings base in health insurance: the payroll tax falls on the entire salary; in contrast, the payroll tax for social security pensions still falls on wages below a limit. Therefore, the very high earners (and their employers) contribute very large amounts to the health accounts. American Medicare is now moving in this direction: Congress in late 1990 set the earnings base for the Hospital Insurance Trust Fund's payroll tax at about double the base for the Old Age, Survivors, and Disability Insurance (OASDI) tax.

Financing health insurance by this method will finally make clear to Americans that their medical care is expensive and they cannot expect "somebody else" to pay for it. The payroll taxes on individuals' earnings—6 percent or more in several European countries, lower than that only if the earnings base is unlimited—will be higher than the premiums in even the most demanding American employment-based contributory schemes. On the other hand, no one need incur the present American expense of individual policies for basic health insurance. The payroll taxes on American employers may be lower than the costs of a generous group plan, and the employers will also be relieved of the administrative burden of the present system. Political skills and a gradual transition will be needed to change from current arrangements to social security financing. Wage adjustments will accompany the shifts of burdens from employers to workers and the addition of the extra social insurance burden on the workers.

The self-employed now pay double the social security rate in the United States—that is, both the workers' and employer's share for OASDI and Medicare—and this would continue in an expanded statutory health insurance. Small businessmen might not resist, since they are already accustomed to paying their own double rate and their share of the payroll tax for their workers. This would seem less burdensome than buying group insurance under the proposed mandates and under the expensive multi-employer pools that they resist. In Europe, the self-employed once opposed their own inclusion under social security, and the compromises allow them lower rates or a lower earnings base.

Tax on Pensions

Once the elderly in Europe paid nothing after retirement but were covered by extra contributions by the economically active and by public subsidies.

But their increasing number and growing costs required substantial contributions. Now they are taxed a proportion of their social security pensions, at rates comparable to the active workers' rates. The need for significant premiums would finally bring to the American elderly a realistic understanding of finance. At present they must pay low premiums for Medicare Part B, but they protest about the size, and Congress nervously avoids substantial increases. The European pensioners pay much more, but their benefits are superior.

A proportionate tax would require lower payments by the low-income pensioners and more money from the richer. The American elderly might cooperate better with a proportionate tax than with the present flat Part B premium. The lower-income elderly have grumbled about the flat premium and have protested against Congress's occasional hesitant attempts to increase it. The richer elderly have lobbied against any attempts to levy extra surcharges on them, and the issue caused the repeal of the Medicare Catastrophic Coverage Act of 1988.

Subsidies

Once all statutory health insurance systems were supposed to break even from payroll taxes, but now nearly all are subsidized by national governments from their general budgets. Money must be found to cover the high costs of the retired, disabled, and poor, when these groups pay low premiums and bring in no payroll taxes from employers. The money goes to the health insurance carrier and not directly to the provider or beneficiary. The patients now are never identified as a special class—unlike categorical programs like Medicaid—and their benefits are never cut back to save money.

Subsidies already exist in American health insurance, and the practice would merely continue. Three-quarters of Medicare Part B now comes from the national treasury. Coverage of the poor under Medicaid depends completely on national and state government contributions.

Subsidies and equalization transfers among sickness funds become the methods of preserving a semiprivate system of health insurance carriers, instead of converting health into a completely government-financed and government-dictated sector. Subsidies are a method of supplementing the proportionate payroll taxes with money derived from the progressive income tax. It is not necessary to replace the present payroll tax by a progressive earnings tax or by a progressive tax on all income.

Insurance Carriers

Since statutory health insurance hews as closely to the private model as possible, and since the legislators avoid antagonizing powerful interests, the preexisting health insurance carriers are retained as fiscal intermediaries. All carriers are eligible to continue, whether they are mutual aid funds sponsored by trade unions or by consumer movements, mutual insurance companies, or stock companies. Only if the private companies withdraw or fail does government replace them with public corporations—as in part of the French market—but, even then, the new entities are autonomous and are not merely government bureaucracies.

The American health insurance market might become more competitive than it is now. Instead of each carrier winning a monopoly from an employer, all carriers could appeal to the group's workers and their families for individual enrollment. Instead of each carrier winning a monopoly of all Medicare or Medicaid business in an area, all carriers could appeal directly to the elderly and poor individuals. The system would use unlimited free choice, available now on a small scale in the Federal Employees Health Benefits Program. Each subscriber's payroll taxes or premiums would go to his carrier. The insurers would strive for the largest number of subscribers yielding the largest revenue. To prevent preferred risk selection, the law would require each carrier to accept any applicant, without medical underwriting and without extra premiums. (This is one of the few regulations of the carriers in statutory health insurance.) Preferred risk selection might also be discouraged by financial equalization transfers between carriers with large profits and carriers with large deficits.

The insurance carriers would become bigger and more important than ever. Their responsibilities in protection of the public interest would increase. They would have to operate within the yield of payroll taxes and public subsidies, they would collaborate with government in setting benefit policies and expenditure targets, and they would be responsible for implementing cost containment. Lest it lose subscribers, each would have to represent its patients in obtaining adequate services and in understanding the delivery system. The carriers would be the principal negotiators with the medical profession in defining work rules and in setting reimbursement. They would participate in hospital rate setting. These roles no longer seem unfamiliar to American health insurers: the Blues have long tried to fulfill them, and the commercial companies too are now trying to become policy leaders and consumer representatives.

Carriers would continue to offer supplementary insurance products.

In mainstream coverage, their discretion over benefits and provider rates would be limited: minimum benefits are set by law, and provider rates are set on an all-payer basis by collective negotiation or by regulation. The carriers' role in statutory health insurance would be that of fiscal administrators, but the American market has already transformed them in this fashion. Employment group health benefits have rapidly become a self-insured system, where the insurance carrier is retained only to administer enrollments and claims. Insurers have been primarily fiscal intermediaries from the start of Medicare.

Paying the Doctor

Statutory health insurance is organized to resemble a private market as much as possible, in large part because the medical profession opposes government control. The doctors themselves remain self-employed businessmen. Since government cannot dictate their working rules and pay, much must be decided by collective negotiations between the health insurance carriers and the medical association. Disagreements over rules and money often become heated, settlements eventually result from compromise or (rarely) from arbitration, government almost never dictates settlements, and patient care then continues with few interruptions (Glaser 1978).

The United States should adopt these methods and abandon the uncertainties, conflicts, and incessant government fine-tuning that has permeated Medicare Part B and that will surely continue under the supposed reforms during the coming years (Glaser 1990). The American medical profession at first will fight proposals that will generalize this experience to all their reimbursement. (See, for example, Adelman's [1992] critique of an early version of this article.) The statutes therefore will include the framework for deciding physicians' working rules and reimbursement. Organized medicine and individual doctors in all countries cooperate (however unhappily) with a system in which they have a voice over their work and income, in which they share responsibility for decisions, but they can block enactment and harmonious implementation of any nationwide arrangements allowing government dictation.

Collective negotiations decide contracts, fee schedules (lists of relative values), and prices (conversion of the relative values into pay rates). Permanent joint committees interpret the fee schedules, review utilization, and perform other tasks. The payer side consists of representatives of all the health insurance carriers. The American medical profession would be represented by a panel from all the medical associations (as in France and Belgium), by a new confederation uniting the AMA and the specialty societies (as in Holland), by the AMA on behalf of all the specialty societies (as in Great Britain), or by a new entity devoted to financial negotiations alone (as in Germany and Quebec).

Negotiations and finances might be managed in one of the following fashions:

- Centralized on a national level: The contract, fee schedule, and financial conversion factor would be settled for the entire country, as in countries with unitary governments, such as France, Holland, and Belgium. America already centralizes Medicare in this manner. Setting the conversion rate becomes complicated in large and sprawling countries like the United States, since revenue and provider costs vary across the country. In Medicare, the Americans exercise their penchant for complicated, controversial, and politically logrolled formulae to vary providers' revenue according to local costs of practice and costs of living. Some large countries (such as France) buy the doctors' cooperation by paying all of them high standard rates throughout the country.

- Nationwide negotiations for the contract and fee schedule: The conversion factor is set at the regional or state level, in negotiations between its insurance carriers and its medical associations. The financial accounts are kept within each region: provider reimbursement is coordinated with the high or low fiscal capacity of each region, without the formulae and political manipulation to vary average national rates. An example is Germany.

- Regional or provincial negotiation of the entire relationship between payers and doctors: Each region or state would have its own contract, fee schedule, prices, and financial accounts. The principal regulators and monitors would be the regional or state governments. Some nationwide similarities would be preserved by regulations and conditional subsidies from the national government. Examples are Switzerland and Canada. The United States conducts Medicaid in this fashion, but greater standardization and patient protection would be necessary under decentralized American statutory health insurance.

Regardless of the form of negotiations, the result is always an all-payer system: all carriers under statutory health insurance pay the same rates according to the same fee schedule. Whether the official fee is always full payment can be one of the options in designing American statutory health insurance. A doctor can extra-bill in a few countries (such as Belgium) but usually charges only a few patients only small amounts of extra cash: the medical professions there are solicitous of their patients (particularly the numerous elderly) and wish to avoid crackdowns by the public and by government. During periods when official fees are being increased slowly, government and the insurance carriers may try to appease the doctors by allowing extra-billing, but (as in France) the concession eventually is withdrawn.

Health maintenance organizations might continue to attract patients as multispecialty groups with superior facilities and high-quality providers. But they can no longer lock in their users, since the statute guarantees freedom of choice. Independent practice associations (IPAs) would no longer be necessary, since the entire system would operate like an all-inclusive IPA with managed care methods.

The medical profession in America—as in other countries—would be better off than before. At first the fees are set at the private market rates, and the negotiations steadily increase them. Doctors have more patients and more work than before (because of universal coverage at full rates), they no longer have bad debts or delays in payment, and administrative costs diminish. Because fees are standardized and predictable, because incomes are secure, and because disputes are fewer, individual doctors would be able to concentrate on clinical work.

Paying the Hospital

The health insurance system is supposed to pay each hospital the costs for adequate performance of its work, with neither profits nor losses. Government and the health insurance carriers need to scrutinize hospitals' financial claims carefully, since the totals make up half of all health spending, since hospitals have been at the root of several countries' cost crises, and since evaluating their needs is very complicated. Hospitals are expected to file accounts of past utilization and spending, and to file prospective budgets for next year's claims. In several countries (such as France, Holland, and Switzerland), these papers are studied by rate regulators expert in hospital operations, equipped with data for peer comparisons, and empowered to examine the hospital's books. After cutting some padded lines, the regulator approves the hospital's budget for next year (Glaser 1987: 119–61).

The health insurance carriers negotiate with the doctors bilaterally, and settle on compromise rates after power bargaining. The rates cover the doctors' costs and as much markup for income as the doctors can win. Investigating hospital accounts to establish the break-even rates to cover all clinical needs is beyond the capacity of sickness funds, so most countries with statutory health insurance rely on respected neutral regulators. The local sickness funds scrutinize the hospital's rate application in France and Holland and advise the rate regulators about the hospital's performance. In Germany, the sickness funds negotiate with each hospital as they do with the medical association, and no rate regulator is used, but this is unusual. In no country with statutory health insurance does government dictate the hospital's rates, as it does in countries with full public financing (such as Canada) or as in American Medicare. During the drafting of American universal statutory health insurance, the hospitals would initially request full payment for the budgets they themselves propose, but they would probably settle for the usual device of screening and approval by a neutral regulator. The method has already been used in several states, such as Maryland, whose methods resemble Holland's.

How to deliver the money to the hospital during the year is one of the options in designing American statutory health insurance. The global budget might be paid in installments, with shares divided among the local sickness funds, according to their shares of the hospitals' admissions. Or, the expected hospital budget is divided by the predicted total number of patient days, and the hospital bills each insurance carrier the resulting per diem, according to that carrier's total patient days.

Reimbursement is an all-payer system. The per diem is an average; the hospital and the insurance carrier gain or lose on individual cases. Unlike present American practice, the hospital management can no longer shift costs from one payer to another: it does not risk deficits from low-paying patients and instead is expected to cover its costs over the year from all patients. European hospitals once could overspend and recover their losses from extra rate increases during the next year, but now they must operate within their budgets. Supplements can be obtained only if the hospital demonstrates unavoidable clinical requirement, such as increases in admissions due to sudden population growth or epidemics.

While some specialist physicians can earn extra cash from a small market of private payers and the privately insured, usually almost the entire revenue of the hospital comes from social insurance. American hospitals would be much better off, since they would be guaranteed their costs and would have no more bad debts. If government and the health insurance funds judge that small rural hospitals are needed, they survive, despite low occupancy. Unintended bankruptcies become rare. The only losers would be the hospital financial departments: their work would be simpler, their staffs would be smaller, and the chief financial officers would become less important.

Every country uses methods that cover each hospital's full costs. None uses standard rates across a class of hospitals, like American diagnosis-related groups. The starting point is each hospital's clinical plan, past performance, and prospective budget. No country follows American Medicare's methods of complicated calculations from a national database, in order to fix an optimum rate for an "efficient" hospital. Efficiency is judged by the sickness funds and by the rate regulator after examining each hospital, not by profits on a balance sheet.

Capital Investment

An important function of government in most countries with statutory health insurance is to provide grants for new buildings and for expensive equipment. New programs are concentrated in a few places, at first in the teaching hospitals. Once their effectiveness is proved, they are placed selectively throughout the country at major hospitals with expert staffs. Patients are brought there, so the staffs have sufficient volume to justify the investment and to develop skills. Expensive programs are not allowed to proliferate throughout the country, with high expenditure, low volume, and an incentive to utilize unnecessarily. In similar fashion, the American government granted money to hospitals in the Hill-Burton program (Glaser 1987: 208–62).

The American method that succeeded Hill-Burton is rarely permitted abroad: the medical staff of a hospital wants the latest in new equipment; it forces the hospital management to buy the new equipment and modernize the building, or it will take its patients to a competing hospital; the hospital borrows in the bond market, with the endorsement of a local government agency; the insurance companies and Medicare automatically agree to the amortization as part of operating costs; the doctors utilize (and overutilize) the new program to enable the hospital to repay the loan and in order to increase their own incomes. Holland once was the only European country to allow this method and costs exploded: now, Dutch planners must approve the new installations, and Dutch rate regulators are stricter in allowing amortization in the prospective operating budget. France and Switzerland allow hospitals to borrow from special capital funds, but their governments and health insurance carriers must approve each application. Ideally, hospital systems planning should set priorities and should govern the capital grants, but Europe's individual hospitals (and their political protectors) have resisted planners, and planning methodology has developed slowly. In order to contain costs and establish a more efficient distribution of increasingly expensive services, public planning is gradually intervening.

Cost Containment

Every statutory health insurance system must operate within limits. Payroll taxes and government subsidies cannot rise indefinitely. Economic downturns in Europe during the late 1970s and 1980s necessitated a halt to the previous cost explosion, which had resulted from a combination of hospital modernization, increases in health personnel, higher wages in health, new technology, higher utilization by both old and young, and so on. Several cost pressures still remain as strong as ever, such as the increase in utilization by an aging population and the greater service intensity for all. Statutory health insurance guarantees access by all and gives doctors discretion to prescribe all recognized therapies. No country tries to limit expenditures by the methods common in American private insurance, namely, reductions in the eligible population, denials of benefits, and large shifts in claims payment to insured patients.

Government monitors the cost problems of statutory health insurance, but it does not dictate limits: the health insurance carriers, the hospitals, and the doctors are autonomous and resist government dictation. The parts of the system must be "coordinated" to control costs, but they are not "centralized" under government. (Even a national health service managed and financed by government is not as "centralized" as one expects.) The providers wish higher remuneration, better facilities, and discretion in giving services; patients wish prompt access to the best services; the taxpayer and budget officers wish to limit taxes and borrowing. A form of negotiations has developed among the interest groups, political parties, and government ministries that are spokesmen and protectors for the social groupings of payers and users. Germany uses a forum that brings the interest groups, insurance carriers, and providers together to agree on policy. Less structured negotiations occur within parliament and among government ministries in all other countries with statutory health insurance, such as France and Holland.

Without a definition of the public interest, the various groups would struggle for maximum self-centered advantage. Consensus has developed that health services must continue to be available and that costs must be consistent with the country's fiscal capacity. An important role of government is to provide trustworthy facts: on the services side, data about trends in morbidity, utilization, technology, and wages; on the revenue side, data about employment, earnings, and inflation in the entire economy. The problem is to develop a consensus about expenditure targets for all health sectors next year, so that adequate care can be delivered without running deficits in the insurance and government accounts, without necessitating excessive increases in taxes and borrowing.

The final consensus is worked out among the ministries representing the different interest groups (health, budget, finance, labor, industry, and social affairs) rather than by parliament. In an American statutory insurance system, the contentious details would be hammered out each year within the executive branch and would not overburden Congress. The guidelines would then be transmitted by the executive agencies to the persons who implement them, that is, the negotiators who set physicians' pay, the administrators of utilization review, the hospital rate regulators, and others. In practice, they hew close to the guidelines, since the sickness funds are reluctant to offer more money, and since the sickness funds and governments no longer automatically cover deficits. Statutory health insurance cannot be kept under fixed caps, because patients are entitled to care on their own initiative and because doctors have discretion in prescribing. But its cost containment methods have achieved nearly the same limits as have the publicly managed systems. Therefore costs can be contained even without full governmentalization.

Costs

A recent tactic by American advocates of inaction is the argument that nothing should be done until America stops the growth in its health care spending. Then, no reform should be enacted unless it is "budget neutral"—that is, spending no more than the status quo. Meanwhile, America's health care analysts find new and profitable employment in simulating the future costs of all the proposed reforms, as in the Advisory Council on Social Security (1991: 379–642).

Unfortunately for this scenario, the United States cannot stabilize the costs of its current uncoordinated arrangements. As the experiences of other countries show, costs cannot be stabilized unless a comprehensive managed system is substituted.

Unfortunately for all attempts to simulate future expenditures, experiences show that every reform initially increases health care spending for several reasons: the doctors' cooperation must be bought with higher fees, access widens, utilization grows, neglected conditions (such as dentistry) are brought to providers on a large scale, and so on. The only reform that would reduce health costs would be the elimination of third-party coverage. Statutory health insurance of the type described in this article would alter the flow of most current spending through new channels and would increase it by expanding access for the uninsured and by improving benefits for the underinsured. Neither I nor anyone else can predict the future spending under this or any other reform. One can only predict that social protection would improve and that cost containment machinery for the long term would be installed.

Private Health Insurance

A private market would remain, depending on the niches left under the statute. Besides administering finance for the mainstream program, the health insurance carriers may also offer private policies. If several classes of persons can opt out of the system—as in Germany today and Holland before 1990—the private companies can sell them as much private coverage as they want.

The principal private market is supplementary coverage for the socially insured. An option in the design of American statutory health insurance is the amount of cost sharing required of patients. Some countries have had little cost sharing, but several of them recently added copayments and coinsurance either to deter waste (as in pharmaceutical prescription charges in many countries) or to reduce the burden on the sickness funds (as in German hospital copayments and Dutch dental coinsurance). Some countries have always had coinsurance as part of their designs (such as France, Belgium, and Switzerland), and both American private insurance and Medicare have required much. So, doubtless American statutory health insurance will have substantial cost sharing, thus creating a market for private supplementary coverage, as in the case of American Medigap and the French *fonds mutuelles*. However, each subscriber's ownership of two policies complicates a system that is supposed to be simple and invites controversy over whether the supplementary coverage destroys the supposed cost-saving deterrent effects from the patients' participation.

If certain benefits are omitted or are limited in statutory health insurance, private policies can be offered for them. Examples are some dentistry, psychiatric visits beyond a maximum number under social insurance, nursing homes, and home care.

Private companies can remain the primary insurers in work accidents and auto accidents.

Political Feasibility

Can the foregoing scheme be enacted? Is the political situation in Washington so confused and are the opponents so powerful that—like other reforms—it cannot be adopted? Or, would it be enacted with so many amendments that it would be unworkable? Every great reform depends on the balance of political forces and on the skill of political leadership.

Forces in Favor

Perhaps the strongest source of support is the widespread exhaustion over health care financing among the general public and policymakers. By 1993 in Washington and elsewhere in the country, one hears intensifying complaints about escalating costs along with disillusionment about the effectiveness of favorite nostrums, such as managed care, competitive markets, and the Canadian model. America adopted a universal system of the European sort to solve the crisis of income security in 1935, and one now hears widespread calls for a "universal" and "comprehensive system" in health. Statutory health insurance of the sort described in this article would be a welcome alternative to the American bugaboos of "nationalization," "centralization," and "dictation by Washington bureaucrats."

Particular interest groups in the population might enlist behind a general reform. The trade unions and political Left in all countries are important forces behind social security and statutory health insurance, and they already are in the United States. They would have to be persuaded to accept substantial payroll taxes in return for an improved system and limits on point-of-service cost sharing. Workers and their families already find their coverage is no longer "free" and must pay mounting contributory premiums.

Interest groups representing the poor and minority groups could also be mobilized. They would be insured with normal benefits, and all providers would accept these persons more readily.

In most countries, Big Businessmen at first oppose social security and statutory health insurance, because they must pay large payroll taxes and because they prefer free markets and self-reliance. However, the financial and administrative burdens of employment-based health benefits have panicked many American business leaders, and they would welcome a substitute capable of limiting their personnel costs, relieving them of responsibility for the increasingly expensive retirees, and transferring all administrative work to the carriers. Business leaders' normal antipathy to government intervention can be overcome, since their preferred solution of decentralized private managed care is unsuccessful, statutory health insurance is more orderly and less expensive than what American business now faces, and an important sector of business (the insurance industry) would administer statutory health insurance.

Threatened with exclusion by the Canadian model, American health insurance companies could become important advocates of statutory health insurance. They would handle more money, would risk fewer deficits, would participate in policy-making, would receive credit from representing the interests of the public and of their subscribers, and would be the principal negotiators with providers. They could still compete for market share, appealing to individual subscribers and no longer wooing the capricious managers of employed groups. The insurance companies could still market supplementary health policies and more profitable lines, such as life insurance.

Certain associations of health providers could be enlisted. Usually an important constituency for the passage of statutory health insurance, the nonprofit and public hospitals would be guaranteed their costs. They would no longer have bad debts, need to shift costs among payers, and experience so many disputes. The inevitable restraint would be rate regulation and capital planning, but the trade-off would be an opportunity to focus on their clinical mission.

Barriers

Ideological objections would have to be overcome. The utopian belief in the efficacy of free markets, in unlimited consumer and provider choice, and in fragmented managed care would finally have to be abandoned. For a decade, the ideology has bewitched the American health policy establishment and the country's medical economists. Confronted by empirical facts and the plight of American patients, much of Washington has begun to look elsewhere during the 1990s.

The philosophy of social solidarity and of social protection would have to be accepted in health—as it previously was in the enactment of other social reforms. Americans would have to accept the levels of payroll taxation and public subsidies necessary to protect the poor, the dissolute, and unpopular minority groups. Such tax and spending increases have already occurred in a half-hearted and chaotic manner during the 1980s. In statutory health insurance and its related reforms, these tax and spending increases would be planned, controlled, and generally understood.

In every country, the medical profession is the principal critic of the first proposals for statutory health insurance. In contrast, American organized medicine is aware of the need for reform and—during the early 1960s, the mid-1970s, and 1990—has proposed its own designs. To American doctors, some system is preferable to the present fragmented administration with multiple payers, bad debts, cost shifting, and guerrilla warfare with government. Doctors prefer the utopia of individual fee setting to the collective rates inherent in universal statutory health insurance. The inevitable compromise is one that American medical associations have long understood, namely, decision-making machinery wherein the medical profession's elected representatives participate in all policies and negotiate with payers over money and working conditions. Under statutory health insurance, the individual American doctor would be pleased with more money, fewer hassles, and the opportunity to focus on clinical care.

Small businessmen would resist statutory health insurance, just as they now oppose mandated group coverage. Their current objections include higher payments, ideological aversion to social protection, and the administrative trouble from special group contracts. Under other American proposals for mandated group coverage, small business would be singled out. However, small businessmen might be induced to accept extension of a program in which they already participate: they now pay social security taxes for their employees and for themselves, statutory health insurance would merely add a few percentage points, payroll taxes are more stable than employment group premiums, and someone else (the carriers) would assume all the administration pursuant to a general public policy.

Several other American provider groups would criticize the statutory health insurance scenario described in this paper. But all must adjust to any effective reform that is better than worsening chaos. American for-profit hospitals have long opposed cost containment and health planning, but they too now suffer from the instabilities and erratic expenditure controls of the present situation. For-profit hospitals operate like all other hospitals in German statutory health insurance, and they can play a similar role in an American program. The pharmaceutical and equipment industries might fear the expenditure limits and plans of an American statutory health insurance, but they can continue to prosper with complete clinical freedom, as their experiences in Europe demonstrate.

The Need for Leadership

One lesson from Europe is that social security and health care are so important and so controversial that a reform requires an all-out effort by the head of government. The president or prime minister must understand all the issues and political forces, must explain the proposal to the country, must mobilize supporters, must disarm opponents, and must expend his political capital in the parliament. Such political skill and determination have been scarce in all sectors of American domestic politics lately. President Bush justified his policy of minimum change in health by misrepresenting the methods of other countries as tyrannical, wasteful, and neglectful of patients (see, for example, Bush 1992). No reform—whether the one described in this paper or any other—is possible without sophisticated understanding and effective leadership by the president. Only a president can do the strategic thinking for a fundamentally new system.

Since effective nationwide health insurance is a public-private partnership, Congress, too, must be willing to understand a complex sector and enact a system requiring it to play a new role. At present, Congress tries to enact complex and logrolled programs and then to micromanage them. Some critics believe that congressmen gain politically by manipulating the legislation and its administration, so they can win the favor of individual constituents and political action committees (Fiorina 1989). Health is one of the intricate, disputatious, and expensive fields where the political costs to a legislator exceed the benefits. To cope with such areas of public policy involving large payments, high costs, complex subject matter, litigation, and overload of Congress—environmental protection, occupational safety, aviation, and nuclear regulation—Congress during the 1980s created "negotiated rule making." Congress sets the guiding principles in a framework law, allows the interested parties to negotiate rules and financial rates, and approves the results with few amendments. The method has been recommended for all government programs where appropriate by the Negotiated Rulemaking Act of 1990, enacted overwhelmingly by all political parties and by all ideological camps (Administrative Conference of the United States 1990). Therefore, a statutory health insurance system managed by the private sector pursuant to law and under public oversight is politically feasible in the United States, as well as urgent.

References

Adelman, Susan H. 1992. Is U.S. Willing to Pay the Price for Health Reform? *American Medical News* 35 (9): 20–21.

Administrative Conference of the United States. 1990. *Negotiated Rulemaking Sourcebook*. Washington, DC: U.S. Government Printing Office.

Advisory Council on Social Security. 1991. *Commitment to Change: Foundations for Reform*. Washington, DC: U.S. Department of Health and Human Services.

Armstrong, Barbara. 1932. *Insuring the Essentials: Minimum Wage plus Social Insurance*. New York: Macmillan.

Beauchamp, Dan E., and Ronald L. Rouse. 1990. Universal New York Health Care. *New England Journal of Medicine* 223 (10): 640–44.

Blendon, Robert J., Karen Donelan, Carol VanDeusen Lukas, Kenneth E. Thorpe, Martin Frankel, Ronald Bass, and Humphrey Taylor. 1992. The Uninsured and the Debate over the Repeal of the Massachusetts Universal Health Care Law. *Journal of the American Medical Association* 267 (8): 1113–17.

Bush, George. 1992. *The President's Comprehensive Health Reform Program*. Washington, DC: The White House.

Clinton, Hillary Rodham. 1993. Speech to the American Medical Association, Chicago, IL, 13 June.

Commissioner of Labor. 1911. *Workmen's Insurance and Compensation Systems in Europe: Twenty-fourth Annual Report*. Washington, DC: U.S. Government Printing Office.

Congressional Budget Office. 1991. *Selected Options for Expanding Health Insurance Coverage*. Washington, DC: U.S. Government Printing Office.

Enthoven, Alain, and Kronick, Richard. 1989. A Consumer-Choice Health Plan for the 1990s. *New England Journal of Medicine*. 320 (1): 29–37, (2): 94–101.

Evans, Robert G., and Greg L. Stoddart. 1986. *Medicare at Maturity*. Calgary: University of Calgary Press.

Feder, Judith, Jack Hadley, and John Holahan. 1981. *Insuring the Nation's Health*. Washington, DC: Urban Institute Press.

Fiorina, Morris P. 1989. *Congress: Keystone of the Washington Establishment*. 2d ed. New Haven, CT: Yale University Press.

Glaser, William A. 1978. *Health Insurance Bargaining*. New York: Gardner.

———. 1981. *Paying the Hospital in Canada*. New York: Columbia University, Center for the Social Sciences.

———. 1987. *Paying the Hospital*. San Francisco, CA: Jossey-Bass.

———. 1990. Designing Fee Schedules by Formulae, Politics, and Negotiations. *American Journal of Public Health* 80 (7): 804–9.

———. 1991. *Health Insurance in Practice*. San Francisco, CA: Jossey-Bass.

Goldberger, Susan A. 1990. The Politics of Universal Access: The Massachusetts Health Security Act of 1988. *Journal of Health Politics, Policy and Law* 15 (4): 857–85.

Himmelstein, David U., and Steffie Woolhandler. 1989. A National Health Program for the United States. *New England Journal of Medicine* 320 (2): 102–8.

Köhler, Peter A., Hans F. Zacher, and Martin Partington, eds. 1982. *The Evolution of Social Insurance 1881–1981*. London: Frances Pinter.

Lewin, John C. 1992. The Implementation of National Health Care Reform: Lessons from Hawai'i. In *Implementation Issues and National Health Care Reform*, ed. Charles Brecher. New York: Josiah Macy Foundation.

Munts, Raymond. 1967. *Bargaining for Health: Labor Unions, Health Insurance and Medical Care*. Madison, WI: University of Wisconsin Press.

Pepper Commission (U.S. Bipartisan Commission on Comprehensive Health Care). 1990. *A Call for Action*. Washington, DC: U.S. Government Printing Office.

Rubinow, I. M. 1916. *Standards of Health Insurance*. New York: Henry Holt.

Sullivan, Louis W. 1990. Speech to the Atlanta Business Roundtable, Atlanta, GA 23 July.

Taylor, Malcolm G. 1978. *Health Insurance and Canadian Public Policy: The Seven Decisions That Created the Canadian Health Insurance System*. Montreal: McGill-Queen's University Press.

U.S. House of Representatives, Committee on Ways and Means. 1990. *Private Health Insurance: Options for Reform*. Washington, DC: U.S. Government Printing Office.

Waldman, Saul. 1976. *National Health Insurance Proposals*. Washington, DC: Office of Research and Statistics, Social Security Administration, Department of Health, Education and Welfare.

Willoughby, William F. 1898. *Workingmen's Insurance*. New York: Crowell.

Index

middle-range reform plans and, 69
policy reform and, 107, 113–15
reform plan presentation to, 70–74
See also Public opinion
U.S. Secretary of Health and Human
Services
Adoption Assistance and Child Wel-
fare Act on, 189, 191
Boren Amendment on, 175, 184,
188n
Estate of Smith v. Heckler on, 169n8,
177n19, 196
1981 Senate Report on, 176
Task Force on Black and Minority
Health, 88–89
U.S. Social Security Administration,
152, 161, 420n. *See also* Social
Security System
U.S. Steel Corporation, 208
U.S. Supreme Court
managerial formalism and, 193
right-privilege distinction and, 171
Rosado v. Wyman and, 172–73
social legislation and, 165, 166n1
Suter v. Artist M. and, 188–90, 192
welfare beneficiary cases and, 174,
183–93
U.S. Treasury Department, 261n
U.S. War Labor Board, 261
U.S. Works Project Administration, 17
USA Today (newspaper), 249n31
Utilization review, 436

Van Guysling, Mark, 424
Vocational Rehabilitation Act, 49
Vocations, 36–37, 117
Voluntarism, 11, 19–21, 24, 327. *See
also* Nonprofit hospitals; Private
charities
Voluntary associations. *See* Membership
associations
Voting rights, 263, 269–70
Voucher plan (Heritage Foundation),
104, 229, 232, 235
Vulnerable groups. *See* Disadvantaged
groups

W. E. B. Du Bois Conference (1976),
82–83
Wages. *See* Employee compensation
Waiting periods, 43n12

Waivers, 43–44, 45, 46
Walker, Jack L., 121–25, 127, 131
Walzer, Michael, 268, 269
War Labor Board, 261
War on Poverty, 98–99, 200
Washington, Harold, 85–86
Washington, D.C., 50
Washington Business Group on Health,
120, 210, 240–42
Washington Post, 339, 377n2
Washington State, 445
Waxman, Henry, 130
Wayman, Frank W., 132
Weber, Max, 150
Weinstein, Jack B., 172n.12
Weitzman, Murray, 326–27
Weld, William, 425, 426
Welfare state, 166, 174, 301, 303–5,
324, 327. *See also* Public welfare
Well-to-do persons, 15, 195–96
altruism of, 326–27, 331n
external identification of, 334
political activism of, 361–62, 363
social welfare attitudes of, 325
vulnerability of, 339–40
See also Middle class
Wennberg, John, 158–59
West German national health insur-
ance. *See* German national health
insurance
*West Virginia University Hospitals v.
Casey* (1989), 185n
White, Byron R., 172, 183n, 192n
Wilder v. Virginia Hospital Association
(1990), 173, 183–85, 188, 191–92,
193
Wilensky, Gail, 229
Williams, Harrison, 128
Wilson, Pete, 432
Wisconsin, 502
Wofford, Harris, 136
American Health Security Plan and,
104
Bush administration and, 387
campaign slogan of, 397
election of, 48, 60, 115, 250, 377
public opinion and, 385–86
Women
actuarial fairness concept and, 28
employment-based insurance and,
264, 284

Contributors

Gary S. Belkin is a physician and associate editor of the Journal of Health Politics, Policy and Law. He has served in a variety of positions in health policy in the New York and Rhode Island state governments. Currently, he is Associate Director of Emergency Services, Department of Psychiatry, Rhode Island Hospital, and in the Department of Psychiatry and Human Behavior, Brown University. He is also completing doctoral studies in the History of Science Department, Harvard University.

Lawrence Brown is professor and head of the Division of Health Policy and Management in the School of Public Health at Columbia University. Previously, he was on the faculty of the University of Michigan and the staff of the Brookings Institution. Brown writes on competitive and regulatory issues in health policy and on the politics of health care policy-making more gnerally. He (and Catherine McLaughlin) evaluated the Robert Wood Johnson Foundation's Community Programs for Affordable Health Care and their Program for the Medically Uninsured. He was editor of the *Journal of Health Politics, Policy and Law* from 1984–89.

Robert G. Evans is professor of economics at the University of British Columbia, where he has held a National Health Scientist award since 1985. Since 1987 he has been a fellow of the Canadian Institute for Advanced Research, and director of its Program in Population Health. He has recently served as a commissioner of the British Columbia Royal Commission on Health Care and Costs, which reported at the end of 1991.

William A. Glaser is professor of health services management at the New School for Social Research in New York. His main research activities have been in cross-national comparative research about health services and other topics. His books on comparative health care include *Paying the Doctor* (1970), *Social Settings and Medical Organization* (1970), *Health Insurance Bargaining* (1978), *Paying the Hospital* (1987), and *Health Insurance in Practice* (1991). From other cross-national research, he has written *The Brain Drain* (1978) and *Teacher Unions and Policymaking* (1993). From research about American government, he has written *Public Opinion and Congres-*

sional Elections (1962) and *Pretrial Discovery and the Adversary System* (1968). In his many research projects, Glaser has prepared reports advising government agencies and private organizations.

Colleen M. Grogan, Ph.D., is currently doing independent research in the People's Republic of China. A recent graduate from the University of Minnesota, her research has focused on health policy at the state level, particularly state Medicaid policy. In addition, she is interested in health policy comparisons among nations and broader issues related to the effect of political systems on health policy.

Robert B. Hackey received a Ph.D. in political science and public policy from Brown University and is an assistant professor of political science at the University of Massachusetts—Dartmouth. His principal teaching and research interests focus on state health policy, trauma systems development, and contemporary democratic theory. Prior to joining the faculty at the University of Massachusetts—Dartmouth, he served as the program manager for trauma system planning at the Rhode Island Department of Health. His research on state hospital rate-setting programs has appeared in *Medical Care Review* as well as in the *Journal of Health Politics, Policy and Law*.

Lawrence R. Jacobs is an assistant professor of political science at the University of Minnesota. He is author of *The Health of Nations* as well as a series of articles on health policy and public opinion, which have appeared in *World Politics* and *Comparative Politics*.

Nancy S. Jecker is an associate professor at the University of Washington School of Medicine, with adjunct appointments in the School of Law and Department of Philosophy. She has been a visiting scholar at the Stanford University Center for Biomedical Ethics (1991), Georgetown University's Kennedy Institute of Ethics (1988) and the Hastings Center (1986) and was awarded Rockefeller fellowships from the University of Texas Medical Branch (1989) and the University of Maryland (1987–88). Dr. Jecker is editor of *Aging and Ethics* (Humana Press, 1991) and has contributed articles to several publications. Currently, she is writing a book (with Lawrence Schneiderman) entitled *The Ends of Medicine: Saying No to Futile Treatment*.

Taeku Lee is a graduate student in the Department of Political Science at the University of Chicago. Lee has an undergraduate degree from the University of Michigan and a master's in public policy from Harvard and specializes in American politics.

Joan M. Leiman is deputy vice president for the health sciences and a senior lecturer in the Faculty of Medicine, School of Public Health (Health Policy and Management) at Columbia University. From 1966 to 1971 she was a program analyst and then an assistant budget director in New York City's Bureau of the Budget, where she worked on the city's health and hospital expenditures. Dr. Leiman received her B.A. from Wellesley College and her Ph.D. from Columbia.

David McBride is professor and head of the Department of African American Studies at The Pennsylvania State University. From 1987 to 1988 he was a Rockefeller Foundation postdoctoral fellow and a visiting scholar at the National Library of Medicine, Division of History. His research and teaching interests concern the medical and public health history of American minorities. Among his publications are two books, *Integrating the City of Medicine: Blacks in Philadelphia Health Care, 1910–1968* (1989) and *From TB to AIDS: Epidemics among Blacks since 1900* (1991).

James A. Morone is an associate professor of political science at Brown University. His most recent book, *The Democratic Wish: Popular Participation and the Limits of American Government* (Basic Books) won the American Political Science Association's 1991 Gladys M. Kammerer award for the best book in the field of American politics and was selected by the *New York Times* as a notable book of 1991. From 1990 to 1993 he was the editor of the *Journal of Health Politics, Policy and Law*. He writes on health issues, social policy, and American political history. Morone was voted the Hazeltine citation for excellence in teaching by the Brown University class of 1993.

Mark A. Peterson (Ph.D., University of Michigan, 1985) is an associate professor of Public Affairs and Political Science in the Graduate School of Public and International Affairs at the University of Pittsburgh. Among his many publications is the book *Legislating Together: The White House and Capitol Hill from Eisenhower to Reagan* (Harvard University Press, 1990). He has been a guest scholar in governmental studies at the Brookings Institution and an American Political Science Association congressional fellow, serving as a legislative assistant on health policy in the office of Senator Tom Daschle, where he helped draft S. 2513, the American Health Security Plan, a comprehensive health care reform initiative introduced by Senators Daschle and Wofford. He is the recipient of the American Political Science Association's E. E. Schattschneider Award and the Midwest Political Science Association's Pi Sigma Alpha Award.

David A. Rochefort is associate professor of political science and public administration at Northeastern University, where he was project administrator and coauthor of the *Insuring American Health for the Year 2000* report. With grant support from the Canadian federal government and the province of Quebec, he is currently researching mental health care under Canadian national health insurance. His latest book, *From Poor Houses to Homelessness: Policy Analysis and Mental Health Care*, was published by Auburn House in the fall of 1993.

Rand E. Rosenblatt is professor of law at Rutgers University Law School—Camden, where he teaches courses on health law; constitutional law; and law, justice, and society. His research interests include legal theory, social justice, and health care delivery, with particular emphasis on the relationships among access, quality, and cost containment. He is coauthor of a legal casebook, *American Health Law* (Little, Brown, 1990) and author of numerous articles on health and social welfare policy, including "Social Duties and the Problem of Rights in the American Welfare State," in *The Politics of Law* (Pantheon, rev. ed., 1990). A member of the National Academy of Social Insurance, the Society of American Law Teachers, and the Conference on Critical Legal Networks, he has consulted for the Hastings Center, the President's Commission on Biomedical Ethics, and the United States District Court in the Agent Orange Products Liability Case.

David J. Rothman is the Bernard Schoenberg Professor of Social Medicine and director of the Center for the Study of Society and Medicine at the Columbia College of

Physicians and Surgeons and professor of history at Columbia University. Trained in social history at Harvard University, he has explored American practices toward the deviant and dependent. *The Discovery of the Asylum* (1971), was cowinner of the Albert J. Beveridge Prize; together with Sheila M. Rothman he has analyzed the process of deinstitutionalization in *The Willowbrook Wars* (1984). In his recent publications, he has addressed issues in the history of drug regulation, the rationing of scarce medical resources, and the relationship between medicine and the state, using Romania and Zimbabwe as case studies. He has also examined the advantages and disadvantages of single disease hospitals for AIDS and, more recently, for milti-drug-resistant tuberculosis. In the spring of 1991, he published *Strangers at the Bedside: A History of How Law and Bioethics Transformed Medical Decisionmaking*.

Joan E. Ruttenberg is an attorney, professor, and consultant in health law. She is currently adjunct assistant professor of legal studies at Brandeis University, where she helped to establish a program in law, medicine, and social policy. Ms. Ruttenberg has taught at the law schools of the University of Chicago and Northeastern University, and was formerly an assistant attorney general in Massachusetts, where she specialized in insurance and health care issues. Ms. Ruttenberg received her law degree from Harvard Law School in 1982.

Mark Schlesinger is associate professor of public health and fellow of the Institute for Social and Policy Studies, Yale University, and a visiting associate professor at the Institute for Health, Health Care Policy and Aging Research at Rutgers. Before this, he taught at the Kennedy School of Government and Harvard Medical School; he has a Ph.D. in economics from the University of Wisconsin. His health policy research includes studies of federal programs for children and the elderly, of for-profit enterprises in health and mental health care, various forms of managed care and utilization management, including their application to managed competition, and public attitudes toward reform. His research on other aspects of social policy includes studies of government contracting with private agencies, public perceptions and attitudes shaping intergenerational tensions and age-targeted social programs, and the comparative performance of private nonprofit, for-profit, and public agencies. Dr. Schlesinger has consulted to a variety of state agencies in Massachusetts and New York and to the General Accounting Office, the Office of Technology Assessment, the Department of Veterans Affairs, the National Institute on Drug Abuse, and the National Institute of Mental Health. He can on occasion be lured into games of volleyball and tennis, as long as the other players forswear any form of cutthroat competition.

Theda Skocpol is professor of sociology at Harvard University. Her first book, *States and Social Revolutions: A Comparative Analysis of France, Russia, and China* (Cambridge University Press, 1979), won the 1979 C. Wright Mills Award and the 1980 American Sociological Association Award for a Distinguished Contribution to Scholarship. For the past decade. Skocpol has been researching U.S. politics and public policies in comparative and historical perspective. In 1988, she published a coedited collection on *The Politics of Social Policy in the United States* (Princeton University Press). Skocpol was a founding member and the 1991–92 president of the History and Politics Section of the American Political Science Association. Her latest book is *Protecting Soldiers and Mothers: The Political Origins of Social Policy in the United States*, published in 1992 by the Belknap Press of Harvard University Press.

Michael S. Sparer is an assistant professor in the Division of Health Policy and Management in the School of Public Health at Columbia University. He received a Ph.D. in political science from Brandeis University and a J.D. from the Rutgers School of Law (at Newark). Sparer spent seven years as a litigator for the New York City Law Department, specializing in intergovernmental social welfare litigation. He now studies and writes about the politics of health care, with an emphasis on the state and local role in the American health care system.

Deborah A. Stone holds the David R. Pokross Chair in Law and Social Policy at Brandeis University. She is the author of three books, *The Limits of Professional Power: National Health Care in Germany* (University of Chicago Press, 1980), *The Disabled State* (Temple University Press, 1984), and *Policy Paradox and Political Reason* (HarperCollins, 1988). She has written widely on topics of health and social policy and served on many government and scientific advisory commissions. Her essay in this volume comes from a work in progress on public and private insurance in the American welfare state.

Kenneth E. Thorpe is deputy assistant secretary for health policy at the U.S. Department of Health and Human Services, on leave from the Department of Health Policy and Administration, University of North Carolina at Chapel Hill, where he is an associate professor. Before moving to UNC, Dr. Thorpe was director of the Program on Health Care Financing and Insurance at the Harvard University School of Public Health. Over the past five years, he has served as an advisor to the Pepper Commission, the Advisory Council on Social Security, the National Leadership Coalition for Health Care Reform, and the New York State Department of Health; he was a gubernatorial appointee to Massachusetts's Universal Health Care Commission; and serves on an Institute of Medicine panel examining the future of employer-sponsored benefits. He has written dozens of articles on health care financing issues, is coauthor of *Competition and Compassion: Conflicting Roles for Public Hospitals*, and is completing an examination of the medical malpractice system.